Visit MediaCenter.Thieme.com
to watch the 70 accompanying videos!

Simply visit MediaCenter.thieme.com and, when prompted during the
registration process, enter the code below to get started today.

B433-BPM3-P5GU-7Z32

	WINDOWS & MAC	TABLET
Recommended Browser(s)	Recent browser versions on all major platforms and any mobile operating system that supports HTML5 video playback. *All browsers should have JavaScript enabled.*	
Flash Player Plug-in	Flash Player 9 or higher. *For Mac users, ATI Rage 128 GPU doesn't support full-screen mode with hardware scaling.*	Tablet PCs with Android OS support Flash 10.1.
Recommended for optimal usage experience	Monitor resolutions: • Normal (4:3) 1024×768 or higher • Widescreen (16:9) 1280×720 or higher • Widescreen (16:10) 1440×900 or higher A high-speed internet connection (minimum 384 Kps) is suggested.	WiFi or cellular data connection is required.

Connect with us on social media

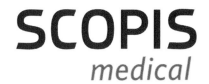

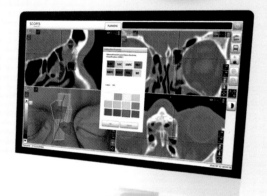

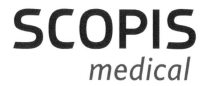
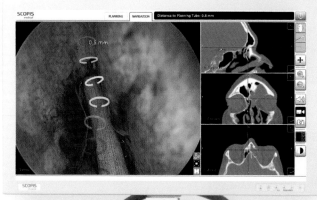

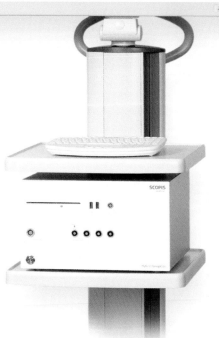

Endoscopic Sinus Surgery

Anatomy, Three-Dimensional Reconstruction, and Surgical Technique

Fourth Edition

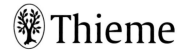

Endoscopic Sinus Surgery

Anatomy, Three-Dimensional Reconstruction,
and Surgical Technique

Fourth Edition

Peter-John Wormald, MD, FRACS, FCS(SA), FRCS(Ed), MBChB
Chairman and Professor of Otolaryngology–Head and Neck Surgery
Professor of Skull Base Surgery
University of Adelaide
Adelaide, South Australia
Australia

Thieme
New York • Stuttgart • Delhi • Rio de Janeiro

Executive Editor: Timothy Hiscock
Managing Editor: J. Owen Zurhellen IV
Editorial Assistant: Mary B. Wilson
Director, Editorial Services: Mary Jo Casey
Production Editor: Heidi Grauel
Editorial Director: Sue Hodgson
International Production Director: Andreas Schabert
International Marketing Director: Fiona Henderson
International Sales Director: Louisa Turrell
Institutional Sales Director: Adam Bernacki
Senior Vice President and Chief Operating Officer: Sarah Vanderbilt
President: Brian D. Scanlan
Printer: Everbest Printing Co.

Library of Congress Cataloging-in-Publication Data

Names: Wormald, P. J., author.
Title: Endoscopic sinus surgery : anatomy, three-dimensional
    reconstruction, and surgical technique / Peter-John Wormald.
Description: Fourth edition. | New York : Thieme, [2018] |
    Includes bibliographical references and index.
Identifiers: LCCN 2017025854 | ISBN 9781626234697 |
    ISBN 9781626234703 (ebook)
Subjects: | MESH: Paranasal Sinuses—surgery | Paranasal Sinuses—
    anatomy & histology | Paranasal Sinus Diseases—surgery | Natural
    Orifice Endoscopic Surgery—methods | Video-Assisted Surgery
Classification: LCC RF421 | NLM WV 340 | DDC 617.5/23—dc23
LC record available at https://lccn.loc.gov/2017025854

Important note: Medicine is an ever-changing science undergoing continual development. Research and clinical experience are continually expanding our knowledge, in particular our knowledge of proper treatment and drug therapy. Insofar as this book mentions any dosage or application, readers may rest assured that the authors, editors, and publishers have made every effort to ensure that such references are in accordance with **the state of knowledge at the time of production of the book.**

Nevertheless, this does not involve, imply, or express any guarantee or responsibility on the part of the publishers in respect to any dosage instructions and forms of applications stated in the book. **Every user is requested to examine carefully** the manufacturers' leaflets accompanying each drug and to check, if necessary in consultation with a physician or specialist, whether the dosage schedules mentioned therein or the contraindications stated by the manufacturers differ from the statements made in the present book. Such examination is particularly important with drugs that are either rarely used or have been newly released on the market. Every dosage schedule or every form of application used is entirely at the user's own risk and responsibility. The authors and publishers request every user to report to the publishers any discrepancies or inaccuracies noticed. If errors in this work are found after publication, errata will be posted at www.thieme.com on the product description page.

Some of the product names, patents, and registered designs referred to in this book are in fact registered trademarks or proprietary names even though specific reference to this fact is not always made in the text. Therefore, the appearance of a name without designation as proprietary is not to be construed as a representation by the publisher that it is in the public domain.

Dedicated with love to Fiona, my wife, without whom this book would not have been possible, and to Nicholas and Sarah, my children who provide my inspiration.

Contents

Menu of Accompanying Videos

Basic Videos

1. Inferior Turbinoplasty
2. Osteotomy to the Head of the Inferior Turbinate
3. Septoplasty 1
4. Septoplasty 2
5. Middle Meatal Antrostomy 1
6. Middle Meatal Antrostomy 2
7. Middle Meatal Antrostomy 3
8. Concha Bullosa 1
9. Agger Nasi Cell
10. Posterior Ethmoidectomy 1
11. Posterior Ethmoidectomy 2
12. Posterior Ethmoidectomy 3
13. Canine Fossa Trephine 1
14. Canine Fossa Trephine 2
15. Canine Fossa Trephine 3
16. Mega-Antrostomy of the Maxillary Sinus

Frontal Videos

17. Mini-Trephine Placement
18. SAC Cell 1
19. SAC Cell 2
20. SAC Cell 3
21. SAC Cell 4
22. SAFC Cell 1
23. SAFC Cell 2
24. SAFC Cell 3
25. Frontal Septal Cell
26. SAC Cell 5
27. SAFC, SBFC
28. Frontal Drillout 1
29. Frontal Drillout 2
30. Frontal Drillout with Pedicled Flaps 1
31. Frontal Drillout with Pedicled Flaps 2

Skull Base Videos

32. Nasal Encephalocele
33. Anterior Cranial Fossa Meningioma 1
34. Anterior Cranial Fossa Meningioma 2
35. Cerebrospinal Fluid Leak Repair 1
36. Cerebrospinal Fluid Leak Repair 2
37. Pituitary Surgery 1
38. Pituitary Surgery 2
39. Clivus Chordoma 1
40. Clivus Chordoma 2
41. Chondrosarcoma
42. Eustachian Tube Tumor

Adjunct Videos

43. Dacryocystorhinostomy 1
44. Dacryocystorhinostomy 2
45. Dacryocystorhinostomy 3
46. Revision Dacryocystorhinostomy 1
47. Revision Dacryocystorhinostomy 2
48. Revision Dacryocystorhinostomy 3
49. Orbital Abscess
50. Orbital Decompression 1
51. Orbital Decompression 2
52. Optic Nerve Decompression
53. Juvenile Nasopharyngeal Angiofibroma
54. Prelacrimal Approach to JNA
55. Medial Maxillectomy with JNA
56. Infratemporal Fossa Tumor
57. Sphenopalatine Artery Ligation 1
58. Sphenopalatine Artery Ligation 2
59. Vidian Neurectomy

Sinus Surgery Videos

60. Left Concha Bullosa Resection
61. Left Middle Meatal Antrostomy
62. Left Agger Nasi and SAC 1
63. Left Agger Nasi and SAC 2
64. Left SAFC
65. Left Posterior Ethmoidectomy and Sphenoidotomy
66. Left Posterior Ethmoid and Sphenoid Dissection
67. Frontal Drillout for Fungal Disease

Tumor Surgery Videos

68. Carcinoma Lacrimal Sac
69. Left Frontal Sinus Inverting Papilloma: Frontal Drillout
70. Clivus Chordoma with Carotid Encasement
71. Tuberculum Sella Meningioma
72. Esthesioneuroblastoma Resection

Preface

This fourth edition of *Endoscopic Sinus Surgery* and its accompanying videos continue to refine and improve the concepts and illustrations of the third edition. With time, surgical techniques are refined and adjusted and these have been added to this edition. Each chapter has been thoroughly revised and although some have required minimal changes, others have undergone extensive revision and adjustment. A recent publication (Wormald PJ, et al. The International Frontal Sinus Anatomy Classification [IFAC] and Classification of the Extent of Endoscopic Frontal Sinus Surgery [EFSS]. *Int Forum Allergy Rhinol* 2016;6[7]:677–696) simplifying the terminology of the cells in the frontal recess (IFAC classification) has resulted in extensive revision of the frontal sinus chapters. This new classification of cells in the frontal recess is both simple and logical and we hope will be adopted as the new world standard for naming of these cells. In addition, there has long been a need for a new classification of the extent of surgery. There has been much confusion about previous classifications with different interpretations for the extent of surgery. The classification of the extent of frontal sinus surgery (EFSS) was also revised in the same publication and again is simple and logical and we hope will become accepted as the world standard for the grading for the extent of surgery. We acknowledge Rowan Valentine's contribution to this book with the high standard of dissection images he has provided. These images were obtained under the guidance of the late Albert L. Rhoton Jr. in the latter's laboratory in Gainesville, Florida. The images in this book reflect the high standard of excellence associated with Rowan's work. In this new edition, we continue to develop and refine surgical techniques. We have added the mega-antrostomy and prelacrimal approaches to the maxillary sinus and adjusted the use of anterior based pedicled flaps for the EFSS grade 6 (frontal drillout) procedure and refined many of the other surgical techniques presented.

This book differs from many others on anatomy and surgical techniques in that its scope is purely anatomical and operative. No attempt is made to cover the pathology or medical treatment of any of the conditions discussed—such information can be found in several excellent texts currently available. Many of the operative techniques presented in this book are novel but the results achieved with them have been carefully audited and published in peer-reviewed journals before they are presented here. It is hoped that the description of the relevant anatomy and surgical techniques in this text are sufficiently clear so that the reader will be able to apply them in his/her everyday practice. The concepts are presented with extensive use of illustrations, CT and MRI scans, and intraoperative and postoperative photographs. In addition, the accompanying videos illustrate the surgical techniques described in the text. This combination of text and videos should reinforce understanding of sinus anatomy and give the surgeon the confidence to tackle the many anatomical variations and technical challenges that may occur during endoscopic sinus and skull base surgery.

Acknowledgments

A book of this nature is an accumulation of all knowledge gleaned from many teachers over many years. However, I would like to single out the late Mike McDonogh as the teacher who had the greatest influence on my career as a rhinologist. Mike was an exceptional person who was highly innovative, and his humor, wit, and intelligence will be greatly missed. His ideas led to the development of the swing-door uncinectomy and the bath-plug closure of cerebrospinal leaks. I will remain forever indebted to him for his teaching, mentoring, and friendship.

Andrew van Hasselt deserves a special mention for his support over many years. In addition, I would like to thank the Australian ENT Society members for making me welcome in Australia and for their ongoing support of the development of academic ENT.

1 Setup and Ergonomics of Endoscopic Sinus Surgery

◆ Introduction

There has been a significant shift from external and headlight sinus surgery to endoscopic sinus surgery (ESS). This dramatic change was initiated by the pioneering studies of Messerklinger in which he demonstrated that each sinus has a predetermined mucociliary clearance pattern draining toward its natural ostium irrespective of additional openings that may have been created into the sinuses.[1] This philosophy of opening the natural ostium of the diseased sinus was then popularized by Stammberger[2] and Kennedy.[3] ESS is now accepted as the surgical management of choice for chronic sinusitis. In addition, as our knowledge of the anatomy of the sinuses has improved, other ancillary techniques such as endoscopic lacrimal surgery[4] and orbital decompression[5] have been developed. The development of specialized instruments has facilitated the endoscopic management of benign endonasal tumors[6,7] and more recently the endoscopic management of malignant tumors[8] of the nose, sinuses, and intracranial cavity. Endoscopic sinus surgery, ancillary nasal and sinus procedures, and, more recently, endoscopic transnasal intracranial surgery requires a broad range of specially designed endoscopic surgical instruments.

◆ Instruments

Disclaimer

A number of instruments that are presented in this book are manufactured and sold by Medtronic ENT and Integra. Those that are identified by an * have been designed by the author and a royalty is received from the sale of these instruments. There are no undeclared financial incentives associated with any of the instruments discussed that do not bear the identifying *.

A complete list of endoscopic sinus surgery instruments used by the author is presented in **Table 1.1**. If the instrument is produced by a number of companies, no manufacturer is named. If a particular instrument is produced by only one company, then the manufacturer is named. The following instruments are important for basic sinus surgery:

- Small rotating backbiting forceps
- Sickle knife
- Small (2.5-mm) straight and 45-degree upturned Blakesley forceps
- Small (2.5-mm) straight and 45-degree upturned through-biting (cutting) Blakesley forceps
- Endoscopic scissors
- Double right-angled ball probe
- Forceps 45- and 90-degree giraffe cup, 45- and 90-degree through-biting giraffe forceps
- Hajek Koeffler forward-biting punch
- Suction Freer's elevator
- Curettes (straight, 45-degree, and 90-degree curette)
- Malleable suction Freer's elevator* (Integra, Plainsboro, NJ)
- Malleable suction curette* (Integra)
- Malleable frontal sinus probe* (Integra)

Powered Microdebriders

Powered microdebriders now form an essential part of the instrumentation required to perform ESS and skull base surgery. These instruments allow the surgeon to remove blood from the operating field with the gate open and then with considerable precision the tissue can be cut by the rotating inner blade of the microdebrider. This precision cutting of mucosa minimizes the potential for stripping of the mucosa and helps to achieve maximum mucosal preservation which should improve postoperative healing and consequently the results of the surgery. These instruments are very effective at removing tissue and if placed in the wrong area, such as the orbit, can create significant damage to the orbital contents in a

Table 1.1   Full list of operating instruments and equipment

Instruments
Jacobson angled 7-inch needle holder
6-inch fine needle holder
Small Luc forceps
Angled Heyman turbinectomy scissors
Tilley Henkel forceps
Tilley packing forceps
Mosquito curved artery clips
Backhaus towel clips
Sponge holder
McIndoe forceps
Adson toothed OR Adson Brown forceps
Adson plain OR tungsten tip forceps
Suture scissors
Iris curved scissors
No. 7 scalpel blade handle
Freer's dissector
Frazier 9 French gauge sucker and stilette
Frazier 10 French gauge sucker and stilette
Dental syringe
Heath's mallet
Small Killian's speculum
Medium Killian's speculum
Large Killian's speculum
Sinoscopy instruments
Medium straight Blakesley forceps
Medium upturned Blakesley forceps
Blakesley forceps straight through cut
Blakesley forceps upturned through cut
Right ostrum punch downcut
Left ostrum punch downcut
Sinus short sucker
Sinus long sucker
Sickle knife
Freer's dissector
Double-ended probe
Kuhn Bolger frontal ostium seeker
Kuhn Bolger frontal sinus curette 55 degrees
Antrum curette
90-degree curette
Sucker Freer's and stiletto
Rotating microbite backbiter
Hajek Koffler sphenoid punch upcut forward
Special instruments
Sinoscopy scissors – straight
Sinoscopy scissors – curved left
Sinoscopy scissors – curved right
Kuhn Bolger giraffe forceps horizontal
Kuhn Bolger giraffe forceps vertical
Kuhn Bolger forceps 60 degrees
Kuhn Bolger forceps 90 degrees
Kuhn Bolger forceps 90 degrees right angled
Kuhn Bolger forceps 90 degrees left angled
Ligature clip carrier
Wormald Sucker Bipolar* Integra
Wormald's suction bipolar forceps – straight*
Wormald's suction bipolar forceps – upturned*
Sterilization case
Bipolar cable
Medtronic ENT frontal trephine set
Medtronic frontal trephine set
Drill guide

Drill pin
Irrigation cannula (reusable; keep six in stock)
Sterilizing tray
Wormald's Malleable Frontal Sinus Instruments* Integra
Wormald malleable frontal sinus probe
Wormald malleable frontal sinus suction
Wormald malleable elevator blunt
Wormald malleable frontal sinus curette
Sterilization tray
Wormald Dacryocystorhinostomy Set* Integra
Sickle knife
Spear knife
Lusk microbite forceps
Wormald MicroFrance Anterior Skull Base and Pituitary
*   Instrument Set* Integra*
5-mm fine scissors: left, right, and straight
5-mm fine scissors: up
8-mm fine scissors: left, right, and straight
8-mm fine scissors: up
1-mm forceps straight and 45 degrees
Malleable probe straight
Malleable probe right-angled hook
Malleable suction dissector
Malleable suction
Malleable suction cage
Malleable small and large 45-degree ring curettes
Malleable small and large 90-degree ring curettes
Bending tool
MicroFrance Medtronic Hemorrhage Control Set* Integra
Clamp straight rotatable
Clamp curved small
Clamp curved long
Clamp 45-degree straight
Clamp 45-degree curved small
Clamp 45-degree curved long
Clip-applying forceps rotatable straight
Clip-applying forceps rotatable 45 degrees
Needle holder rotatable
Equipment
Camera system
STORZ HD digital camera SPIES
0-degree endoscope (4 × 11 mm Hopkins)
30-degree endoscope
45-degree endoscope
70-degree endoscope
Lens washer
Medtronic Endoscrub II
Consumables
0-degree Endoscrub II sheath
30-degree Endoscrub sheath
Microdebrider
Medtronic IPC (integrated power console)
M5 handpiece
Midas Rex Stylus handpiece
Skull base burs
Solutions
Topical
Cocaine solution (10% – 2 mL)
Adrenaline (1:1000 × 1 mL)
Normal saline (0.9 × 3 mL)

*Instruments identified by an asterisk were designed by the author.

very short space of time.[9,10] Due to its soft consistency, orbital fat can be sucked into the blade opening and cut by the rotating inner blade at a frightening rate. If the surgeon is unaware of having penetrated the orbital periosteum with microdebrider, significant damage can occur within a few seconds. There are numerous case reports in the literature in which powered microdebriders have caused inadvertent injury to the orbital contents and to the medial rectus muscle.[9,10]

The blade is used in oscillate mode for the majority of the surgery. Most of the instruments have a default setting that will allow the blade to oscillate at 3000 or 5000 revolutions per minute. The foot pedal will also usually have a switch to allow the surgeon to select either variable or full speed when the pedal is depressed. Variable mode allows the surgeon to slow the speed whereas full speed will result in the blade turning at 3000 or 5000 rpm immediately as the pedal is depressed. It is important to understand that the speed at which the blade turns determines the amount of tissue that is cut. The higher the speed the less time the port is open and the less tissue is able to be sucked into the blade before the turning blade cuts the tissue. Conversely, the slower the speed the more tissue is sucked in and the more aggressively the blade cuts. **Fig. 1.1a** shows the blade in open mode and **Fig. 1.1b** shows tissue being sucked into the port of the blade before rotation of the blade cuts the tissue.

In forward and reverse mode the revolutions may vary from 3000 to 12,000 rpm and consequently the blade is open for only a very short period of time. Tissue cutting in this mode is thus severely limited. Forward mode is usually used for the various bur attachments that can be used in place of the blade. However, forward mode can also be used for very gently shaving bony septations on the lamina papyracea or skull base. This needs to be done with absolute knowledge of the anatomy and great care as inadvertent penetration of either structure can be disastrous. When this is done, the septations are brushed with the rotating blade without any use of pressure.

Endoscopic High-Speed Drills

Medtronic ENT (Minneapolis, MN) has a microdebrider base box that takes both a microdebrider handpiece with power range up to 30,000 rpm and all standard microdebrider blades and burs. The new burs designed to be run at 30,000 rpm come in a variety of angles as well as cutting or diamond options. This high-speed bur is very efficient at

removing large amounts of bone quickly and has resulted in much shorter operating times for procedures requiring bone removal. A caution must be added that the efficiency of these burs and the high speed at which they function may contribute added risk to the surgery as quick bone removal may result in breach of the skull base and intracranial penetration or orbital penetration. Experience and care is required when using the high-speed burs. In addition, this base box also takes an electronic endoscopic high-speed drill (Stylus) with curved irrigated diamond and cutting burs with power range up to 60,000 rpm. The surgeon can switch between the standard hand piece with drill (M5) and the high-speed electric drill by simply touching the button on the foot pedal. This high-speed electric drill, although irrigated, does not have in-built suction like a normal microdebrider drill and therefore is more suitable in a two-surgeon setup where the second surgeon can provide suction during drilling.

Endoscope Cleaners

A large number of companies manufacture endoscope cleaners or scrubbers. These are designed to wash the lens of the endoscope should it become obscured with blood. If the surgical field is bloody, the endoscope cleaner keeps the scope lens clear of blood and allows the operation to proceed without the need to remove the endoscope from the nose and manually clean it. The endoscope cleaner speeds up the operation and improves the safety of the surgery by maintaining visibility and decreasing the surgeon's frustration level by allowing the surgery to progress more rapidly.

Cameras and Monitors

Surgery was originally performed by the surgeon looking through the eye piece of the endoscope but this traditional technique is seldom used anymore. Currently, most surgeons connect a video camera to the endoscope which enables the surgeon to operate using the view on the monitor. A significant advantage of operating from the monitor is the ergonomic advantage this affords the surgeon as he or she can sit or stand next to the patient and not have to bend either their back or neck to obtain a view of the nasal cavity. This is especially valuable if the frontal recess is being operated upon as the surgeon viewing the procedure through the eyepiece

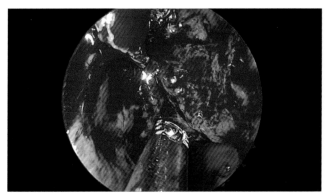
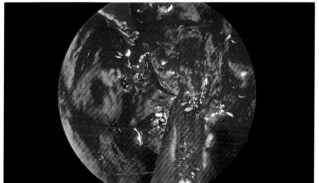

a   b

Fig. 1.1 (**a**) The blade open and (**b**) with tissue being sucked into the blade prior to rotation of the inner blade and severing of the tissue.

may have to almost have their head on the patient's chest to obtain an adequate view. In addition, if a large instrument such as the microdebrider is been used at the same time, this instrument may touch the surgeon's head when it is being manipulated into tight spaces. The monitor provides a large magnified image that can be advantageous for delicate work (e.g., optic nerve, skull base, and intracranial surgery) and it allows two surgeons to operate together (pituitary, infratemporal fossa, and intracranial surgery). Another major advantage of operating from the monitor is that it allows a senior surgeon to monitor the trainee's surgery and allows the trainee (and all in the operating room) to watch the senior surgeon operate. The nurse can anticipate the surgical instrument required for the next step and the anesthetist can monitor the operating field and undertake anesthetic interventions to improve the surgical field as required. If the surgeon is operating from the monitor, a high definition digital camera is required with a powerful light source and medical grade monitor. Analog cameras generally do not cope well with blood in the surgical field and depth perception and tissue contrasts can be lost. If inferior cameras are used, visibility and orientation become increasingly difficult for the surgeon and the risk of complications increases.

◆ Position of the Patient and the Surgeon

My preference is to sit at the right-hand side of the patient. The surgeon may stand but if his or her elbow is not resting on the operating table, the monitor image tends to move excessively, reflecting the instability of the hand holding the endoscope. The patient should be supine and the operating table tilted a minimum of 15 degrees up to 30 degrees anti-Trendelenburg. The patient's head should be in a neutral position (neither flexed nor extended). This allows the surgeon to operate in a plane parallel to the skull base, which diminishes the risk for skull base injury by decreasing the

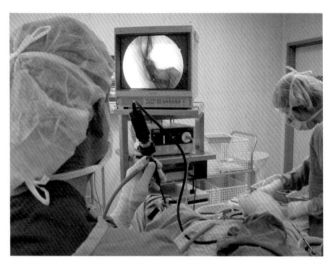

Fig. 1.2 Picture of the operating setup with the surgeon, the patient's head, and the video monitor all in a straight line. The scrub nurse stands opposite the surgeon which allows a view of the monitor and facilitates the handing of instruments to the surgeon.

angle of approach. The video monitor should be positioned so that the surgeon, the patient's head, and the monitor are in a straight line (**Fig. 1.2**).

A thin arm board is placed next to the patient's head to widen the upper part of the operating table so that the surgeon can comfortably rest their elbow on the arm board. If this position is too low and extra height is needed, sterile drapes folded into a square are placed on the arm board to build this up. The patient's head can also be turned toward the surgeon which decreases the height at which the elbow needs to be supported. The scrub nurse should position his or her instrument table so that the far edge of the table is parallel with the head of the operating table. This allows the monitor stack to be placed in a straight line with the patient's head and surgeon (**Fig. 1.3**).

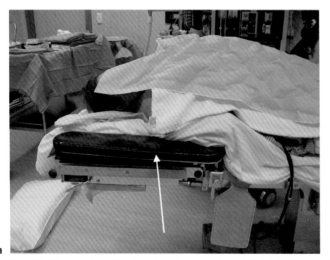

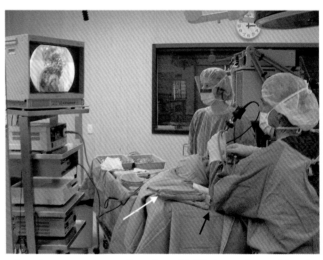

a

b

Fig. 1.3 The arm board is placed on the operating table (**a**) (*white arrow*) to allow the surgeon to rest their elbow (**b**) (*black arrow*) to stabilize the camera. This allows the surgeon's forearm and wrist to be straight which is ergonomically comfortable for the surgeon. It also ensures that the monitor picture is stable (**b**). The height of the elbow can be adjusted with sterile towels (*white arrow*) as required.

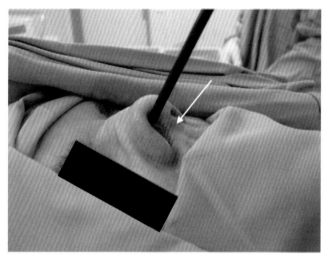

Fig. 1.4 The scope is used to tent the nasal vestibule superiorly creating space below the endoscope (*white arrow*) through which the instrument is passed into the nose.

◆ Principles of Endoscope Placement and Instrument Placement during ESS

With the surgeon's elbow resting on the added arm board, the endoscope is slid into the nose. The endoscope should then be pushed as far superiorly as possible. This should distort the nasal vestibule by placing the endoscope high in the nasal vestibule. This creates a space in the nasal vestibule below the endoscope through which all instruments are placed (**Fig. 1.4**).

The endoscope and the instruments should never cross during surgery. It is only very rarely when dissecting in the frontal sinus with a 70-degree endoscope that the endoscope needs to be placed below the instrument. When this is done, the surgeon loses sight of the tip of the instrument and accurate and careful dissection is no longer possible. The 0-degree endoscope should be used whenever possible

and in the techniques described in the following chapters it is used unless otherwise stated. This makes the surgery as simple as possible and decreases the risk of unnecessary injury to the adjacent or surrounding mucosa during passage of the endoscope and instrument. It also limits the risk of disorientation that can occur when using angled endoscopes. If angled endoscopes are used, instruments need to be curved so that the tip of the instrument can be manipulated in the center of the endoscope view (see Chapter 7). The greater the angle of the endoscope, the longer the curve needs to be on the instrument. The greater the angle of the endoscope and curve of the instrument, the greater the degree of difficulty of dissection so it is best to use the angled endoscopes (especially the 70-degree endoscope) as infrequently as possible during surgery.

References

1. Messerklinger W. Endoscopy of the nose. Munich: Urban and Scharzenberg; 1978:52–54
2. Stammberger H. Endoscopic endonasal surgery—concepts in treatment of recurring rhinosinusitis. Part I. Anatomic and pathophysiologic considerations. Otolaryngol Head Neck Surg 1986;94(2):143–147
3. Kennedy DW. Functional endoscopic sinus surgery. Technique. Arch Otolaryngol 1985;111(10):643–649
4. Wee DTH, Carney AS, Thorpe M, Wormald PJ. Endoscopic orbital decompression for Graves' ophthalmopathy. J Laryngol Otol 2002;116(1):6–9
5. Wormald PJ. Powered endoscopic dacryocystorhinostomy. Laryngoscope 2001;112:69–72
6. Wormald PJ, Ooi E, van Hasselt CA, Nair S. Endoscopic removal of sinonasal inverted papilloma including endoscopic medial maxillectomy. Laryngoscope 2003;113(5):867–873
7. Wormald PJ, Van Hasselt A. Endoscopic removal of juvenile angiofibromas. Otolaryngol Head Neck Surg 2003;129(6):684–691
8. Knegt PP, Ah-See KW, vd Velden LA, Kerrebijn J. Adenocarcinoma of the ethmoidal sinus complex: surgical debulking and topical fluorouracil may be the optimal treatment. Arch Otolaryngol Head Neck Surg 2001;127(2):141–146
9. Graham SM, Nerad JA. Orbital complications in endoscopic sinus surgery using powered instrumentation. Laryngoscope 2003;113(5):874–878
10. Bhatti MT, Giannoni CM, Raynor E, Monshizadeh R, Levine LM. Ocular motility complications after endoscopic sinus surgery with powered cutting instruments. Otolaryngol Head Neck Surg 2001;125(5):501–509

2 The Surgical Field in Endoscopic Sinus Surgery

◆ Introduction

The presence of significant bleeding in the surgical field is a critical factor in the potential success or failure of endoscopic sinus surgery (ESS).[1–4] When significant bleeding is present, recognition of anatomical landmarks becomes difficult.[2–4] Bleeding obscures surgical planes and makes the identification of the drainage pathways of the sinuses difficult. Cell walls become difficult to distinguish from the lamina papyracea or skull base and the risk of causing complications increases.[3,4] If the patient has significant inflammation of the sinuses, from chronic infection or the presence of pus/fungal debris, increased vascularity will often contribute to more bleeding.[2,5] If the surgeon attempts to manipulate an instrument in the surgical field after the discernable anatomy is covered in blood, the risk of a complication increases. In addition, greater surgical trauma may occur, cells may be left behind, and there is an increased likelihood of postoperative scarring and failure of the surgical procedure. It is therefore critical to optimize the surgical field and in so doing make the surgical dissection as easy as is possible.[2–4]

Our department has a special interest in this aspect of ESS and has conducted a number of double-blind randomized controlled studies in an attempt to establish which maneuvers to reduce bleeding are worthwhile. To date, not all maneuvers have been scientifically evaluated but where there is evidence for a specific maneuver this is presented. The first important issue to address is a grading system for bleeding in the surgical field. Boezaart and van der Merwe described and validated a grading system of five grades presented in **Table 2.1**.[3]

Although this grading system is valuable, we have found that the majority of surgical fields are around grade 3 with some grade 2 and some grade 4.[2] Only on rare occasions are grade 1 and 5 fields encountered. This tends to compress the grading system and makes differentiation of more subtle changes difficult. Grade 3 may need to be further divided to allow variation within grade 3 to be discerned.[2] We have recently developed and validated an endoscopic sinus surgical field score, which separates the middle grades and allows more accurate grading of the surgical field (**Table 2.2**).

◆ Local versus General Anesthetic

Local anesthetic has the advantage of not inducing generalized vasodilatation. Increased circulating catecholamines may also improve the surgical field by continuing to act on the prearteriolar and precapillary sphincters. However, there are a number of limitations to local anesthetics:

- Patient anxiety and sudden patient movement during delicate surgery can be problematic
- Surgery takes between 1 and 2 hours. Some patients (especially older patients) have difficulty remaining still for this length of time
- Appropriate anesthesia needs to be achieved in all the sinuses and the nasal cavity,
- If the procedure is bloody the patient may have difficulty dealing with the volume of blood trickling into the pharynx. If the patient is sedated aspiration can occur.
- Water from the scope scrubber may add to the secretions in the pharynx that the patient needs to deal with
- Teaching of residents can be more difficult when the patient is awake

In our department, local anesthetic is offered to patients having limited ESS confined to the middle meatus. We prefer general anesthesia for ESS that involves the frontal recess and/or posterior ethmoids and/or sphenoids.

◆ Standard Nasal Preparation for ESS

Laryngeal Mask versus Endotracheal Intubation

It is our current practice to use laryngeal masks rather than endotracheal intubation for all our patients undergoing

Table 2.1 Boezaart and van der Merwe grading system for bleeding during endoscopic sinus surgery[3]

Grades	Surgical field
Grade 1	Cadaveric conditions with minimal suction required
Grade 2	Minimal bleeding with infrequent suction required
Grade 3	Brisk bleeding with frequent suction required
Grade 4	Bleeding covers surgical field after removal of suction before surgical instrument can perform maneuver
Grade 5	Uncontrolled bleeding; bleeding out of nostril on removal of suction

sinus surgery. The rationale for this is that it allows the patient to be kept under a lighter general anesthetic with less vasodilatation and less intraoperative bleeding. In addition, the patient does not cough and strain on the endotracheal tube as they recover from the anesthetic, avoiding the venous congestion and subsequent hemorrhage often associated with such straining. One of the potential downsides of a laryngeal mask is the possibility of contamination of the upper airway by blood. This is prevented by the placement of a small throat pack above the laryngeal mask in the back of the throat to catch any blood from the nasal cavity. Another possible downside is the potential difficulty with ventilation of the patient during surgery. Our standard protocol is total intravenous anesthesia (TIVA) with a laryngeal mask in a nonparalyzed patient. The remifentanil infusion (part of TIVA) suppresses spontaneous ventilation and allows the patients to be ventilated through the laryngeal mask. The lack of paralysis provides additional safety against intraoperative awareness because the patient should move if the level of anesthesia becomes too light.

Table 2.2 The Wormald grading system for bleeding during endoscopic sinus surgery

Grade	Surgical Field
0	No bleeding
1	1–2 points of ooze (no blood in the sphenoid)
2	3–4 points of ooze (no blood in the sphenoid)
3	5–6 points of ooze (slight blood accumulation in the sphenoid)
4	7–8 points of ooze (moderate blood accumulation of sphenoid—fills after 90 seconds)
5	9–10 points of ooze (sphenoid fills after 60 seconds)
6	> 10 points of ooze, obscuring surface (sphenoid fills between 40 and 60 seconds)
7	Mild bleeding/oozing from entire surgical surface with slow accumulation of blood in post nasal space (sphenoid fills by 40 seconds)
8	Moderate bleeding from entire surgical surface with moderate accumulation of blood in post nasal space (sphenoid fills by 30 seconds)
9	Moderately severe bleeding with rapid accumulation of blood in post nasal space (sphenoid fills by 20 seconds)
10	Severe bleeding with nasal cavity filling rapidly (sphenoid fills in < 10 seconds)

Positioning the Patient

The positioning of the patient is described in Chapter 1. It is important to have the patient 30-degrees head up so that the venous return from the head and neck is facilitated. This puts the patient's head above the chest, which lowers the arterial pressure and prevents venous congestion, and thereby improves the surgical field.[6]

Topical Vasoconstriction

In a study recently published, we showed that any packing material placed in the nasal cavity tends to cause damage to the nasal mucosa.[7] The more abrasive the packing, the worse the trauma.[6] Taking this into consideration, the least abrasive packing material is used, namely the neurosurgical Cottonoid patties (Codman, Boston, MA) or a standard Merocel (Medtronic ENT, Minneapolis, MN) nasal pack cut into six pieces. The anesthetist is consulted to ensure there is no contraindication to the use of cocaine. If there is a concern, then 1% oxymetazoline is used in place of cocaine. In an adult patient, a mixture of 2 mL of 10% cocaine, 1 mL of 1:1000 adrenaline, and 4 mL of saline is divided into two portions, with half used to soak six neuropatties or Merocel pieces. These six pieces are placed in the nose once the patient is anesthetized. The other half of the cocaine mixture and, if a standard 10 neuropattie pack was used, the remaining four neuropatties are kept sterile on the instrument trolley for later use during surgery if required. Three Cottonoids/pieces are placed on each side directly after intubation using a Freer's elevator to manipulate them gently into place. The first is placed in the sphenoethmoidal recess, the second under the middle turbinate, with the third being placed over the axilla of the middle turbinate (**Fig. 2.1**). If there is a concha bullosa or significantly lateralized middle turbinate, the Cottonoid is placed along the inferior margin of the middle turbinate. No force is used to position the Cottonoid in the middle meatus.

As only half the solution is used at the beginning of surgery, the total dose of cocaine that the patient is exposed to is about 100 mg. The toxic dose of cocaine is 3 mg/kg without

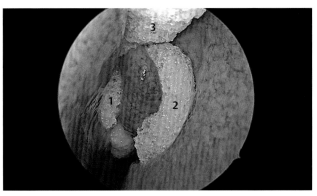

Fig. 2.1 Placement of the Merocel pieces in the left nasal cavity prior to surgery. A Merocel piece is in the sphenoethmoidal recess (1), another is in the middle meatus (2), and another is in the region of the axillary flap (3).

the simultaneous use of adrenaline. It has also been shown that the presence of adrenaline inhibits mucosal absorption and that a proportion of the solution will remain in the pack. This decreases the amount of cocaine that the patient is exposed to and the doses used are well below the toxic dose in adult patients. The dose needs to be appropriately adjusted in children.

Local Infiltration

A 2% solution of lidocaine (lignocaine in the UK and Australia) with either 1:80,000 or 1:100,000 adrenaline is administered with a dental syringe and needle. The injections are given after the patient has been draped and the camera and endoscope are available. Under endoscopic guidance, the area above the middle turbinate is infiltrated. This is followed by infiltration into the anterior end of the middle turbinate. Note that the area anterior to the uncinate is not infiltrated as bleeding from an injection site can obscure the uncinate during its removal. In some patients, where there is an expected increased likelihood of bleeding, a third injection is given into the back end of the middle turbinate in the region of the sphenopalatine artery. A spinal needle is used as the dental needle is usually not long enough to reach this area. **Fig. 2.2** illustrates the routine infiltration points used.

Preoperative Antibiotics and Steroids

Inflammation increases the vascularity of tissues and when surgery is conducted on highly inflamed tissues, increased bleeding results. Patients with acute sinusitis, who have an infective complication requiring surgery, will often have a very bloody surgical field. It therefore stands to reason that

using antibiotics in patients with a significant infection preoperatively should improve the surgical field. However, most of our patients undergoing ESS have had extended medical therapy which normally includes numerous courses of antibiotics and often systemic steroids, and therefore rarely have an acute infection present. The value of using antibiotics preoperatively in this elective patient group is unknown as there are no well-designed studies addressing this issue. The important questions that remain unanswered are the type of antibiotic, the length of time it should be used before surgery, and the patient group most likely to benefit from preoperative use. Currently, I do not routinely place patients on antibiotics preoperatively.

It has been suggested that patients with significant nasal polyposis may benefit from a course of preoperative steroids.[8] The theory is that steroids should decrease the size of the polyps and the vascularity associated with these polyps. A recently published study evaluated the effect of preoperative steroids on the degree of bleeding during sinus surgery.[8] In this study prednisone, 30 mg daily was given for 5 days preoperatively and the results showed a significant improvement in a visual analog grading of the surgical field during surgery.[8] However, it remains unclear what doses of steroids should be given, for how long, and to which patient groups. Empiric treatment regimens range from 30 mg[8] to 50 mg of prednisone daily for between 3 and 7 days preoperatively, and is usually only utilized in nasal polyposis patients.

The Blood Pressure during ESS

One of the critical factors that the anesthetist can control during surgery is the blood pressure. This is usually presented as the mean arterial pressure (MAP) and calculated by MAP = diastolic pressure + 1/3(systolic pressure–diastolic pressure). Hypotensive anesthesia (defined as a MAP of 50–70 mm Hg) is a well described technique and frequently used in cardiac, orthopaedic, and spine surgery.[9,10] Its use in ESS procedures has also been described[9] but its value has been controversial with risk often considered to outweigh benefit.[9,10] Although a recent article showed benefit of hypotensive anesthesia in ESS, it is was still unclear as to what the optimal MAP is during ESS and if such a MAP is safe with regard to the perfusion of vital organs during the procedure. In our department, we designed a study to firstly assess if hypotensive anesthesia benefits the surgical field during ESS[11] and secondly at what MAP levels this is best achieved and, by using middle cerebral artery perfusion to assess organ perfusion, what MAP levels can be used with relative safety.[12] In the first study, although there was a clear statistical improvement in surgical fields with lower MAPs, most of the readings tended to be at lower MAPs which skewed the data as there were few MAPs at the higher end to show that the bleeding did get worse at higher MAPs.[11] The second study was designed so that the MAP was artificially elevated during surgery on one side then lowered into the hypotensive range for the second side.[12] Sides were randomized and the observers blinded to the MAP manipulations. In addition, in this study the cerebral perfusion as measured by an extracranial Doppler placed over the middle cerebral artery was measured

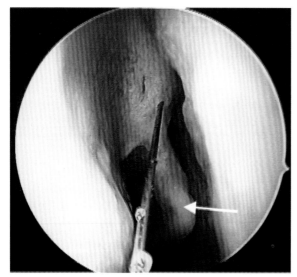

Fig. 2.2 Injection sites in the right nasal cavity for local anesthetic prior to endoscopic sinus surgery. The needle is in the region of the axillary flap and the *white arrow* indicates the injection site on the anterior end of the middle turbinate.

during the changes in blood pressure. These studies have conclusively shown that the most significant manipulation affecting the surgical field is the blood pressure and that the anesthetist should aim in a healthy patient without comorbidities for a MAP of around 65 mm Hg. Cerebral blood flow was minimally affected at a MAP of above 60 mm Hg and was considered safe. Although there were further improvements in the surgical field at MAPs of below 60 mm Hg, these were small and did not warrant the risk associated with the potential hypoperfusion of vital organs. Therefore, our current protocol is to ask the anesthetist to keep the MAP around 65 mm Hg. The methodology by which this is achieved is also important and detailed here.

Total Intravenous Anesthesia and Inhalational Agents

Inhalational agents used during general anesthesia cause peripheral vasodilatation by relaxing of the prearteriolar muscle sphincters.[6] This significant peripheral vasodilatation usually results in mild hypotension.[3,4,6] Peripheral vasodilatation with paralysis of the arteriolar and precapillary sphincters may result in significant bleeding if surgery is performed when the tissues of the nose and sinuses are inflamed.[3,4,6] Any maneuver that attempts to lower the MAP using vasodilatation results in a poor surgical field. General anesthesia results in vasodilatation and the extent of the vasodilatation is to a certain extent dependent upon the type and quantity of inhalational agent used.[6] Halothane gives significant vasodilatation and should not be used.[6] Isoflurane and sevoflurane produce less vasodilatation but if they are used to deepen the level of anesthesia with the intention of lowering the blood pressure, significant vasodilatation can occur.[6] Total intravenous anesthesia (TIVA) is usually given by utilizing a constant infusion of propofol. Propofol induces anesthesia by enhancing the action of GABA neurotransmitter on the GABA receptor, which allows the chloride channels to be opened causing hyperpolarization and reduced excitability of the cell.[13] Propofol is short acting and needs to be administered as a constant infusion. Although it does depress the heart, this response is not dose-dependent and increasing the infusion rate of propofol will not result in an increasing suppression of pulse rate and cardiac output. It, however, does not affect the muscle tone of the prearteriolar and precapillary sphincters and does not cause vasodilatation and increased bleeding. This allows inhalational agents to be avoided. If bleeding during ESS continues to be problematic despite the patient receiving TIVA, other drugs such as β-blockers or clonidine can be added. In a recent study in our department, we performed a randomized controlled single-blinded (to the surgeon) study using TIVA and isoflurane. This study showed that the surgical fields were better if TIVA was used.[14] All other factors were kept constant during the surgery. The pulse rate, when analyzed independently, again correlated to the surgical field, emphasizing the importance of the pulse rate on the surgical field. Some anesthetists are uncomfortable using TIVA as it can be difficult to judge the depth of anesthesia so it is a good idea to discuss the merits of use of TIVA with the anesthetist before surgery. Our protocol does not use a muscle relaxant. The remifentanil infusion sufficiently depresses the patient's respiration and allows the patient to be ventilated during the procedure. However, should the propofol become disconnected or infusion rate be inappropriate, then the patient wakes up and, because the patient is not paralyzed, it is obvious to all that the TIVA is no longer working.

β-Blockers

If vasodilatation occurs during general anesthesia the body attempts to compensate for this reduced venous return and low cardiac output by increasing the heart rate in an attempt to improve the cardiac output.[3,4,6] In a seminal paper, Boesak and van der Merwe showed that vasodilatation induced by sodium nitroprusside caused a significant worsening in the surgical field despite the lowered blood pressure.[3] What they also showed was that esmolol, a highly selective β1 β-blocker, improved the surgical field with a much smaller drop in blood pressure.[3] Esmolol is a short-acting cardioselective β adrenergic receptor-blocking drug that has a fast onset and short half-life. In contrast to a drug such as sodium nitroprusside, which although effectively lowering the blood pressure results in a compensatory increase in heart rate, esmolol is highly effective at depressing cardiac output and results in a slowing of the pulse rate despite a fall in blood pressure.[6] Esmolol is given by a constant IV infusion and has a very short half-life (around 3 minutes) so its effect can be closely controlled. Although this can be a very worthwhile maneuver, it is a very expensive drug and there is some resistance (based on cost) against using it as a regular or routine part of ESS anesthesia. The expense of this drug stimulated our department to conduct a double-blind placebo controlled prospective study in the effects of metoprolol taken orally 20 minutes before general anesthetic, as compared to a vitamin B placebo.[2] This study showed that patients who received the β-blocker (metoprolol) had a significantly lower pulse rate (mean of 59) than the placebo group (mean of 69). There was no significant difference in blood pressure or surgical fields in the two groups. However, what was interesting was the significant correlation between heart rate in the overall patient group with surgical grade.[2] Thus, irrespective of whether a β-blocker is given to the patient, if the heart rate of the patient can be kept below 60 beats per minute, the surgical field was usually good.[2] Therefore, we recommend the use of a β-blocker (atenolol, metoprolol, or esmolol) in patients who at induction of anesthesia have a pulse rate significantly above 60 beats per minute and who do not have a contraindication (such as asthma) as a worthwhile manipulation that can improve the surgical field. However, asthma is a common comorbidity in patients with chronic sinusitis and alternatives are needed. In this group of patients we use clonidine.

Clonidine

Clonidine is a centrally active alpha agonist that initially results in an elevation of blood pressure before depressing the cardiac output by inhibiting the central cardiac regulatory mechanism. It should be used with caution and should be given in small increments, as the effect is not easily reversible. It also results in mild postoperative sedation and its effects on the blood pressure are usually seen in the initial few hours after surgery. This is beneficial for the majority of patients as this mild hypotension allows the small blood vessels in the nose to coagulate with a reduced chance of postoperative epistaxis. There are now good studies in the literature that show that patients in whom clonidine has been used have significantly better surgical fields than those who do not. I therefore highly recommend the use of clonidine as part of the anesthetic technique to control MAP.

◆ Additional Maneuvers for Optimizing the Surgical Field in ESS

Suction Bipolar Cautery* of Isolated Bleeding Areas

It is common to see isolated bleeding vessels in the surgical field during ESS. These result from the transection of small blood vessels and may continue to ooze into the surgical field, significantly adding to the volume of blood that may obscure the surgical field.[4] In addition, such an ooze may obscure the end of the endoscope requiring either the endoscope scrubber to be used or the endoscope to be removed from the nose to be cleaned. If the axillary flap approach to the frontal recess is used (Chapter 7), the cut mucosal edge may bleed and this can be controlled by the use of the suction bipolar cautery. Other common areas where bleeding is seen are the posterior region of the maxillary sinus, the sphenopalatine region of the lateral nasal wall, and from the anterior wall of the sphenoid below its ostium. The suction bipolar allows the bleeding vessels to be accurately identified and cauterized. Not having to remove the instrument from the nose after the suction clears the blood allows for identification of the bleeding point, which is a significant advantage of this instrument (**Fig. 2.3**).

The Anatomy of the Greater Palatine Canal and Local Anesthetic Infiltration of the Pterygopalatine Fossa

Injection of local anesthetic into the pterygopalatine fossa does improve the surgical field.[15,16] The maxillary artery and its terminal branches make up the main blood supply of the nose. There are two approaches; the less reliable approach is direct infiltration into the region of the sphenopalatine foramen. The needle is introduced just under the posterior end of the middle turbinate. Sometimes the needle can be felt to slip into the sphenopalatine foramen but in most cases location of the foramen is difficult and the injection is given into the general region of the foramen. This should cause vasospasm of the vessels exiting the foramen. However, because the foramen is not easily located, the resulting vasoconstriction achieved may not be as great as injecting the pterygopalatine fossa through the greater palatine canal.

The second more reliable approach is to inject the pterygopalatine fossa through the greater palatine foramen and canal. First, the greater palatine foramen needs to be located on the hard palate (**Fig. 2.4**). The greater palatine foramen is located just anterior to the posterior edge of the hard palate opposite the second molar tooth.[16] It is usually halfway between the tooth and the midline of the hard palate. The opening of the foramen into the canal is funnel-shaped and the canal is angled at about 45 degrees to the hard palate.

In a cadaver study performed in our department to evaluate the anatomy of the greater palatine canal, 20 cadaver heads were CT scanned in the axial plane at 0.5 mm.[16] Parasagittal reconstructions were performed in the plane of the greater palatine canal. The length of the canal and depth of the soft tissue overlying the canal were measured. In addition, needles were bent at 10, 20, and 30 mm and inserted into the greater palatine canal prior to CT scanning to demonstrate the degree of penetration into the pterygopalatine fossa in four cadavers (**Fig. 2.5**).

This was done to ascertain the likelihood of damage to the contents of the fossa (branches of the maxillary nerve, maxillary artery, and pterygopalatine ganglion) and the orbit. Note that the bend in the needle stops at the soft tissue overlying the hard palate and that this soft tissue had a mean thickness of 6.9 mm (95% CI = 6.2–7.6) (**Fig. 2.6**). The mean length of the greater palatine canal was 18.5 mm (95% CI = 17.9–19.1) and the mean height of the pterygopalatine fossa was 21.6 mm (95% CI = 20.7–22.5).[16] Therefore, to perform an effective infiltration of the pterygopalatine fossa, the needle should be bent at 25 mm from the tip at an angle of 45 degrees.[16] This will result in the tip of the needle just penetrating the pterygopalatine fossa without putting any of the contents of the fossa at risk.[16]

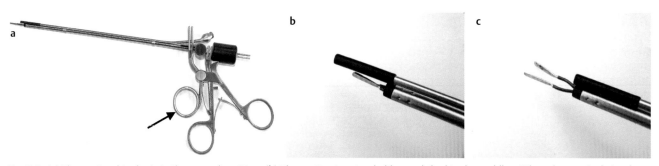

Fig. 2.3 (**a**) The suction bipolar is in the normal position. (**b**) The suction is extended beyond the bipolar paddles. When the manipulating lever (*black arrow*) in (**a**) is relaxed the suction retracts behind the bipolar paddles (**c**).

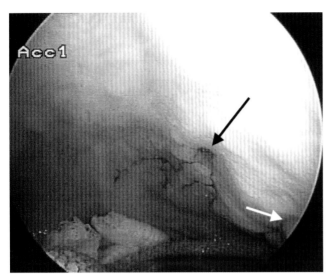

Fig. 2.4 Blood staining can be seen from where the needle was introduced into the greater palatine canal (*black arrow*) of the left hard palate. The second molar tooth is marked with a *white arrow*.

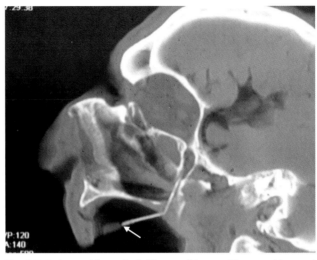

Fig. 2.5 Cadaver with needle (*white arrow*) bent at 20 mm and inserted into the greater palatine canal after which the CT scan was performed.

The greater palatine canal has an hourglass shape, dilating as it enters the pterygopalatine fossa. This funnel-shaped entrance into the greater palatine canal means that it can be difficult to determine exactly where the pterygopalatine fossa ends and the greater palatine canal begins (*white arrow*) (**Fig. 2.6**).

The easiest way to locate the greater palatine foramen is by palpating the palate with the finger. This is performed by placing a tongue depressor in the mouth and holding down the tongue, then passing a finger and the endoscope into the mouth together. The finger first locates the posterior free edge of the hard palate and then slides anteriorly over this ridge onto the hard palate. The foramen should be felt as a depression directly anterior to the free edge about midway between the second molar tooth and the midline of the palate. Visualize the finger palpating the foramen on the monitor and identify the spot on the palate as the finger is withdrawn from the mouth. With the needle bent at 25 mm and at a 45-degree angle, insert the needle into the spot that you had visually marked on the palate. If the needle strikes bone then a small amount of lidocaine is infiltrated, the needle is withdrawn, and an adjacent spot is tried. The assumption is that the needle had just missed the foramen and that a slight adjustment needs to be made before the foramen is located. If repeated attempts to introduce the needle fail, then the landmarks for the foramen (the midpoint between the second molar tooth and midline of the palate) are reassessed and the finger and endoscope are replaced into the mouth and the foramen relocated. The needle is reintroduced until the foramen is located by the needle advancing into the greater palatine canal without any resistance up to the bend in the needle. After aspirating (to ensure that the needle is not in a blood vessel), the pterygopalatine fossa is infiltrated with 2 mL of 2% lidocaine and 1:80,000 adrenaline.

Our department has conducted a double-blind randomized controlled trial in which the effects of local anesthetic and adrenaline infiltration of the pterygopalatine fossa were assessed on the surgical field in 55 patients.[17] To be included in the study the patient required bilateral ESS with similar procedures being performed bilaterally. A surgeon not involved in the surgery randomly infiltrated one fossa transorally so that the operating surgeon would not be aware of which side had been infiltrated. The surgeon then alternated the surgery on the patient and assessed the surgical field on each side. Statistical analysis showed that the side that had received the pterygopalatine fossa injection had significantly better surgical field (mean surgical grade of 2.59) than the control side (mean surgical grade of 2.99; $p < 0.01$).[17]

◆ General Guidelines for the Maneuvers for Improving the Surgical Field

The ideal surgical field is grade 2 on the Boezaart scale and grades 1–4 on the Wormald scale. However, the majority of

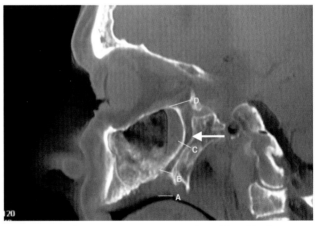

Fig. 2.6 The soft tissue measurement was from (**a**) to (**b**), the greater palatine canal from (**b**) to (**c**), and the height of the pterygopalatine fossa from (**c**) to (**d**). The funnel-shaped opening of the greater palatine canal into the pterygopalatine fossa is indicated with a *white arrow*.

our patients fluctuate between grade 2 and 3 on the Boezaart scale and 2–6 on the Wormald scale. Operating in more bloody conditions can be aided by the use of suction dissection instruments* (see Chapter 1) such as the suction curette* and suction Freers*. These instruments allow the blood to be cleared from the surgical field during the dissection and obviate the need to change from a dissecting instrument to a suction in order to clear the surgical field.

Surgical Field Change from Boezaart Grade 3 to Grade 4 or 5

Please note surgery should not be performed if the surgical field is grade 5 or Wormald grade 8–10.

- Check positioning of the patient
- Check that you have properly infiltrated the lateral wall of the nose with lidocaine and adrenalin
- Place neuropatties soaked with cocaine and adrenaline in the surgical field
- Check the patient's pulse rate and, if greater than 60, ask the anesthetist to adjust this to below 60 (using β-blockers if not contraindicated)
- If the patient is hypertensive, ask the anesthetist to bring the mean blood pressure down to around a mean of 65 mm Hg without increasing the inhalational agent (consider the use of a β-blocker or clonidine).

Re-check Your Surgical Field

- If there is a specific bleeder, cauterize it with the suction bipolar.*
- If the bleeding is emanating from the posterior region of the nasal cavity, consider replacing the neuropatties and performing a pterygopalatine fossa block.
- If bleeding is still not controlled or is coming from the anterior aspects of the nose, then consider asking the anesthetist to further lower the pulse rate with small incremental doses of clonidine. Remember to stay within the safe range of MAP (>60 mm Hg[6,11,12]), especially when considering the age of the patient and the previous mean blood pressure of the patient. If the patient was known to suffer from hypertension this figure should be higher.
- Consider changing patient from inhalational anesthesia to TIVA.

References

1. Stankiewicz JA. Complications of endoscopic intranasal ethmoidectomy. Laryngoscope 1987;97(11):1270–1273
2. Nair S, Collins M, Hung P, Rees G, Close D, Wormald PJ. The effect of beta-blocker premedication on the surgical field during endoscopic sinus surgery. Laryngoscope 2004;114(6):1042–1046
3. Boezaart AP, van der Merwe J, Coetzee A. Comparison of sodium nitroprusside- and esmolol-induced controlled hypotension for functional endoscopic sinus surgery. Can J Anaesth 1995;42(5 Pt 1):373–376
4. Boezaart AP, van der Merwe J, Coetzee AR. Re: Moderate controlled hypotension with sodium nitroprusside does not improve surgical conditions or decrease blood loss in endoscopic sinus surgery. J Clin Anesth 2001;13(4):319–320
5. Mortimore S, Wormald PJ. Management of acute complicated sinusitis: a 5-year review. Otolaryngol Head Neck Surg 1999;121(5):639–642
6. van Aken H, Miller ED. Deliberate Hypotension. In: Miller RD, ed. Anesthesia. Vol. 2. New York, NY: Churchill Livingstone; 1994:1481–1503
7. Shaw CL, Dymock RB, Cowin A, Wormald PJ. Effect of packing on nasal mucosa of sheep. J Laryngol Otol 2000;114(7):506–509
8. Sieskiewicz A, Olszewska E, Rogowski M, Grycz E. Preoperative corticosteroid oral therapy and intraoperative bleeding during functional endoscopic sinus surgery in patients with severe nasal polyposis: a preliminary investigation. Ann Otol Rhinol Laryngol 2006;115(7):490–494
9. Condon HA. Deliberate hypotension in ENT surgery. Clin Otolaryngol Allied Sci 1979;4(4):241–246
10. Cardesin A, Pontes C, Rosell R, et al. A randomised double blind clinical trial to compare surgical field bleeding during endoscopic sinus surgery with clonidine-based or remifentanil-based hypotensive anaesthesia. Rhinology 2015;53(2):107–115
11. Ha TN, van Renen RG, Ludbrook GL, Valentine R, Ou J, Wormald PJ. The relationship between hypotension, cerebral flow, and the surgical field during endoscopic sinus surgery. Laryngoscope 2014;124(10):2224–2230
12. Ha TN, van Renen RG, Ludbrook GL, Wormald PJ. The effect of blood pressure and cardiac output on the quality of the surgical field and middle cerebral artery blood flow during endoscopic sinus surgery. Int Forum Allergy Rhinol 2016;6(7):701–709
13. Sonner J, Zhang Y, Stabernack C, Abaigar W, Xing Y, Laster M. GABAA receptor blockade antagonizes the immobilizing action of propofol but not ketamine or isoflurane in a does-related manner. Anesth Pharm 2003;96(3):706–712
14. Wormald PJ, van Renen G, Perks J, Jones JA, Langton-Hewer CD. The effect of the total intravenous anesthesia compared with inhalational anesthesia on the surgical field during endoscopic sinus surgery. Am J Rhinol 2005;19(5):514–520
15. Wormald PJ, Wee DTH, van Hasselt CA. Endoscopic ligation of the sphenopalatine artery for refractory posterior epistaxis. Am J Rhinol 2000;14(4):261–264
16. Douglas R, Wormald PJ. Pterygopalatine fossa infiltration through the greater palatine foramen: where to bend the needle. Laryngoscope 2006;116(7):1255–1257
17. Wormald PJ, Athanasiadis T, Rees G, Robinson S. An evaluation of effect of pterygopalatine fossa injection with local anesthetic and adrenalin in the control of nasal bleeding during endoscopic sinus surgery. Am J Rhinol 2005;19(3):288–292

3 Imaging in Endoscopic Sinus Surgery

◆ Introduction

It is fortunate that the development of endoscopic sinus surgery (ESS) has coincided with major advances in computed tomography (CT) scanning technology. Before CT scanning was available, the extent of sinus disease and anatomy of the nose and sinuses were assessed on plain X-rays. Plain X-rays are no longer used in this role as they do not provide sufficient anatomical detail or accurate information on the extent of nasal and sinus pathology. The CT scan has allowed the detailed anatomy of the sinuses to be evaluated and, in this textbook, CT scans are used extensively to reconstruct the anatomy of the sinuses, thereby enabling a surgical plan to be made before surgery begins. The surgical philosophy of this textbook is underpinned by the availability of high quality CT scans in three planes.

◆ Computed Tomography Scans

The Value of Scans in Three Planes

CT scans are used as an aid for both the diagnosis of chronic sinusitis and for the planning of the surgery. However, there is a significant incidence of mucosal abnormalities seen in completely asymptomatic patients.[1] Thus, it is important that the patient has undergone adequate medical treatment for the nasal and sinus condition before a CT scan of the sinuses is performed.[2] The coronal scan is the primary scan used to assess the anatomy of the sinuses.[3] These scans should be sufficiently close together so that an identified cell can be followed from one slice to the next. This allows a three-dimensional image of the anatomy to be reconstructed from the scans.[4–6] The axial scan is of particular value in determining the drainage pathway of the frontal sinus. This is important when deciding where the curette or probe is going to be slid during the dissection of the frontal recess. Our department published a study evaluating the value of the parasagittal scan in assessing the frontal recess and in the understanding and planning of the surgery.[7] We found that the parasagittal scan significantly improved the surgeon's ability to assess the frontal recess and improved the understanding of the anatomy by a mean of 57% on a 10-point visual analog scale. The parasagittal scan also altered the surgical plan for the patient in over 50% of patients studied. We therefore recommend that the all patients undergoing ESS have a high definition helical 64 multislice CT scan of the sinuses with the scans presented in all three planes. An example of the quality of the CT scans that should be expected using this protocol is shown in **Fig. 3.1**.

Disclaimer

Software that allows the CT scan to be simultaneously viewed in all three planes and that allows the anatomy of the cells to be reconstructed was developed in conjunction with Scopis®. The author received royalties from the sale of this software.

Scanning Protocol

Good quality CT scans are critical to the ability of the surgeon to reconstruct the anatomy and drainage pathways of the sinuses. Ideally, images should be in the coronal, axial, and parasagittal plane and should be relatively close together so that a cell can be followed from one scan to the next. Our current CT scan imaging protocol on a 64 multislice CT helical scanner requires scans to be performed in the axial plane at 0.5-mm to 1-mm intervals with coronal and parasagittal reconstruction. Images in all planes are printed for the surgeon and available for digital download and used on the Scopis software for viewing and detailing of the anatomy (see disclaimer). The windows of the scan are set at between 1500 and 2000 with a center of +100 to +300 for highest bony definition. If there is a suspicion of fungal sinus disease, the

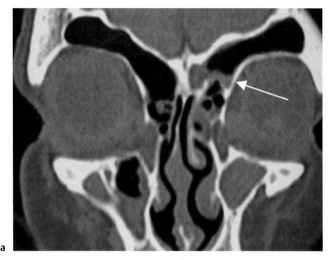

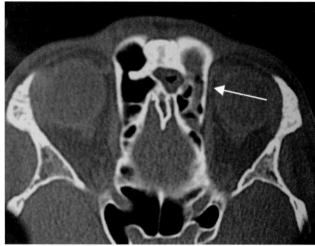

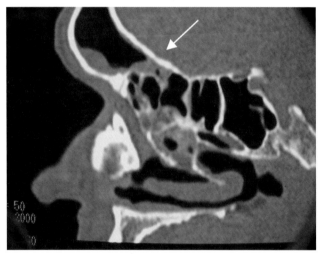

Fig. 3.1 Computed tomography scans with slices in the (**a**) coronal, (**b**) axial, and (**c**) parasagittal planes. The disease in the left frontal recess (*white arrow*) can be evaluated and the cellular structure better understood if all three planes are available.

window settings are changed to soft tissue settings. This allows the opacified sinuses to be assessed for double densities that are often present in chronic fungal sinus disease.

Three-Dimensional Views and the Concept of Building Blocks

Some CT scanners have software where cursors can be moved through a series of scans in one plane while at the same time the views of where the cursor is in the other planes is simultaneously displayed. Software that does the same thing can be purchased independently if not available on the scanner. Scopis software is available for download (http://planning.scopis.com) and is suitable for both PCs and MACs. It allows DICOM images from CT scanners to be loaded and will create images in all three planes with movable crosshairs. In addition, all computer-aided surgical (CAS) systems also have this facility. With these systems, the CT scans can be scrolled in a particular plane and the other views change depending upon where the cursor is placed on the scan being viewed. Scopis software is able to draw a building block over each cell and place a drainage

pathway along the frontal sinus drainage pathway. This allows the surgeon not only to fully understand the anatomy of the frontal recess but also to carefully plan each surgical step of the dissection. An example of such a reconstruction is shown in **Fig. 3.2**.

A central theme throughout this book is the utilization of high quality CT scans in three different planes to build a three-dimensional picture of the anatomy of the sinuses. In this book, I use Scopis software to place a building block on each cell. **Fig. 3.2** shows a red building block placed on the agger nasi cell. Note how each corner of the building block has a circle in each of the planes. The surgeon chooses which plane would be best to manipulate the block and then grabs these corners to change the block in one plane. Once this is done, the circles on the corners of the other blocks disappear but the sides of the block can still be manipulated. In **Fig 3.3** the axial plane block has been manipulated to better fit the CT scan. In **Fig. 3.4** the supra agger cell (*green box*) has been manipulated in the parasagittal plane. In **Fig. 3.5** the frontal septal cell (*blue box*) has been manipulated in the axial plane and in **Fig. 3.6** the supra bulla cell (*pink box*) has been manipulated in the parasagittal plane. The final cell of the frontal recess (*light blue box*) completes the anatomical

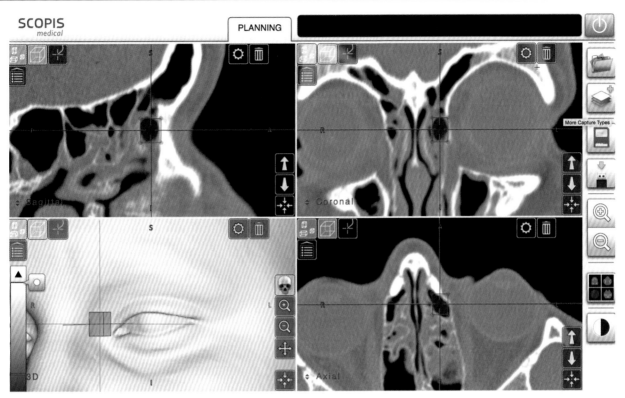

Fig. 3.2 The red building block is placed over the left agger nasi cell. In all three planes the corners of the building block are circles. The surgeon can choose which plane to manipulate the corners.

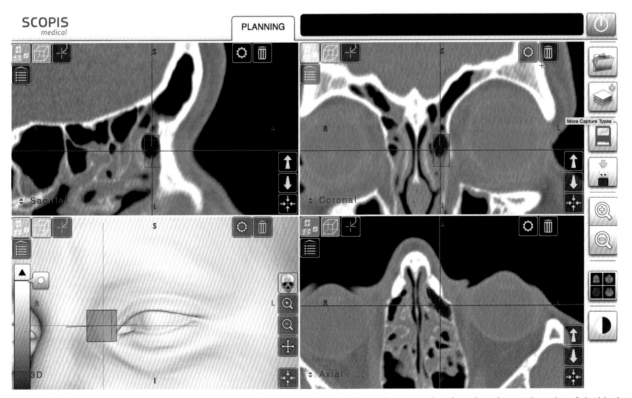

Fig. 3.3 The building block has been manipulated in the axial plane so the circles have disappeared in the other planes. The sides of the blocks in the other planes can be manipulated but only the corners in the axial plane.

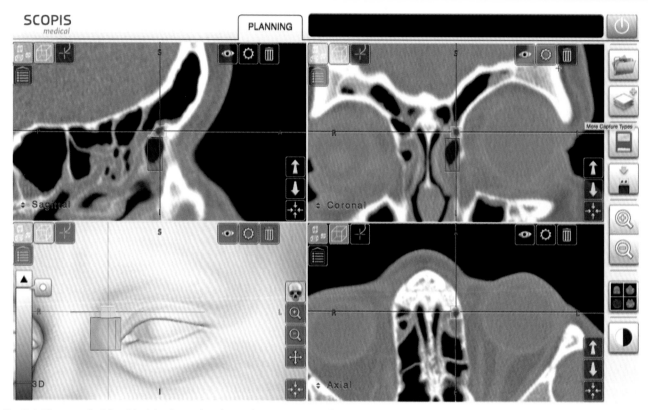

Fig. 3.4 The green building block has been placed over the supra agger cell and manipulated in the parasagittal plane.

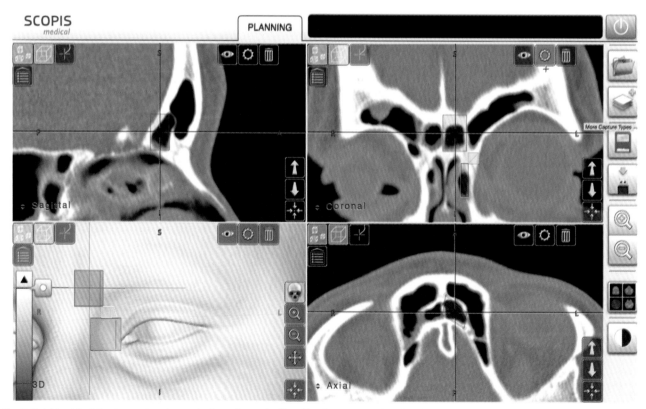

Fig. 3.5 A blue block has been placed over the frontal septal cell and has been manipulated in the axial plane.

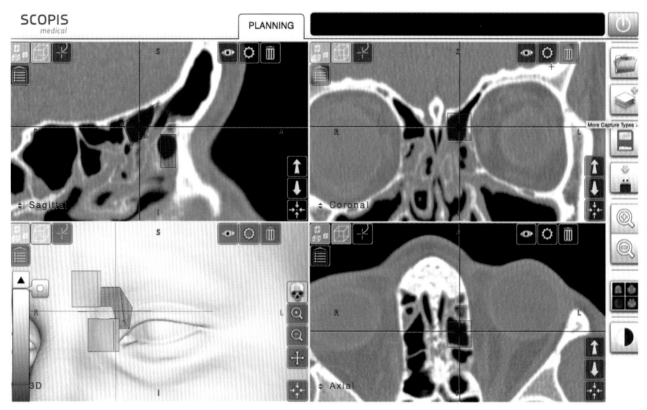

Fig. 3.6 The pink block has been placed over the supra bulla cell and has been manipulated in the parasagittal plane.

configuration of this patient's frontal recess (**Fig. 3.7**). In the bottom left box of **Fig. 3.7**, all the cells can be seen that make up the anatomy of the frontal recess. **Fig. 3.8** shows the frontal sinus drainage pathway that has been placed among the cells. Note how the drainage pathway passes lateral to the frontal septal cell but posteromedial to the supra agger cell and agger nasi cell and in front of the supra bulla cell and bulla ethmoidalis. This ability to understand both the cells and the frontal drainage pathway is especially important in understanding the anatomy of the frontal recess (Chapter 6). After completion of the frontal recess, the process can be repeated in the posterior ethmoids and sphenoid (Chapter 8). The concept of three-dimensional anatomical reconstruction using building blocks to re-create the anatomical formation in the frontal recess and posterior ethmoids and then to surgically establish the drainage pathways is the central theme of this textbook.

◆ **Magnetic Resonance Imaging Scans**

Magnetic resonance imaging (MRI) scans are not routinely used for the assessment of patients undergoing ESS as they do not provide bony definition. In addition, MRI scans are very sensitive to mucosal thickening of the nasal or sinus mucosa (especially of a vascular region such as the inferior turbinate). Normal mucosa may enhance and in some patients even appear pathological even though it is normal.

However, the MRI scan can be very useful in a number of situations. We routinely request a MRI scan in patients who have previously undergone an osteoplastic flap with obliteration who have ongoing symptoms.[8,9] In these patients, the MRI can differentiate sepsis or mucocele formation from those with healthy fat in their obliterated frontal sinuses. All patients who have an intranasal tumor are assessed with an MRI scan.[10] In these patients, we are primarily interested in whether an opacified sinus is filled with tumor or retained mucous and whether a breach or invasion of the dura or orbital periosteum has occurred. An example of the usefulness of a MRI in surgical planning is shown in **Fig. 3.9**. This patient had an adenocarcinoma with opacified frontal sinuses and right maxillary sinus on CT scanning. On the MRI, it can clearly be seen that the left frontal sinus and right maxillary sinus are filled with mucus not tumor.

Our protocol to assess these patients is to perform a T1-weighted fat saturation gadolinium-enhanced scan and a T2-weighted scan. The tumor enhances on the T1 gadolinium-enhanced scan but the fluid in the sinuses does not. If the T2-weighted scan is reviewed, fluid (mucus) usually enhances significantly. In scans (c) and (d) of **Fig. 3.9**, the lamina papyracea and skull base are eroded. However, it appears that the orbital contents have been pushed laterally by the tumor rather than the tumor invading into the orbit. In this patient both orbits were preserved and there was a good surgical plane between the tumor and the orbital periosteum. The tumor also appears to push the dura superiorly rather than eroding through the dura. Again, we were

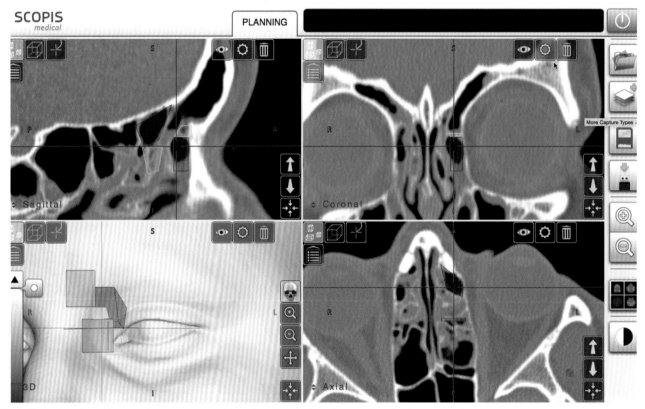

Fig. 3.7 The light blue block has been placed over the bulla ethmoidalis and manipulated in the parasagittal plane.

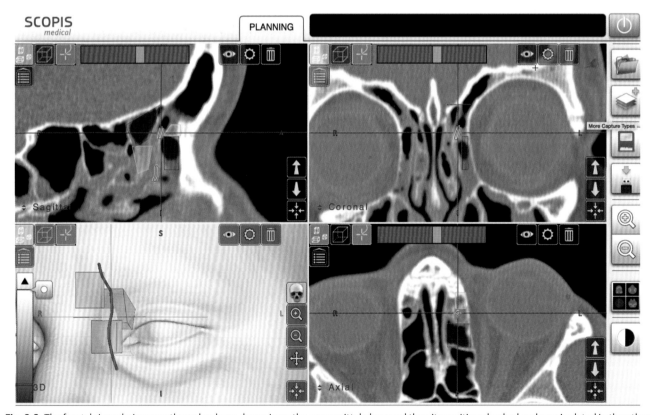

Fig. 3.8 The frontal sinus drainage pathway has been drawn in on the parasagittal plane and then its position checked and manipulated in the other planes until the pathway was correct.

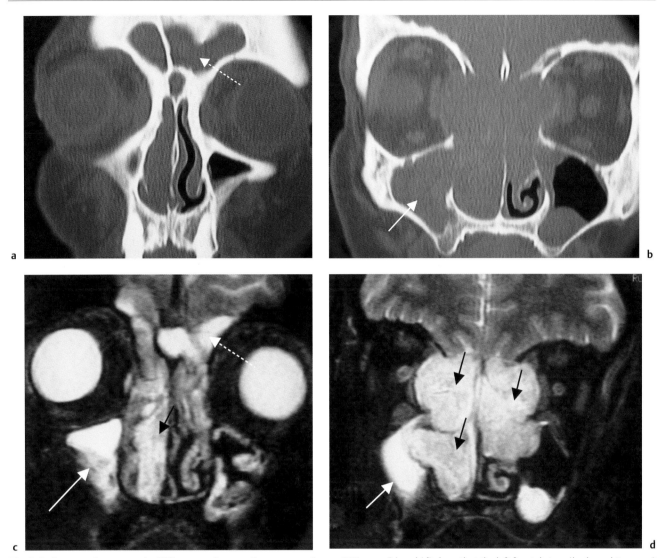

Fig. 3.9 Computed tomography (CT) scan and magnetic resonance imaging (MRI) scan of a patient with adenocarcinoma. CT scans (**a**) and (**b**) show opacification of the frontal sinuses (*broken white arrow*) in (**a**) and the right maxillary (*solid white arrow*) in (**b**). The T2-weighted MRI scans (**c**) and (**d**) show that the left frontal sinus (*broken white arrow*) (**c**) and that both maxillary sinuses (*solid white arrow* for right sinus) contain fluid and not tumor (right frontal unclear on this scan).

able to establish a good surgical plane between the tumor and the dura and achieve a complete macroscopic resection of the tumor without resection of the dura. The patient had postoperative radiotherapy and continues to be tumor free 3 years after the surgical procedure.

MRI scans are also useful in the assessment of complications of sinusitis, particularly for orbital complications with subperiosteal abscess formation and intracranial complications.[11] MRI scans are used as first-line assessment for pituitary tumors and for extended skull base lesions such as clival tumors.

◆ Angiography

Angiography is useful in patients who have a suspected vascular tumor and an attempt is to be made to remove this tumor endoscopically.[12] It is of great importance that the vascularity of the tumor be reduced as far as possible to facilitate endoscopic removal. Vascular tumors that have not been embolized can bleed so profusely during endoscopic resection that the procedure needs to be abandoned. Although a number of tumors can benefit from preoperative embolization, this intervention is of particular value in angiofibroma[12] (**Fig. 3.10**).

◆ Dacryocystogram and Lacrimal Scintillography

A dacryocystogram (DCG) can be very useful for assessing the anatomy of the nasolacrimal system.[13,14] It is important to identify patients with a significant stricture of the

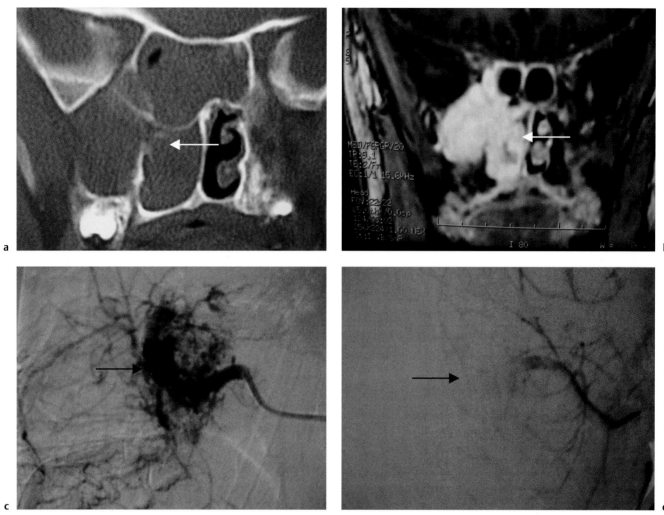

Fig. 3.10 The computed tomography scan (**a**) shows an angiofibroma (*white arrow*) filling the posterior nasal cavity with extension into the pterygopalatine and infratemporal fossas. The tumor (*white arrow*) extent is better seen on the magnetic resonance image (**b**). The digital subtraction angiogram (**c**) illustrates in the intense vascularity of the tumor (*black arrow*) before embolization while the effectiveness of embolization is illustrated in (**d**) where no tumor blush can be seen (*black arrow*).

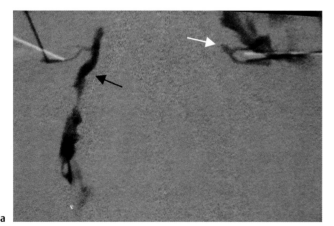

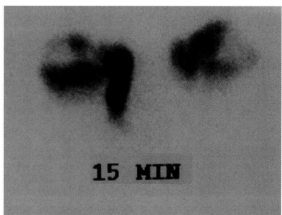

Fig. 3.11 (**a**) The dacryocystogram: the right side is normal with the normal lacrimal sac (*black arrow*) and canaliculi clearly seen. On the left side, the superior, inferior, and common canaliculi can be seen but dye does not penetrate the lacrimal sac (*white arrow*) and there is no filling of the lacrimal sac. This represents a common canaliculus obstruction. (**b**) The corresponding lacrimal scintillogram for the patient in (**a**). A normal scintillogram can be seen on the right. There is some isotope filling of the left lacrimal sac but no nasal penetration. This indicates probable kinking of the common canaliculus as it enters the sac.

common canaliculus as these patients are not suitable for dacryocystorhinostomy.[13,14] In some patients with significant epiphora, a DCG reveals a free flow of dye from the canaliculus to the nose. A DCG is not a physiological test as abnormally high pressures are generated in the nasolacrimal system during injection of the dye. In these patients, lacrimal scintillography can be very useful as the placement of a radioisotope in the tear lake with subsequent detection of its passage into the nasolacrimal system and nose provides important information regarding the function of the system (**Fig. 3.11**). These tests are fully elaborated upon in Chapter 11.

References

1. Flinn J, Chapman ME, Wightman AJA, Maran AGD. A prospective analysis of incidental paranasal sinus abnormalities on CT head scans. Clin Otolaryngol Allied Sci 1994;19(4):287–289

2. Lusk RP, Muntz HR. Endoscopic sinus surgery in children with chronic sinusitis: a pilot study. Laryngoscope 1990;100(6):654–658

3. Kennedy DW, Zinreich SJ. The functional endoscopic approach to inflammatory sinus disease: current perspectives and technique modifications. Am J Rhinol 1988;2:89–96

4. Wormald PJ. The agger nasi cell: the key to understanding the anatomy of the frontal recess. Otolaryngol Head Neck Surg 2003;129(5):497–507

5. Wormald PJ. The axillary flap approach to the frontal recess. Laryngoscope 2002;112(3):494–499

6. Wormald PJ, Chan SZX. Surgical techniques for the removal of frontal recess cells obstructing the frontal ostium. Am J Rhinol 2003;17(4):221–226

7. Kew J, Rees G, Close D, Sdralis T, Sebben R, Wormald PJ. Multiplanar reconstructed computed tomography images improves depiction and understanding of the anatomy of the frontal sinus and recess. Am J Rhinol 2002;16(2):119–123

8. Wormald PJ, Ooi E, van Hasselt CA, Nair S. Endoscopic removal of sinonasal inverted papilloma including endoscopic medial maxillectomy. Laryngoscope 2003;113(5):867–873

9. Wormald PJ. Salvage frontal sinus surgery: the endoscopic modified Lothrop procedure. Laryngoscope 2003;113(2):276–283

10. Wormald PJ, Ananda A, Nair S. The modified endoscopic Lothrop procedure in the treatment of complicated chronic frontal sinusitis. Clin Otolaryngol Allied Sci 2003;28(3):215–220

11. Mortimore S, Wormald PJ. Management of acute complicated sinusitis: a 5-year review. Otolaryngol Head Neck Surg 1999;121(5):639–642

12. Wormald PJ, Van Hasselt A. Endoscopic removal of juvenile angiofibromas. Otolaryngol Head Neck Surg 2003;129(6):684–691

13. Tsirbas A, Wormald PJ. Endonasal dacryocystorhinostomy with mucosal flaps. Am J Ophthalmol 2003;135(1):76–83

14. Wormald PJ. Powered endoscopic dacryocystorhinostomy. Laryngoscope 2001;112:69–72

4 Powered Inferior Turbinoplasty and Endoscopic Septoplasty

◆ Powered Endoscopic Inferior Turbinoplasty

Turbinectomy is seldom required in patients with significant chronic sinusitis as successful surgical management of the sinuses will, in most cases, result in normalization of the mucosa of the inferior turbinates. The inflammatory cytokines and cells contained within the mucus emanating from the diseased sinuses causes an inflammatory response from the mucosa of the inferior and middle turbinates. Once the sinuses are properly aerated and this inflammatory exudate resolves, the edema of the turbinate mucosa subsides. However, in patients with ostiomeatal complex disease or minimal maxillary mucosal thickening as their only computed tomography (CT) findings, who have nasal obstruction as their main nasal symptom, turbinoplasty with mini functional endoscopic sinus surgery (FESS) may be needed to resolve these patients' symptoms. In addition, there are some patients without sinus disease who have intractable inferior turbinate hypertrophy (nonresponsive to treatment), and in which turbinate reduction can improve the patient's nasal airway and quality of life. There have been many techniques described for inferior turbinate reduction and these include submucous turbinoplasty, partial turbinectomy, complete turbinectomy, and diathermy (usually performed in the submucosal plane).[1-5] Arguments against complete removal of the inferior turbinates cite the risk of the patient developing atrophic rhinitis, especially in hot and dry climates.[1] In addition, amputation of the turbinate flush with the lateral nasal wall will inevitably result in a significant bleed at the time of surgery as the branch of the sphenopalatine artery to the inferior turbinate is cut[6] (**Fig. 4.1**). This may require diathermy of the bleeder and this again increases the amount of necrotic tissue and results in significant postoperative crusting. Partial turbinectomy may also result in significant bleeding and require diathermy for control. Submucosal turbinoplasty and diathermy, although initially effective, does not appear to have the same long-term success as partial or complete turbinectomy.[1,7] In addition we are all aware of the patients who have undergone turbinectomy and have a capacious nasal airway but still have the sensation of nasal obstruction.[1] This may be due to the removal or destruction of airflow receptors on the medial and superior aspect of the inferior turbinate. However, this remains to be proven. The other significant problem patients suffer from after turbinectomy or diathermy (not submucous turbinoplasty) is crusting on the cut surface of turbinate.[6-8] This problem increases if diathermy has been used to control bleeding. These crusts can be uncomfortable and cause nasal obstruction. In addition, hemorrhage may occur when they either fall off or are removed.[1,3] In the group of patients undergoing submucosal diathermy and to a lesser extent submucosal turbinoplasty, they have significant postoperative swelling of the inferior turbinate which obliterates the nasal cavity and makes the first 3 weeks after surgery very uncomfortable for the patient, who is usually unable to breathe through their nose.[7]

Powered inferior turbinoplasty was designed to preserve the medial wall of the inferior turbinate thereby preserving the airflow receptors. In addition, the technique allows the inferior turbinate to be reduced in size by about 50% without leaving a raw surface for crusts to form in the postoperative period.

◆ Internal Nasal Valve

The most significant airflow limiting area in the nose is the internal nasal valve (**Fig. 4.2**). The valve is formed by a combination of anatomical structures made up by protruding leading edge of the upper lateral nasal cartilage, the nasal septum, and the head of the inferior turbinate. Collapse of the upper lateral cartilage during inspiration can significantly contribute to the sensation of airway obstruction. To determine the component contribution by the upper lateral cartilage, the patient is asked to perform Cottle's maneuver; the skin adjacent to the nasal alar is pulled up and laterally supporting

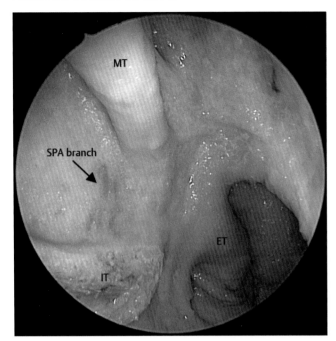

Fig. 4.1 Cadaveric dissection of the right posterior lateral nasal wall demonstrating the inferior turbinate (IT) branch of the sphenopalatine artery (SPA). Note, the posterior attachment of the middle and inferior turbinates and the sphenopalatine foramen is to the palatine bone.

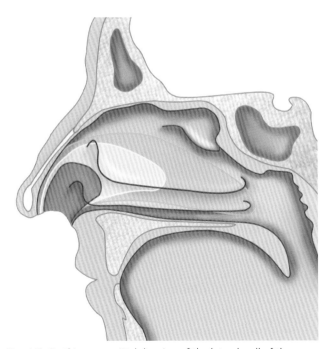

Fig. 4.2 On this parasagittal drawing of the lateral wall of the nose, the red color indicates the region of highest airflow and consequently the narrowest part of the nasal cavity which includes the internal nasal valve. The most prominent structure in the internal nasal valve is the head of the inferior turbinate. The yellow region has a lower air flow and the green region lower again when compared to the red area.

the upper lateral cartilage and the patient is asked to assess the impact on the airway. A significant improvement in airway may require the surgeon to suggest grafts to support the airway. If there is little improvement in airway patency, the surgeon needs to assess the role of the septum and head of the inferior turbinate. Septal deviation in the region of the valve needs to be assessed as well as prominence of the head of the inferior turbinate. Low septal deviations can be managed by standard septoplasty techniques, as described later, but high septal deviations often require more advanced techniques such as an external rhinoplasty approach to the septum. In these patients, surgically reducing the head of the inferior turbinate may be an easier and more attractive option. In most patients, the standard inferior turbinoplasty as described will suffice. However, in some patients with a very narrow nose and with a narrow internal nasal valve where further septal surgery will not improve the valve, an inferior turbinate shoulder osteotomy and turbinate reduction is an excellent alternative. This is described after the standard technique.

◆ Surgical Technique of Inferior Turbinoplasty

Under general or local anesthetic, the anterior end of the inferior turbinate is infiltrated with lidocaine 2% and 1:80,000 or 1:100,000 adrenaline. A spinal needle attached to a 2-mL syringe is used to infiltrate along the posterior inferior border of the inferior turbinate. The most important part of the inferior turbinate contributing to nasal valve obstruction is the head of the inferior turbinate (**Fig. 4.3**). Note that even after decongestion the nasal airway is compromised (*red double arrow*). The microdebrider is used to shave the

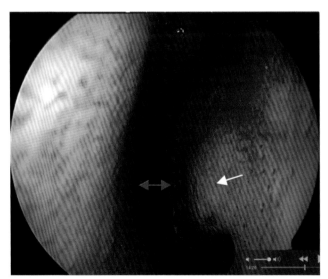

Fig. 4.3 This image of the internal nasal valve shows how the head of the inferior turbinate (*white arrow*) is the largest contributor to the narrow nasal airway (*double red arrow*). In this patient, the septum is straight.

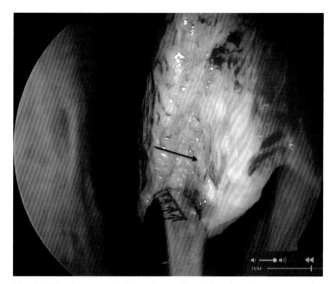

Fig. 4.4 The first step in the endoscopic turbinoplasty is to remove the mucosa over the bone of the head of the inferior turbinate with the microdebrider, making sure that bone is exposed (*black arrow*).

mucosa of the head of the inferior turbinate, making sure to expose the underlying bone (**Fig. 4.4**). The inferior border (**Fig. 4.5a**) and lateral surface of the rest of the inferior turbinate is then shaved, again making sure the bone is exposed (**Fig. 4.5b**). This is done until the posterior end of the inferior turbinate is approached but stopped about 1 cm from the posterior end so as not to cut the arteries that enter the posterior end and supply blood to the turbinate. A sharp dental elevator is used to identify and establish the subperiosteal plane to gain access to the bone of the inferior turbinate (**Fig. 4.6**). Initially the medial mucosa is elevated off the inferior turbinate bone over the top of the turbinate and progressively more posterior. Usually the dorsal inferior turbinate branch of the inferior turbinate artery is seen in its

canal and dissected free of this canal. The vessel is usually found at the junction of the vertical and horizontal portions of the turbinate. Once this mucosal flap has been elevated, the lateral mucosal flap is established at the anterior end of the inferior turbinate bone. As this flap is elevated, the inferolateral branch of the inferior turbinate artery is seen in its bony canal. This bony canal is often complete at the posterior end of the turbinate and the vessel may need to be torn if it does not dissect free of this bony canal. These two vessels are identified with every inferior turbinoplasty (**Fig. 4.7**) so that after removal of the vertical inferior turbinate bone; they are individually cauterized with the suction bipolar forceps (**Fig. 4.8**). This cauterization of both vessels prevents postoperative bleeding. With the bone removed and the major feeding vessels cauterized, the medial mucosal flap can now be rolled laterally to produce a new turbinate that is usually about half the size of the original turbinate (**Fig. 4.9a**). This highly effective turbinoplasty preserves the medial functional mucosa of the inferior turbinate while still creating a significant airway. The rolled medial mucosal flap is held in place by a thin strip of Surgicel (Ethicon, Somerville, NJ) (**Fig. 4.9b**). This technique gives very good long-term nasal patency without compromising the function of the turbinate as the entire medial mucosal surface (the functional part of the turbinate) is preserved. In **Fig. 4.10**, a 1-year postoperative view demonstrates the continued patency of the nasal airway but still with a functional turbinate.

◆ Inferior Turbinate Shoulder Osteotomy for Internal Nasal Valve Obstruction

This approach is very similar to the prelacrimal approach described in Chapter 5. The initial incision runs along the insertion of the inferior turbinate into the lateral nasal wall and anteriorly up to the bony piriform aperture (**Fig. 4.11**,

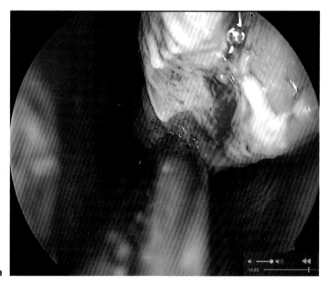

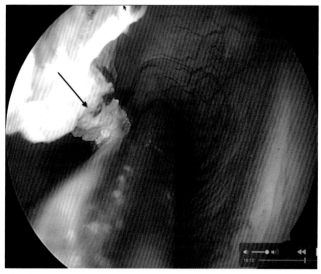

a   b

Fig. 4.5 (**a**) The bone along the inferior edge of the turbinate is exposed. (**b**) The endoscope and microdebrider are placed in the inferior meatus lateral to the inferior turbinate and the mucosa is removed off the lower lateral portion of the inferior turbinate (*black arrow*).

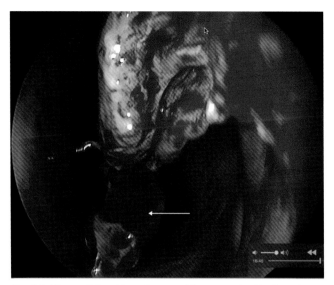

Fig. 4.6 The medial and lateral mucosal flaps are raised in the subperiosteal plane and the vertical bone of the inferior turbinate (*white arrow*) dissected free from the turbinate and removed.

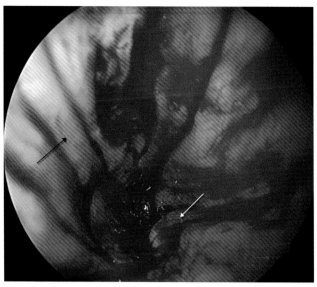

Fig. 4.7 This image was taken after bone removal with the medial and lateral mucosal flaps splayed to reveal the constant vasculature seen supplying the inferior turbinate. There are always two major vessels: a medial superior vessel (*black arrow*) and a lateral inferior vessel (*white arrow*). These two branches are the major inferior turbinate arterial supply from the branch of the sphenopalatine artery that feeds the back end of the inferior turbinate.

white arrow). The malleable suction Freer is used to elevate the mucosal flap in the subperiosteal plane over the head of the inferior turbinate (**Fig. 4.12**, *black arrow*), exposing the bone of the head of the inferior turbinate and continuing this elevation posteriorly for about 2 cm (**Fig. 4.12**). The bone of the vertical portion of the inferior turbinate is exposed (**Fig. 4.12**, *white arrow*) and removed from the turbinate. Depending upon the prominence of this bone, it can be removed from the entire length of the turbinate or just from the anterior 2 to 3 cm of the turbinate. A 4-mm osteotome is used to create osteotomies from the piriform aperture posteriorly by removing the bone anterior to the head

of the inferior turbinate posteriorly until the entire head of the turbinate is removed (**Fig. 4.13**). This bony removal continues posteriorly until the region of the nasolacrimal duct. If prominent, then the bone around the nasolacrimal duct can be removed to allow further lateralization of the inferior turbinate. The mucosa that had previously been over the head and anterior end of the turbinate is replaced and a suture placed to hold the mucosa in place (**Fig. 4.14**). The mucosa is pushed laterally and the displaced turbinate held in place

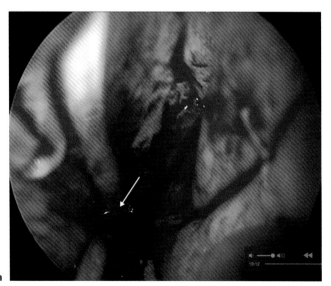

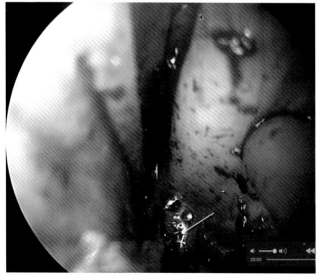

a   b

Fig. 4.8 (**a,b**) Each of the vessels are individually cauterized with the bipolar forceps.

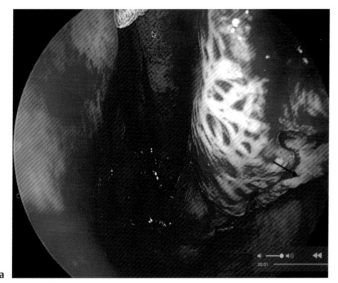

a

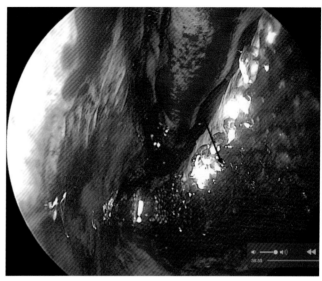

b

Fig. 4.9 (**a**) The medial inferior turbinate flap is rolled laterally to cover any exposed tissue; this increases the nasal airway, preserves the functional medial wall of the turbinate, and prevents postoperative crusting.

(**b**) A strip of Surgicel has been placed over the rolled turbinate to hold the medial flap in place.

by a strip of Surgicel. Note how the internal nasal valve is now significantly larger due to the underlying bone removal although the anatomy of the valve and turbinate remains largely unchanged.

◆ Postoperative Care

The patient starts saline nasal douche within a few hours of the surgery. This is continued for a month postoperatively. After a day, the patient is allowed to very gently blow their

nose after saline wash. Systemic antibiotics are given for 5 days. The patient is seen for follow-up after 2 weeks.

◆ Results of Inferior Turbinoplasty

To evaluate the effectiveness of inferior turbinoplasty, a prospective randomized comparative study was performed where patients were randomized to undergo powered

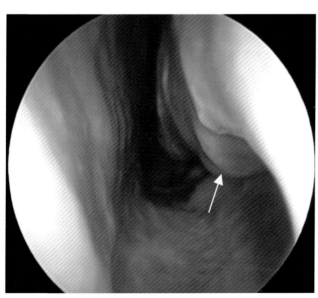

Fig. 4.10 This picture demonstrates the size of the turbinate after 1 year (*white arrow*).

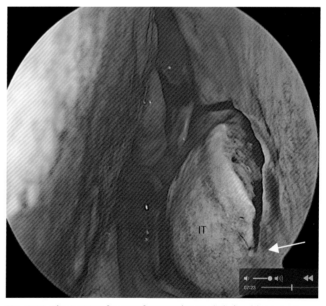

Fig. 4.11 The incision for an inferior turbinate (IT) shoulder osteotomy extends from the natural ostium of the maxillary sinus along the insertion of the inferior turbinate onto the lateral nasal wall (*white arrow*) and then curves over the head of the inferior turbinate onto the piriform aperture.

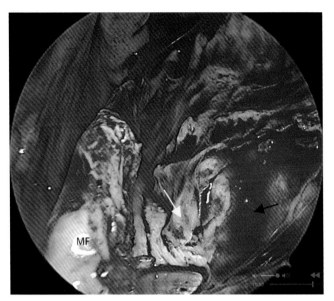

Fig. 4.12 The mucosa of the inferior turbinate is elevated off the bone of the inferior turbinate to form a medial flap (MF). The head of the inferior turbinate is exposed (*black arrow*) with the dissection continuing onto the vertical portion of the inferior turbinate bone (*white arrow*). The dissection is then taken posteriorly depending upon the amount of inferior turbinate bone to be resected.

inferior turbinectomy on one side and submucous diathermy on the other. Nineteen patients were assessed by a pre- and postoperative symptom score, endoscopic grading of turbinate hypertrophy, and acoustic rhinometry. The symptoms were scored individually for each side. This showed a significant improvement in symptoms of nasal patency on the powered turbinoplasty side in the immediate (first 3 weeks) postoperative period. The submucous diathermy

side continued to have nasal obstruction during this period. Objectively, there was also a statistically significant decrease in nasal crust formation at 3 weeks. After 3 weeks, objective nasal patency improved on the side that had undergone submucous diathermy but the difference in symptomatic and objective nasal patency was maintained on the powered turbinoplasty side at 1, 3, and 6 months but was not present at 1 year. There was no difference in postoperative hemorrhage rates. Long-term follow-up was performed at 5 years and this showed that turbinate hypertrophy had recurred on the submucous diathermy side but not on the powered turbinoplasty side when the nasal cavity was assessed endoscopically and with acoustic rhinometry.

Fig. 4.10 shows a typical view of an inferior turbinate in a patient who had undergone powered inferior turbinectomy.

◆ Endoscopic Septoplasty

A significant percentage of patients have septal deviation that impedes adequate access to the middle meatus or to the axillary region of the middle turbinate. Following the surgical principle that exposure is one of the keys to successful surgery, we recommend having a fairly low threshold in straightening such a deflection and thereby improving the access to the middle meatus and to the frontal recess. As the surgeon has the endoscopes all set up and ready to go, there seems little sense in using a headlight to perform an operation that is straightforward to perform with the endoscope. In addition, performing the surgery using the monitor allows all observers in the theatre to view the surgery and has the significant advantage of allowing the surgeon to teach the operative steps to the junior resident. It is very difficult for the resident to follow the surgical steps if the surgeon

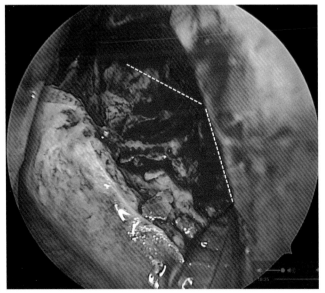
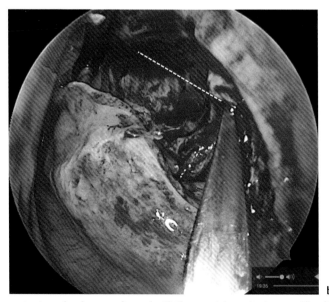

a

b

Fig. 4.13 (a) The osteotome is just medial to the piriform aperture and the direction of the osteotomy to remove the bone of the head of the inferior turbinate is illustrated with the *white dotted line*. **(b)** Half the osteotomy has been performed with the remaining osteotomy outlined with the *white dotted line*.

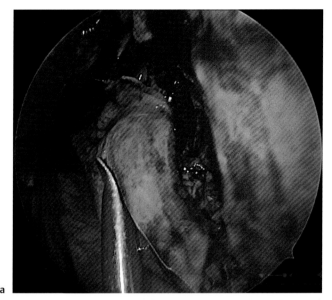
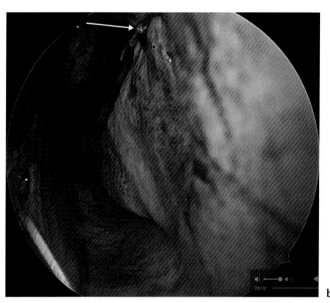

a
b

Fig. 4.14 (**a**) After removal of the bone of the head of the inferior turbinate, the medial flap is replaced. (**b**) the flap is secured with a single suture (*white arrow*). Note the significant improvement is the size of the airway at the region of the internal nasal valve (head of inferior turbinate).

performs the surgery utilizing the headlight and speculum. The key to successful endoscopic septoplasty is instrumentation. A suction Freer elevator helps to keep the surgical field clear of blood and it is extremely helpful to have an endoscope lens cleaner to remove any blood that may blur the end of the endoscope. If the septal deviation is to one side only then it is advisable to perform the ESS on the widely patent side and then perform the septoplasty with the incision on the side through which surgery had been performed. This decreases the likelihood of contaminating the endoscope as it is introduced through the nose.

◆ Surgical Technique

The principle of endoscopic septoplasty is to preserve as much of the quadrilateral cartilage as possible. This is done by only elevating the mucosa off one side of the cartilage and leaving the other attached. In a large number of patients, the septum is too long and dislocates off the maxillary crest creating an anterior septal spur. As the cartilaginous septum is often too long, it bows and deviates, aggravating the contralateral nasal obstruction. If there is a dislocation of the caudal end of the cartilaginous septum and the end of the septum protrudes into one of the nasal vestibules, this should be addressed with a hemi-transfixion incision rather than a Killian's incision. If the deviation starts in the region of the lower border of the upper lateral cartilage, then a Killian's incision is performed just beyond this landmark. The back of the scalpel is used to lift the presenting edge of the upper lateral cartilage. The vertical incision is started as high on the septum as possible, progressing to the floor of the nose and curving posteriorly as it reaches the floor of the nose (**Fig. 4.15a**). A suction Freer elevator is used to elevate the mucosal flap in the subperichondrial plane (**Fig. 4.15b**).

The flap is raised in a posterior direction before the dissection proceeds to the floor of the nose. Once the floor is reached, the flap is separated from the maxillary crest from posteriorly to anteriorly. If the cartilaginous septum is too long and is dislocated off the maxillary crest, a strip of cartilage needs to be removed from its lower insertion into the maxillary crest. The subperichondrial flap is brought down to the presenting edge of the spur but the flap is not raised over this deflection as it is likely to tear. Rather, using the sharp end of a regular Freer elevator, a horizontal incision is made above the spur through the cartilage from the bony cartilaginous junction about 2 to 3 mm above the maxillary crest up to the anterior Killian's incision (**Fig. 4.16**).

The subperichondrial flap is raised on the opposite side of this inferior segment down onto the maxillary crest. This segment of cartilage is then elevated out of the maxillary crest starting anteriorly and working under the cartilage in the groove of the crest. In this manner, the mucosa over the anterior spur can often be preserved. If the maxillary crest is large or has a bony spur (**Fig. 4.17**), this can be trimmed back using a chisel. Usually only the half of the crest that is protruding into the nasal cavity is removed because damage to the nerves that supply the incisor teeth is more common if the whole maxillary crest is removed.

To manage the posterior bony septum, the bony and cartilaginous junction is disarticulated up to the roof of the nose (**Fig. 4.17**). The suction Freer is used to develop the subperichondrial flap on the other side of the bony septum. Bony deviations are removed with special attention given to the bony septum directly under the nasal bones which is often cancellous and quite thick. A great view of this is obtained with the endoscope and deviated bone is resected as this bone will often obstruct the view of the insertion of the middle turbinate onto the lateral nasal wall—the so-called axilla of the middle turbinate. No attempt is usually made to preserve

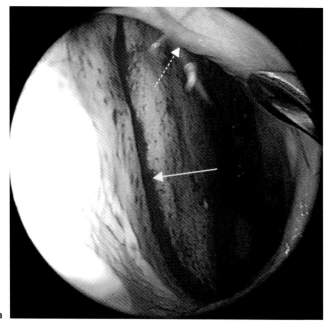

a

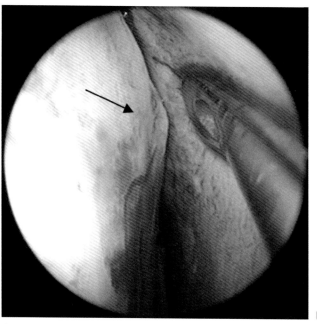

b

Fig. 4.15 (**a**) A Killian's incision (*white arrow*) has been performed just behind the leading edge of the upper lateral cartilage (*broken white arrow*). (**b**) The mucoperichondrial flap has been raised with a suction Freer elevator and the deviation at the junction of the cartilaginous and

bony septum is seen (*black arrow*). Note the pearly white appearance of the cartilage indicating that the mucoperichondrium has been elevated in the correct plane.

bone in the posterior septum. The cartilaginous septum at this point has only had the lower 2 to 3 mm resected from it where it was dislocated from the maxillary crest. It still has the mucosal flap attached to one side and a subperichondrial flap raised on the opposite side. Superiorly, the cartilaginous septum is attached to the under surface of the upper lat-

eral cartilages. The cartilage has a free lower and posterior margin and if free of inherent bends or twists, should hang relatively straight.

Management of the remaining quadrilateral cartilage depends upon there being any visible residual deviations within the cartilage. If there is a fracture line through the

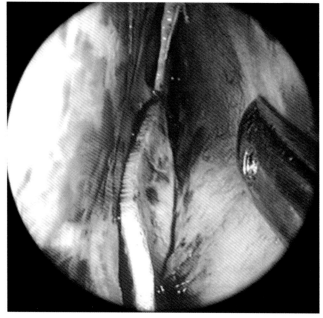

a

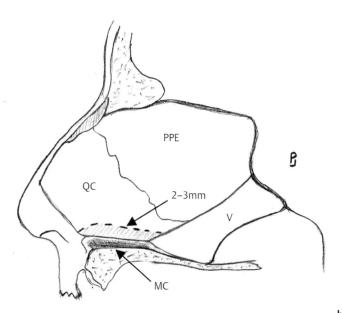

b

Fig. 4.16 (**a**) The horizontal incision 2 to 3 mm above the maxillary crest has been made. This cartilage is gently elevated out of the groove of the maxillary crest starting anteriorly and moving posteriorly.

(**b**) The quadrilateral cartilage (QC), perpendicular plate of the ethmoid (PPE), vomer (V), and maxillary crest are demonstrated. The 2 to 3 mm of cartilage to be excised above the maxillary crest is shaded.

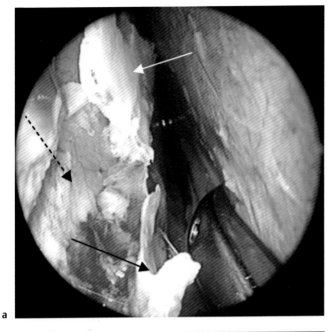

a

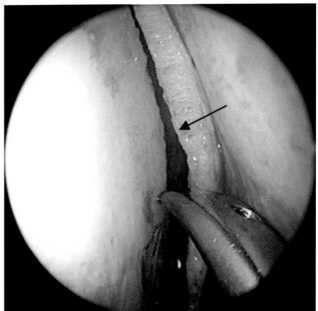

b

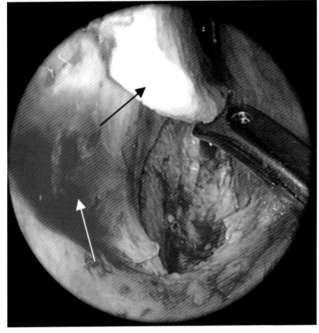

c

Fig. 4.17 (**a**) The 2- to 3-mm strip of cartilage forming the lower border of the quadrilateral cartilage has been resected (*broken black arrow*). The maxillary crest is seen (*black arrow*) and the bony septum is indicated with a white arrow. (**b**) The cartilaginous septum has been dislocated from the posterior bony septum (*black arrow*). (**c**) The inferior bony septum has been resected (*white arrow*) and the thick upper bony septum remains (*black arrow*) and should be resected up to the roof of the nose.

cartilage, this can be excised and the remaining cartilage should then be straight. If, however, the cartilage has a bend or twist, the exposed surface is weakened with multiple incisions. The most difficult cartilaginous deviations are high anterior bends. This should be identified prior to surgery and the incision and flap elevation planned so that the concave surface of such a deviation is exposed during surgery. This allows multiple incisions and, if necessary, powered debridement with the microdebrider blade or septoplasty bur set on forward at a minimum of 12,000 rpm.

If no tear of either mucosal flap has occurred, the scalpel is used to make a posterior 2- to 3-cm horizontal incision on the floor of one of the mucosal flaps to ensure that no blood accumulates within the septum in the postoperative period.

After the ESS has been performed, a quilting suture is placed through the septum to hold the flaps together and to prevent hematoma formation. A 3-0 Vicryl (Ethicon) on a cutting needle is used. A standard needle holder holds the needle with the shaft of the needle positioned between the jaws of the needle holder (**Fig. 4.18**). A knot is made at the end of the suture and the needle is passed through the septum from one nasal cavity to the other (**Fig. 4.19**).

Counterpressure is often required with the endoscope to allow the needle to pass from one nasal cavity to the other. The stitch is pulled through the septum until the

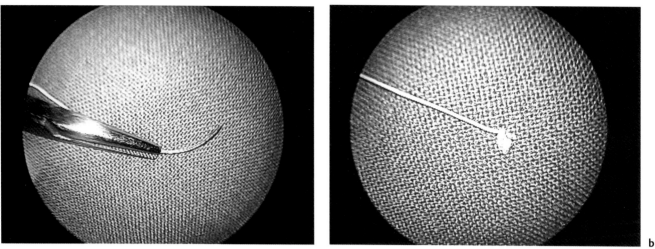

Fig. 4.18 (a) Image shows the shaft of the needle down the length of the needle-holding forceps. (b) Image demonstrates the knot at one end of the suture.

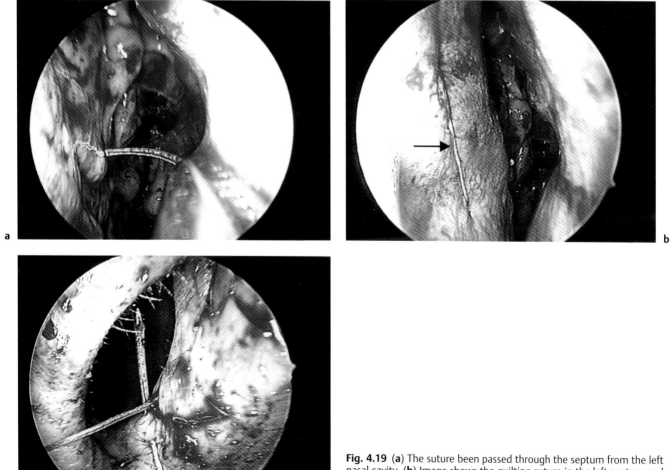

Fig. 4.19 (a) The suture been passed through the septum from the left nasal cavity. (b) Image shows the quilting suture in the left septum and (c) the suture catching a small bite of skin so it can be tied on itself in the right nasal vestibule.

knot reaches the mucosa in the other nasal cavity and prevents further passage of the suture. The suture is then placed some distance from its exit point through the septum into the other nasal cavity. This results in a quilting suture that keeps the two mucosal flaps of the septum apposed. The suture is used to appose the mucosal edges of the incision and then tied on itself through the vestibular skin (**Fig. 4.19**).

References

1. Clement WA, White PS. Trends in turbinate surgery literature: a 35-year review. Clin Otolaryngol Allied Sci 2001;26(2):124–128

2. Lippert BM, Werner JA. Long-term results after laser turbinectomy. Lasers Surg Med 1998;22(2):126–134

3. Warwick-Brown NP, Marks NJ. Turbinate surgery: how effective is it? A long-term assessment. ORL J Otorhinolaryngol Relat Spec 1987;49(6):314–320

4. Gupta A, Mercurio E, Bielamowicz S. Endoscopic inferior turbinate reduction: an outcomes analysis. Laryngoscope 2001;111(11 Pt 1):1957–1959

5. Kawai M, Kim Y, Okuyama T, Yoshida M. Modified method of submucosal turbinectomy: mucosal flap method. Acta Otolaryngol Suppl 1994;511(suppl 511):228–232

6. Berenholz L, Kessler A, Sarfati S, Eviatar E, Segal S. Chronic sinusitis: a sequela of inferior turbinectomy. Am J Rhinol 1998;12(4):257–261

7. Elwany S, Harrison R. Inferior turbinectomy: comparison of four techniques. J Laryngol Otol 1990;104(3):206–209

8. Moore GF, Freeman TJ, Ogren FP, Yonkers AJ. Extended follow-up of total inferior turbinate resection for relief of chronic nasal obstruction. Laryngoscope 1985;95(9 Pt 1):1095–1099

5 Uncinectomy and Middle Meatal Antrostomy Including Canine Fossa Puncture

◆ Introduction

Uncinectomy is the first step undertaken during ESS. If poorly performed, it may result in failure of the ESS procedure[1-3] and may result in orbital or lacrimal complications.[4,5] It is important that the anatomy of the uncinate and ethmoidal infundibulum are properly understood. The uncinate is a sickle-shaped bone extending from the frontal recess superiorly and attaching to the inferior turbinate inferiorly. If the uncinate is viewed in the parasagittal plane, the upward extension of the uncinate into the frontal recess cannot be seen. The middle and horizontal portions of the uncinate form a sickle-shaped bone attaching to the lacrimal bone and the ethmoidal process of the inferior turbinate and lying below the bulla ethmoidalis (**Fig. 5.1**).

The middle third of the uncinate arises from the lacrimal bone and frontal process of the maxilla.[6] It projects posteriorly forming a gutter (the infundibulum) on its lateral aspect. It has a free edge that creates a space between this free edge and the bulla ethmoidalis.[6] This space is known as the hiatus semilunaris as it is crescent shaped (**Fig. 5.1**). **Fig. 5.2** illustrates the orbital attachment of the uncinate process, the infundibulum, and the hiatus semilunaris.

When viewed with an endoscope only, the medially projecting middle portion of the uncinate can be visualized (**Fig. 5.3**).

The superior portion of the uncinate that extends into the frontal recess is considered in detail in Chapter 6. The attachment of the horizontal portion of the uncinate to the ethmoid process of the inferior turbinate is by a series of feet (**Fig. 5.4**). This can clearly be seen in **Fig. 5.4** where the horizontal portion of the uncinate has been dissected free. Posteriorly, it may have a free end or it may attach to the palatine bone.

◆ Uncinectomy

The Swing-Door Technique of Uncinectomy[4]

Removal of the Middle Part of the Uncinate

This technique was devised in an attempt to achieve a complete removal of the midsection of the uncinate process and, in so doing, expose the natural ostium of the maxillary sinus. If there is doubt about the position of the free edge of the uncinate, a ball-tipped right-angled probe can be used to palpate its free edge confirming its position (**Fig. 5.3**). The mid part of the uncinate is incised superiorly and inferiorly. The superior incision is performed with a sickle knife just under the axilla of the middle turbinate (**Fig. 5.5**). The tip of the sickle knife cuts the soft bone of the uncinate from its posterior free edge until the tip of the knife can be felt to strike the hard bone of the frontal process of the maxilla. In this area, the uncinate attaches directly to the hard bone of the frontal process of the maxilla usually above the lacrimal bone (**Fig. 5.1**). It is highly unlikely that this incision will penetrate the lacrimal sac or lamina papyracea and expose orbital fat.

The pediatric backbiter is passed into the middle meatus and opened (**Fig. 5.6**). It is gently wriggled into the hiatus semilunaris so it engages the free edge of the uncinate process. It is easier to introduce the backbiter about midway up the middle portion of the uncinate before it is slid down the free edge until it comes to rest on the transition of the middle and horizontal parts of the uncinate. The uncinate is cut using sequential bites of the backbiter.[4] Usually (depending on the length of the uncinate and the size of the tooth of the backbiter), two to three bites are necessary. If the backbiter can still palpate residual uncinate, then a final bite is made. The backbiter should be turned upward to an angle of 45 degrees before this final bite is made. This brings the

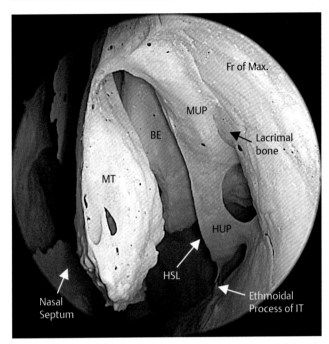

Fig. 5.1 Endoscopic image taken from a dry skull on the left side demonstrating the middle (*MUP*) and horizontal (*HUP*) portions of the uncinate attaching to the lacrimal bone and ethmoidal process of the inferior turbinate (*IT*). The uncinate lies beneath the bulla ethmoidalis, and the hiatus semilunaris (*HSL*) can be visualized between the free edge of the uncinate process and the bulla ethmoidalis (BE). *MT*, Middle turbinate. *Fr of Max*, frontal process of maxilla.

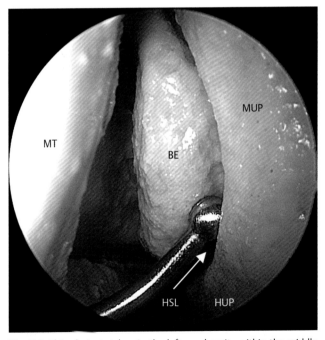

Fig. 5.3 This photo is taken in the left nasal cavity within the middle meatus. The middle (*MUP*) portion of the uncinate and horizontal (*HUP*) of the uncinate is visualized. The ball probe has been placed within the hiatus semilunaris (*HSL*), and lies between the free edge of the uncinate and the bulla ethmoidalis (*BE*).

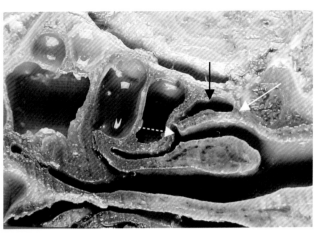

Fig. 5.2 This cadaver dissection specimen of the left nasal cavity is cut in the axial plane with the anterior aspect of the specimen on the right. The *white solid arrow* indicates the uncinate attachment, the *black arrow* the infundibulum, and the *broken white arrow* the hiatus semilunaris (entrance to the infundibulum).

tooth of the backbiter medial to the nasolacrimal duct and protects it from injury. In patients with a lateralized uncinate, care needs to be taken so that the tooth of the backbiter does not penetrate the lamina papyracea during positioning of the tooth on the uncinate. In these patients, the proximity of the uncinate and lamina papyracea can result in the tooth penetrating the lamina papyracea as the tooth is opened and while open it is pulled anteriorly to engage the uncinate. To avoid this, the tooth is used to gently medialize the uncinate before the tooth is pulled anteriorly to engage the uncinate.

Next a right-angled ball probe or curette is slid through the inferior incision behind the uncinate process fairly closely to the uncinate's insertion into the lateral nasal wall. The probe is pulled anteriorly and the uncinate is fractured at its insertion to the lateral nasal wall[4] (**Fig. 5.7**).

The posterior blade of a 45-degree upturned through-cutting Blakesley forceps is placed through the inferior cut in the uncinate and the forceps pushed against the lateral nasal wall, bringing the forceps hard up against the frontal process of the maxilla. The middle section of the uncinate is then removed flush with the lateral nasal wall (**Fig. 5.8**).

In most circumstances, the mid portion of the uncinate can be removed in one piece (**Fig. 5.9**). In **Fig. 5.9** the superior, inferior, and anterior cuts as well as the free edge are labeled.

A number of surgeons remove the middle third of the uncinate with a microdebrider blade. This is *not* advocated as the lamina papyracea that lies directly behind the uncinate is the thinnest part of the medial orbital wall. Turning the microdebrider blade laterally and working onto the lamina with limited visualization of the lamina may end with inadvertent penetration of the lamina with the microdebrider with significant orbital complications.

Removal of the Horizontal Portion of the Uncinate

The zero-degree endoscope is changed for a 30-degree endoscope. This allows better visualization of the middle meatus

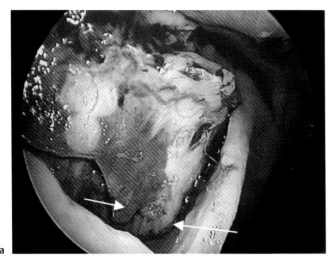

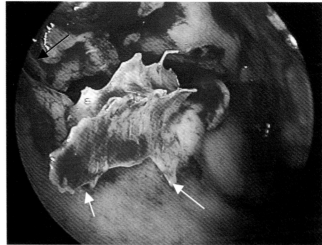

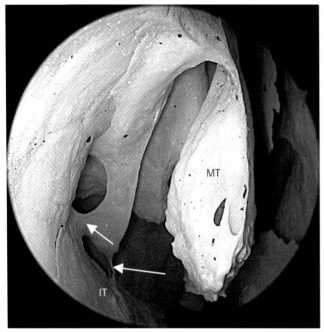

Fig. 5.4 (**a**) The uncinate bone is displayed in situ (right nasal cavity) with the medial mucosal flap dissected away from the bone in picture. (**b**) The horizontal portion of the uncinate has been removed from between the two layers of mucosa. (**c**) Image demonstrates these feet-like process in a dry skull specimen. The feet-like attachments are indicated with *white arrows*. These feet attach to the ethmoidal process on the inferior turbinate (*IT*). *MT*, middle turbinate.

and greater precision in the dissection. The next step is to dissect the horizontal portion of the uncinate bone out from between its two mucosal layers (**Fig. 5.10**).

The double right-angled ball probe is used to elevate the mucosa off the medial aspect of the uncinate (**Fig. 5.10**). The bone is then fractured medially and the ball probe used to elevate the mucosa over the lateral aspect of the bone. Removal of this bone allows the mucosa covering the natural ostium to be delicately trimmed downward with the microdebrider exposing the natural maxillary ostium (**Fig. 5.11**). Note that the microdebrider blade here is positioned inferiorly so that it is working away from the orbit toward the nasal floor. Using the microdebrider allows these edges to be trimmed so that they lie directly opposed to each other without exposed bone separating these edges. This results in these mucosal edges healing by primary intention without scarring (**Fig. 5.11**).

If there is any doubt as to the location of the natural ostium, the right-angled ball probe or right-angled olive tip suction can be placed directly behind the cut edge of the middle portion of the uncinate in the ethmoidal infundibulum. The probe or suction is slid down this natural gutter; it must enter the natural ostium of the maxillary sinus. In this way, the natural ostium of the maxillary sinus should always be able to be located.

◆ **Results with the Swing-Door Technique[4]**

As part of the study comparing the swing-door and traditional techniques of uncinectomy, we examined the results of 636 consecutive swing-door uncinectomies. There were

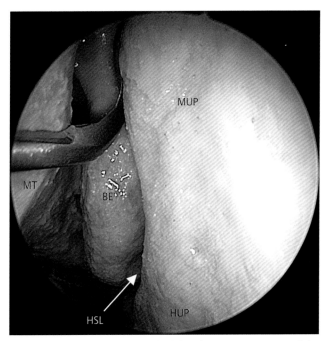

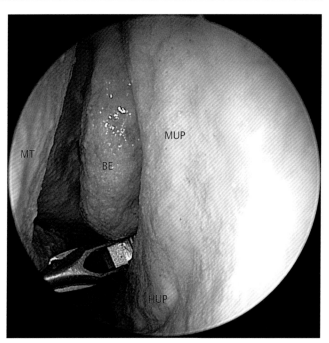

Fig. 5.5 Cadaver dissection on the left side. Superior incision of the middle portion of the uncinate process (*MUP*) is made with a sickle knife placed directly under the axilla of the middle turbinate (*MT*). *BE*, bulla ethmoidalis; *HSL*, hiatus semilunaris; *HUP*, horizontal portion of the uncinate.

Fig. 5.6 A pediatric backbiter is introduced and the lower cut is made. *BE*, bulla ethmoidalis; *HUP*, horizontal portion of the uncinate; *MT*, middle turbinate; *MUP*, middle portion of the uncinate.

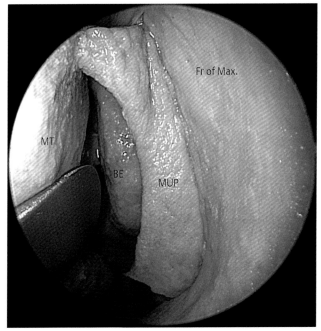

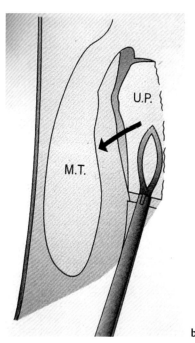

a

b

Fig. 5.7 (**a**) Insertion of a curette or ball probe behind the uncinate has allowed the middle portion of the uncinate (*MUP*) attachment to the lateral nasal wall to be fractured anteriorly in a swing-door technique for uncinectomy. (**b**) The 45-degree through-biting Blakesley used to cut the uncinate flush with the lateral nasal wall. *BE*, bulla ethmoidalis; *Fr of Max*, frontal process of maxilla; *MT*, middle turbinate; *UP*, uncinate process.

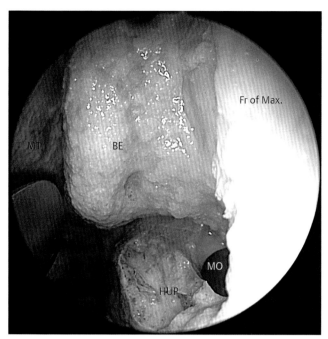

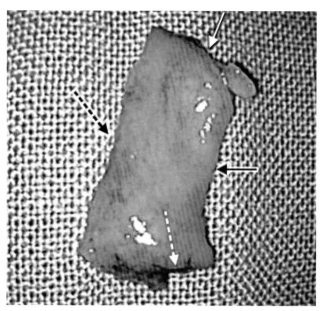

Fig. 5.9 The middle section of the uncinate with superior (*white arrow*), inferior (*broken white arrow*), anterior cut edges (*black arrow*), and free edge (*broken black arrow*) labeled.

Fig. 5.8 Removal of the middle third of the uncinate process reveals the natural maxillary ostium (*MO*), with the remaining horizontal portion still in place. *BE*, bulla ethmoidalis; *Fr of Max*, frontal process of maxilla; *HUP*, horizontal portion of the uncinate; *MT*, middle turbinate.

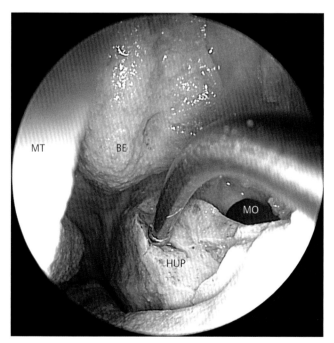

Fig. 5.10 A double right-angled ball probe dissecting the bone of the horizontal portion of the uncinate process (*HUP*). *BE*, bulla ethmoidalis; *MO*, maxillary ostium; *MT*, middle turbinate.

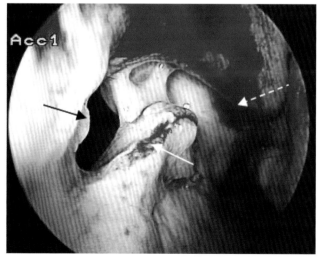

Fig. 5.11 Intraoperative picture of the right maxillary ostium (*black arrow*) after removal of the horizontal portion of the uncinate with apposition of the mucosal edges (*white arrow*). The final common drainage pathway is indicated by the *broken white arrow*.

no orbital penetrations with fat exposure and all natural ostia of the maxillary sinuses were identified. However, there were four patients in whom the nasolacrimal duct was exposed and not opened and one patient in whom the nasolacrimal duct was opened. The important outcome was the ability of the surgeon to identify the natural ostium of the maxillary sinus in all 636 uncinectomies.

To compare the swing-door technique with the traditional technique of uncinectomy, a further 636 uncinectomies were performed using the traditional technique described below.[7] The traditional technique for uncinectomy starts with the identification of the uncinate's free edge. While the free edge is palpated, the surgeon attempts to gauge the site of the uncinate's insertion into the lateral wall of the nose. This decision is critical. If the surgeon starts too close to the uncinate insertion, the first incision may penetrate the lamina papyracea with a resultant prolapse of orbital fat. Surgeons tend to allow for such an error and tend to leave a few millimeters of uncinate behind incising distal to its insertion (**Fig. 5.12**).

If too much uncinate remains, the ostium may remain hidden behind this residual uncinate. In this situation, the ostium should be sought behind the anteroinferior residual uncinate (**Fig. 5.13**).

In 636 consecutive traditional uncinectomies, we were unable to locate the natural ostium of the maxillary sinus in 42. There were six cases of orbital fat exposure and no cases of nasolacrimal duct injury. In our hands the swing-door technique was more reliable to identify the natural ostium of the maxillary sinus and was less likely to result in penetration of the orbit.

Complications of Uncinectomy

The two areas at risk during uncinectomy are the orbit and the nasolacrimal duct.[4,5] To date, penetration of the orbit has not occurred with the superior horizontal incision of the middle part of the uncinate. This is due to the insertion of this part of the uncinate on the thick bone of the frontal process

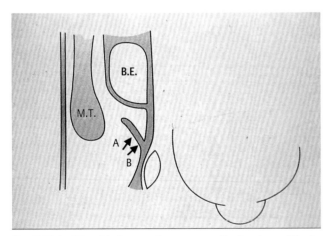

Fig. 5.12 In this axial diagram the surgeon will often have difficulty deciding exactly where the uncinate attaches to the lateral nasal wall and will usually make the incision into the uncinate as indicated by the *A arrow* as this gives a margin of safety when compared to the incision in the region of the *B arrow*, which may traverse the lamina papyracea and expose orbital fat.

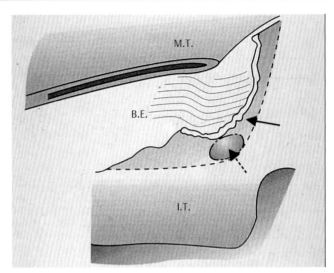

Fig. 5.13 After the uncinectomy has been performed, 2 to 3 mm of residual uncinate remains (*solid black arrow*). This obscures visualization of the natural ostium (*broken black arrow*) and may not be located by the surgeon. This may result in a posterior fontanelle ostium being created. *B.E.*, bull ethmoidalis; *I.T.*, inferior turbinate; *M.T.*, middle turbinate.

of the maxilla. The traditional technique of uncinectomy has a higher risk of orbital penetration. This is due to the knife penetrating the orbit during the anterior incision made into the uncinate at its insertion onto the lateral nasal wall.[4] This may result in the prolapse of orbital fat. Frequent palpation of the globe should be performed throughout the surgery. If inadvertent entry into the orbit or removal of the lamina papyracea has occurred, palpation of the globe will either cause a prolapse of orbital fat or cause the orbital periosteum to move. If orbital periosteum is exposed, care should be taken in this region during the rest of the surgery. If penetration of the orbit has occurred and orbital fat prolapse is seen, this should be left alone and not manipulated. The microdebrider should not be used in an area where orbital fat has prolapsed as it can be sucked very rapidly into the blade with rapid removal of fat and damage to the medial rectus muscle. Damage to the nasolacrimal duct is less likely with the traditional technique than the swing-door technique as there is less utilization of the backbiter and therefore less risk to the nasolacrimal duct. If the nasolacrimal duct is opened, any small bony pieces are removed and the opening left as it is. Normally no symptoms will result as the duct has not been obstructed. A crush injury of the duct has a worse prognosis as this may result in scar tissue formation within the duct with subsequent obstruction of the duct.

The surgeon should also be aware that collapse of the uncinate onto the lamina papyracea (so-called atelectatic uncinate) puts the orbit at greater risk of damage.[8] This occurs with complete opacification of the maxillary sinus with absorption of all gas within the sinus and resultant negative pressure sucking the uncinate laterally onto the lateral nasal wall. If this is long-standing, expansion of the orbit may occur with enophthalmos—the so-called silent sinus syndrome (**Fig. 5.14**). Anterior incisions into an atelectatic uncinate will result in a high incidence of orbital penetration and should not be used. The retrograde removal of the uncinate (swing-door technique) is preferred.

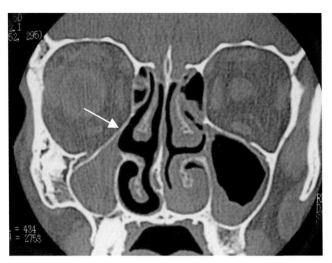

Fig. 5.14 CT scan of a patient with a right atelectatic uncinate (*white arrow*). The uncinate is plastered against the lamina papyracea over a considerable length.

◆ Posterior Fontanelle or Accessory Ostium

An accessory ostium is located within the posterior fontanelle of the maxillary sinus behind the natural ostium. Cadaveric studies have shown that 10% of the general population have an accessory ostium.[9] In addition, failure of the surgeon to locate the natural maxillary sinus ostium at surgery may result in the creation of a posterior fontanelle ostium. This is a common cause for ESS failure.[1–3] The presence of an accessory or posterior fontanelle ostium may result in the circular flow of mucus from the natural ostium of the maxillary sinus into the posterior fontanelle ostium with resultant recurrent chronic sinusitis symptoms (**Fig. 5.15**).

Patients who present with recurrent symptoms of sinusitis after ESS should have an endoscopic examination and, after appropriate medical treatment, a computed tomography

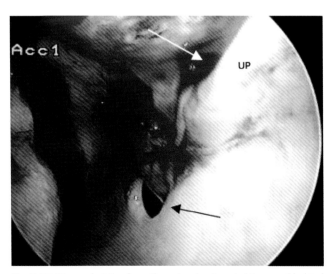

Fig. 5.15 Mucus draining from the natural ostium (*white arrow*) behind the uncinate process (*UP*) into an accessory ostium (*black arrow*).

(CT) scan. On clinical examination, the presence of a posterior fontanelle and circular flow of mucus should be sought. This can often be seen on endoscopy with a 30-degree endoscope. In addition, the CT scans of the patient should be closely scrutinized for presence of a natural ostium and a posterior fontanelle ostium or accessory ostium (**Fig. 5.16**).

If a posterior fontanelle ostium or accessory ostium is identified, this should be surgically joined to the natural ostium to prevent ongoing circular flow of mucus. This can be done by inserting a backbiter into the accessory ostium and coming forward to the natural ostium. After creating this tissue edge, the microdebrider is used to trim away excessive tissue.

◆ Enlarging the Maxillary Ostium

Currently there is debate as to whether enlarging the maxillary sinus ostium can be detrimental to the long-term health of the sinus.[10] The debate centers on the role of nitric oxide (NO) in the sinuses.[10] NO is produced by nitric oxide synthase (NOS) in the mucosa of the sinuses.[11,12] There are three types of NOS with type II thought to be most important in the production of NO in the sinuses.[11–14] Type II is found in various cells in the nasal mucosa and is induced by bacterial inflammation.[14–17] NO is believed to play an important role in the local innate defense of the nasal sinus mucosa by stimulating ciliary motility and by inhibiting infection by bacteria, viruses, and fungi.[17] In the early stages of the development of ESS, many surgeons advocated enlargement of the maxillary ostium toward the posterior fontanelle.[18,19] This results in a very large maxillary ostium. Recently, there have been contrary opinions expressed where surgeons have argued that the proximity of the uncinate to the maxillary ostium results in a narrow transitional space that becomes easily obstructed and that removal of the uncinate alone is sufficient to restore the health of the maxillary sinuses.[20,21] Unfortunately, there is little data published to support either argument. Kennedy et al[18] described the natural size of the maxillary ostium to be 5 mm by 5 mm which raises the possibility that significantly enlarging the ostium routinely may in some patients cause sufficient dilution of the sinus NO concentration to allow colonization of the sinus by bacteria with subsequent disease. Our department recently published a study in which we measured the size of the maxillary sinus ostium and correlated this to the concentration of NO found in both in the maxillary sinus and nasal cavity.[10] There were 52 sinuses in the study with 22 sinuses having enlarged ostia and 30 sinuses having ostia less than 5 × 5 mm. This study showed that there was a significant decrease in NO concentration in sinuses and nasal cavities with large maxillary sinus ostia (greater than 5 × 5 mm). This does not mean that the study showed that a lower NO concentration predisposed patients to recurrent infections but only that a large maxillary ostium lowers the concentration of NO in the maxillary sinus and nasal cavity.[10] The association between large maxillary ostia and recurrent infections still needs to be formally studied. An example of a patient with recurrent maxillary sinus infection with a large maxillary antrostomy is presented in **Fig. 5.17**.

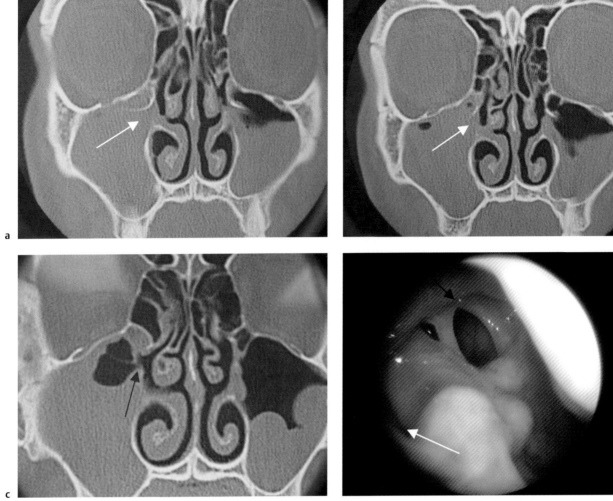

a   b

c   d

Fig. 5.16 The endoscopic picture and corresponding series of sequential coronal computed tomography scans reveal a partially obscured natural ostium (**a, b**, *white arrow*) and two accessory ostia (**c**, *black arrow*). (**d**) The natural ostium (*white arrow*) and the accessory ostia (*black arrow*) in the postfontanelle region.

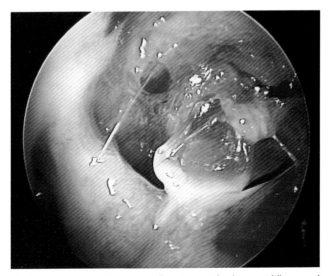

Fig. 5.17 Secretions filling a maxillary sinus with a large middle meatal antrostomy on the left side.

An additional consequence of removal of the posterior fontanelle during enlargement of the maxillary ostium may be dumping of secretions from the frontal sinuses and anterior ethmoids into the maxillary sinus. The natural drainage pathway of the frontal sinus and anterior ethmoids is above the natural ostium of the maxillary sinus along the base of the bulla ethmoidalis before crossing the posterior fontanelle and under the eustachian tube to the nasopharynx. In **Fig. 5.18** secretions can be seen coming from the frontal recess and anterior ethmoids across the natural ostium of the maxillary sinus.

Currently, the decision as to whether the maxillary ostium is enlarged or not is dependent upon the degree of disease within the maxillary sinus. If the maxillary sinus has minimal disease with only mucosal thickening present on the CT scan (**Fig. 5.19**), then only the uncinate is removed.

If the surgeon wishes to view the maxillary sinus then the ostium is enlarged until the dimensions are about 10 mm by 10 mm. After removal of the horizontal bone of the uncinate, the mucosa is lowered onto the insertion

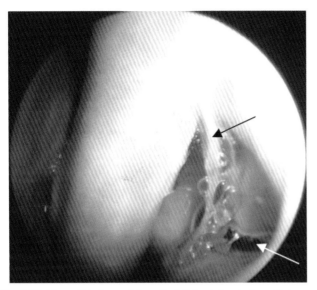

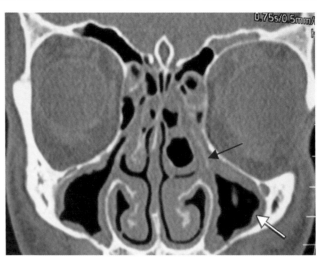

Fig. 5.19 CT scan of a patient with bilateral mucosal thickening in the maxillary sinus (*black arrow*) with an obstructed ostiomeatal complex (*white arrow*).

Fig. 5.18 Mucus (*black arrow*) from the left frontal and ethmoid sinuses moving over the left small maxillary ostium (*white arrow*).

of the inferior turbinate. In most cases, this is sufficient to view the majority of the maxillary sinus with a 70-degree telescope. If there is submucosal abscess formation or polyps and mucus that need removal from the sinus, curved instruments and malleable suctions are used through this natural but enlarged ostium to achieve this. This sinus is still seen as having reversible mucosal disease or grade 2 maxillary sinus disease. If, however, the sinus has grade 3 disease where there is extensive polyp formation within the maxillary sinus or large amounts of thick and viscid secretions, particularly fungal mucin, a canine fossa trephine

is performed and the maxillary ostium is opened into the posterior fontanelle and maximally enlarged with removal of the posterior fontanelle (**Fig. 5.20**). In patients with Sampter's triad and cystic fibrosis, the ostium is always enlarged to its maximum size. This allows maximal penetration of nasal douching usually with topical medication into the maxillary sinus.

In **Fig. 5.21a**, a polyp pedicled on the roof of the maxillary sinus is seen. Polyps that are based on the posterior roof and posterior wall of the maxillary sinus can usually be removed through an enlarged maxillary ostium. If the majority of polyps or mucin remains after attempted removal through the large ostium, then a canine fossa trephine is performed as described below.

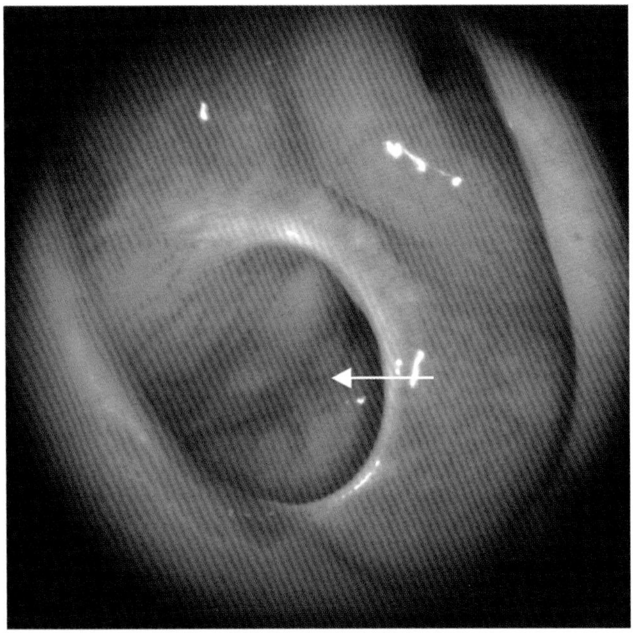

◆ **The Severely Diseased Maxillary Sinus**

Grading the Maxillary Sinus

To date, when dealing with a severely disease maxillary sinus, emphasis has been placed on the creation of the maxillary antrostomy and ensuring that natural ostium is incorporated into any antrostomy created.[3,4] While establishment of a patent maxillary ostium is a vitally important part of the management of the severely diseased maxillary sinus, management of the sinus and its contents should not be ignored.[3] The diagnosis of the severely diseased maxillary sinus should be suspected if the maxillary sinus is completely opacified on the CT scan.[18] **Fig. 5.22** shows examples of severely diseased maxillary sinuses.

However, the diagnosis can only be confirmed on endoscopy during surgery as the opacification may well be mucus which is easily cleared through the natural maxillary ostium. The first step at surgery is to perform an uncinectomy and middle meatal antrostomy. A 70-degree endoscope is used

Fig. 5.20 A patient with a large right maxillary antrostomy (*white arrow*) after having extensive sinus disease.

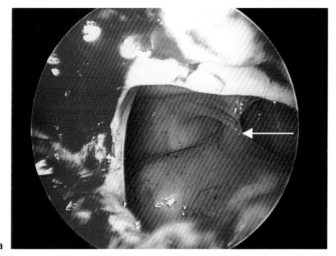

a

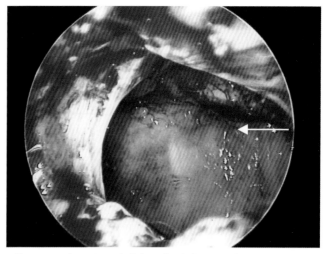

b

Fig. 5.21 (**a**) A large polyp on a twisted pedicle (*white arrow*) and (**b**) the maxillary sinus after removal of the polyp (*white arrow*).

to visualize the natural ostium and contents of the maxillary sinus. The extent of disease affecting the maxillary sinus should be graded according to **Table 5.1**.

Grades 1 and 2 are reversible with adequate clearance of mucus and aeration of the maxillary sinus but grade 3 is irreversibly diseased (**Fig. 5.23**) and therefore the polyps and especially the thick eosinophilic mucus should be cleared before adequate re-epithelialization and eventually re-ciliation will occur.

If standard ESS techniques and instruments are used, the polyps and mucus from the posterior region of the maxillary sinus can be removed with angled microdebrider blades and curved forceps.[18] However, due to the two fulcrums that a microdebrider blades and instruments have when passed through the maxillary antrostomy or inferior meatal antrostomy, polyps in the anterior, inferior, and medial regions cannot be reached. The anterior fulcrum is the nasal vestibule and the posterior fulcrum is the antrostomy or inferior meatal antrostomy site. If the blade or instrument is passed through the anterior wall of the maxillary sinus, it only has

one fulcrum so a much greater degree of manipulation of the blade is possible (**Fig. 5.24**).

In current teaching, the maxillary sinus is managed by creating a large antrostomy and then removing whatever can be removed through the maxillary antrostomy. Polyps and thick tenacious mucus in the anterior region or floor of the nose require removal (**Fig. 5.23c**). In patients with severe and aggressive sinus disease such as allergic fungal sinusitis, nonallergic eosinophilic fungal disease (**Fig. 5.23c**), and nonallergic nonfungal eosinophilic disease, leaving eosinophilic mucin in the maxillary sinus may contribute to a rapid recurrence of disease.[18,19] Whether this is due to a continuing exposure to fungus in the eosinophilic mucus or due to ongoing inflammation from the toxic substances within the mucus such as superantigens, major basic protein and other substances released by the eosinophils is unclear. In other patient groups, such as Sampter's triad and severe recurrent polyposis, it appears that if the maxillary sinus is left filled with polyps that these polyps do not resolve with only a maxillary antrostomy.

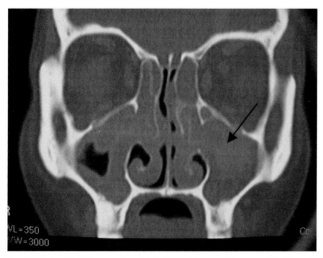

a

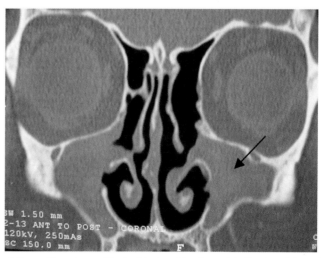

b

Fig. 5.22 (**a, b**) CT scans in which there is complete opacification of the left maxillary sinus with double densities (*arrow*) indicative of fungal sinusitis. (**b**) Previous surgery had cleared the ethmoid cavity on the left and this remains disease free.

Table 5.1   Grading and management of the diseased maxillary sinus

Grade	Endoscopic findings	Suggested surgery of maxillary ostium
1	Normal or slightly edematous mucosa (reversible disease)	Uncinectomy alone with visualization of the natural ostium
2	Edematous mucosa with small polyps (reversible disease) without significant eosinophilic mucus	Enlargement of the maxillary ostium to about 1 × 1 cm to allow suction clearance of maxillary, mucociliary clearance, and aeration
3	Extensive polyps and tenacious mucus (nonreversible disease)	Canine fossa puncture (CFP) or trephine (CFT) with complete clearance of polyps and mucus and creation of a large antrostomy

Is it Necessary to Remove Polyps and Thick Mucin from a Severely Diseased Maxillary Sinus?[18–22]

We performed a study to establish whether this philosophy of clearing the polyps and mucus in a grade 3 maxillary sinus improved patient outcome.[18] All patients who had undergone ESS in the department over the prior 3 years were identified and their CT scans reviewed. If there was complete opacification of the maxillary sinus or sinuses they were included in the study. The researcher at that stage was not aware what surgical procedures had been performed or what the current status of the patient sinuses were. This was therefore an unselected patient cohort. The surgical notes were reviewed and the patients were placed into two groups depending upon whether the patient had undergone a large middle meatal antrostomy with clearance of all accessible polyps through the antrostomy or whether a canine fossa puncture/trephine (CFP/T) had been performed. If a trephine

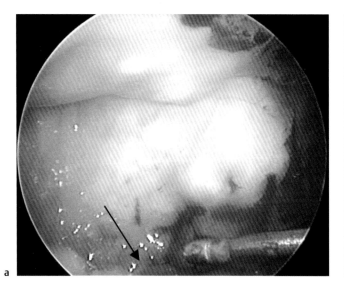

a

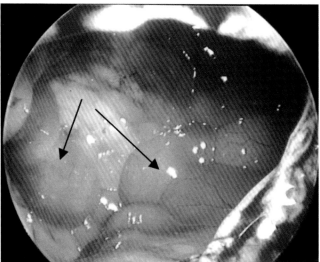

b

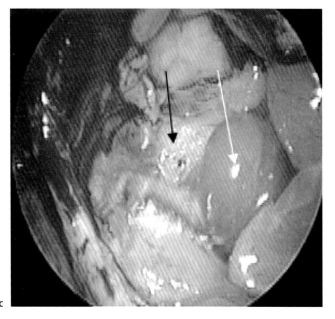

c

Fig. 5.23 The following pictures of the left maxillary sinus are taken after a maxillary antrostomy has been performed and illustrate the grades of disease. (**a**) Grade 1: the mucosa is cobblestoned in the floor of the antrum (*arrow*) with edema of the residual sinus mucosa. (**b**) Grade 2: maxillary disease, the polyps are seen in the floor and posterior wall of the maxillary sinus (*arrows*) and could be left and should reverse with medical treatment provided there is no eosinophilic mucus around the polyps. If mucus was present, a canine fossa trephine (CFT) should be performed. (**c**) Grade 3: the maxillary sinus is completely filled with polyps (*white arrow*) and eosinophilic mucus (*black arrow*) and should be managed with a CFT.

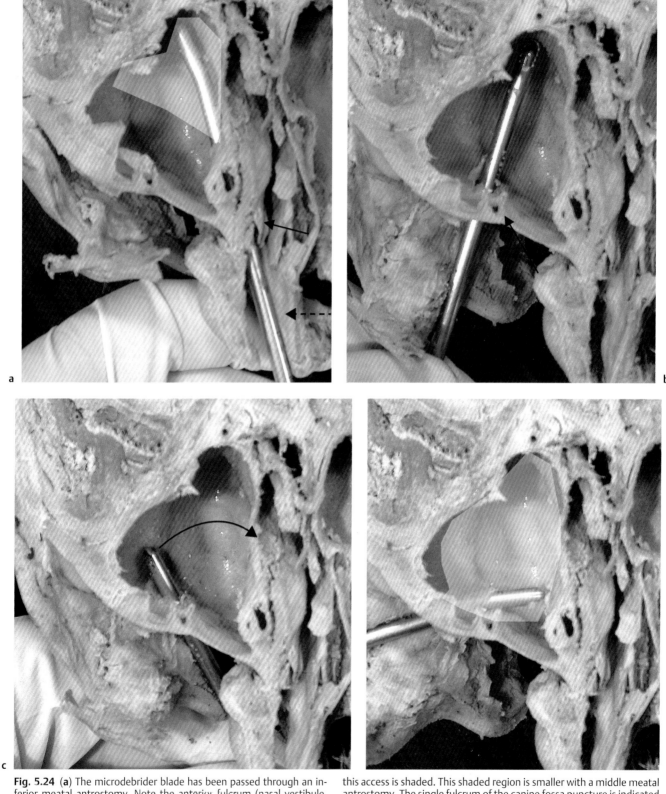

Fig. 5.24 (**a**) The microdebrider blade has been passed through an inferior meatal antrostomy. Note the anterior fulcrum (nasal vestibule, *broken arrow*) and the posterior fulcrum (inferior meatal antrostomy, *arrow*). The region of the maxillary sinus that can be cleared through this access is shaded. This shaded region is smaller with a middle meatal antrostomy. The single fulcrum of the canine fossa puncture is indicated in (**b**), (**c**), and (**d**), illustrating how the entire maxillary sinus can be accessed as the blade only has a single fulcrum.

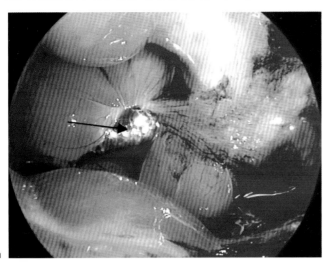
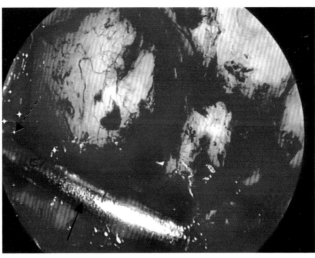

a   b

Fig. 5.25 (**a**) The microdebrider blade has been passed through a canine fossa trephine site in the anterior face of the maxillary sinus (*arrow*).
(**b**) The polyps have been removed from the sinus without stripping the
basement membrane from the sinus (note no exposed bone). The debrider blade can be seen entering the sinus through the anterior wall
(*broken arrow*).

or puncture was performed, our standard practice is to place
a microdebrider blade through this puncture/trephine site
and perform a complete clearance of polyps under visualization of a 70-degree endoscope placed at the middle meatal
antrostomy (**Fig. 5.25**).

The polyps and thick mucus were removed from the sinus
under direct visualization with the 70-degree endoscope.
Care was taken not to strip the mucosa from the maxillary sinus. Only the polyp was taken while the base layer
of mucosa underlying was preserved. This allowed rapid
re-epithelialization after surgery and diminished crusting
and secretion retention.

The patients in this study[18] underwent a magnetic resonance imaging (MRI) scan at a mean time since surgery of
19.9 months. On the MRI, scan the maxillary sinus was
graded as normal, mucosal thickening less than 4 mm, mucosal thickening >4 mm but the sinus still aerated or a completely opacified sinus (**Fig. 5.7**). This grading was confirmed
on nasal endoscopy. In addition, the patients were asked to
grade their sinus symptoms on a visual analog scale and to
complete the Chronic Sinusitis Survey (CSS) quality of life
questionnaire. In the CFP group, the sinuses were normal
in 62% of the patients compared to 12% in the patients that
had undergone routine middle meatal antrostomy and as
much maxillary sinus polyp resection that could be achieved
through the natural ostium. The CSS symptom subscore and
symptom score were statistically better in the CFP group indicating better symptom control in this group. If the preoperative overall disease burden was compared between the
two groups using the Lund and Mackay score, it was found
to be higher in the CFP group (Lund and Mackay = 10.3) as
compared to the group undergoing standard ESS techniques
(8.6). In addition, all the other sinuses were treated in exactly
the same manner with complete removal of all polyps and
mucin from these sinuses and exposure of the natural ostium
of the sinuses. This study confirmed the clinical perception
that complete clearance of the severely diseased maxillary
sinus plays a major role in the control of the disease and decreases the overall incidence and severity of recurrence of
the disease.[18] In addition, we have shown the benefit of CFT
in patients with severely disease maxillary sinus[20] and in
Samter's triad patients.[21]

◆ Technique and Complications of the Old Technique of Canine Fossa Puncture[22]

The old standard technique for CFP was as follows[22]: The lip
of the patient was elevated and the canine tooth identified
(there are two front teeth either side of the midline before
the canine tooth). The root of this tooth was traced with
the finger under the lip until the canine fossa was palpated.
One milliliter of 1:80,000 2% lignocaine and adrenaline was
infiltrated in this region. A canine fossa trocar (Karl Storz)
was placed in the fossa and directed posteriorly. The trocar
was introduced with a rotating forward motion. When the
bone was too thick, a couple of firm taps with the palm of
the hand were usually sufficient to drive the trocar through
the bone. However, in some patients in whom the bone
was thicker, the trocar needed to be tapped with a mallet. After the tip of the trocar was felt to fully penetrate
the sinus, it was withdrawn and the microdebrider blade
was introduced through the mucosal and bony hole into
the maxillary sinus. The blade was kept closed during introduction to prevent soft tissues from been sucked into
the debrider during passage into the maxillary sinus. Once
the blade was in the maxillary sinus, the 70-degree endoscope is introduced into the nasal cavity and the gate of
the blade is opened. This helps remove most of the blood
from within the sinus and allows the blade to be visualized
within the sinus (**Fig. 5.25a**). This needs to be done before
the blade is used to remove polyps. This visualization ensures that the blade is within the sinus and not in the orbit
or soft tissues.

Complications[22]

The incidence of complications with the old CFP technique performed at the same time as ESS was 75%.[22] A telephonic survey revealed that the most common complications were cheek swelling, cheek pain, and facial pain. Most of these symptoms resolved within the first month after surgery. If the symptoms associated with the soft tissue dissection were removed, 28% of patients experienced a persistent significant complication of facial tingling, numbness, or continued pain. This incidence is similar to other studies where numbness of the upper lip and/or the upper teeth was seen in up to 38% of patients.[23] These persisting complications were thought to be a result of injury to branches of the infraorbital nerve. The infraorbital nerve divides before it exits the infraorbital foramen into the anterior superior alveolar nerve (ASAN) and the middle superior alveolar nerve (MSAN). These nerves traverse the anterior maxilla and supply sensation to the upper lip and teeth. Placement of the trocar through the anterior wall of the maxilla can injure these nerves and result in paresthesia and numbness of the upper lip and teeth. The risk of injury to this nerve increases if the trocar is placed too medially and cranially.[22,23] In most cases (91%) the paresthesia and numbness recovers within 12 months as the nerves either regrow or the area is re-innervated by nerves close by.[22,23] The area of numbness gradually shrinks then disappears.

The Neural Anatomy of the Anterior Maxilla[24]

In order to determine the best way to avoid injury to these nerves, a cadaver-based study was undertaken in our department on 20 cadavers.[24] The soft tissue overlying the maxillae was removed and the underlying pattern of the ASAN and MSAN determined. The ASAN and the MSAN both run in the bone of the anterior face of the maxilla. The infraorbital nerve divides prior to exiting the infraorbital foramen (IOF) within the maxillary sinuses. The ASAN usually enters the anterior face of the maxilla just below the IOF and then traverses across the anterior face of the maxillary sinus. There were six patterns of branching of the ASAN and MSAN (types 1 to 6). The most common pattern was a single trunk of the ASAN (75%) with no branches (30%, type 1) (**Fig. 5.26a**) followed by multiple branches (25%, type 2) (**Fig. 5.26b**) and a single branch (20%, type 3). Type 4 was a double trunk with no branches (10%) (**Fig. 5.26c**) and type 5 a double trunk with multiple branches (15%). The MSAN was present only as a single trunk with no branches (10%) (type 6) and with multiple branches (13%) (type 7) (**Fig. 5.26d**).

Landmarks for New Technique of Canine Fossa Puncture or Trephine[25]

In order to determine the region where neurological injury would least likely occur, landmarks were determined on the cadavers as to the safest place to place the trephine.[24] The landmarks chosen were the intersection of the mid-pupillary line and a horizontal line drawn through the floor of the nose (**Fig. 5.27**). Canine fossa punctures were then performed on all 40 sides of the cadavers. In only 5 of the 40 punctures performed was there injury to one of the minor branches of the ASAN or MSAN confirming that these landmarks were the safest to perform a canine fossa puncture or trephine.

Canine Fossa Trephine[20–25]

Rationale

One of the problems associated with CFP is that the trocar is placed in a blinded manner. Although the soft tissue is dissected off the anterior face of the maxilla, the area through which the trocar is placed is not visualized and the ASAN or the MSAN could be damaged. In addition, placement of the trocar may cause fracture of the thin bone of the anterior wall of the maxilla around the puncture site. This is especially true if the trocar is not rotated with minimal pressure so that the edges of the trocar act as a drill as it penetrates the maxilla. If significant pressure is applied to the trocar a fracture of the surrounding bone will often occur. This enlarges the area of trauma and in so doing increases the risk of possible associated neurological injury. Also, the currently available canine fossa trocar (Karl Storz, Germany) is 4 mm in diameter. When a 4-mm debrider blade is placed through this opening the fit is very snug and when the blade is manipulated within the maxillary sinus this may cause fracture of the surrounding maxillary bone, again increasing the potential risk of neurological damage. In order to overcome these problems, an endoscope sheath* was developed with an extension to hold away the soft tissues (Medtronic ENT, Minneapolis, MN).

Technique[25]

An approximately 6-mm incision is made in the gingivobuccal sulcus above and slightly lateral to the apex of the canine tooth. A suction Freer elevator is used to elevate the soft tissues off the anterior face of the maxilla in a subperiosteal plane. Once this plane is achieved the endoscope soft tissue sheath* (Medtronic ENT) is placed over the zero-degree endoscope and is placed into the incision and the soft tissues held away from the bone allowing the surgical plane to be endoscopically visualized (**Fig. 5.28**).

Dissection is continued in a superior and superolateral direction, exposing the canine fossa and the region lateral to the fossa where the mid-pupillary line and line through the nasal floor intersect. If any nerve or branch of one of the nerves is seen (**Fig. 5.29**), further dissection is performed to create space so that the nerve can be avoided.

The canine fossa drill guide* (Medtronic ENT) is then placed on the anterior face of the maxilla at the intersection of the previously described lines. The canine fossa drill* (Medtronic ENT) is attached to the microdebrider handpiece and irrigation to the back of the drill guide. This allows irrigation of the bur during trephination. The drill should be used at 12,000 rpm for best results (lower revolutions may result in the bur sticking in the bone). A 5-mm diameter hole is neatly

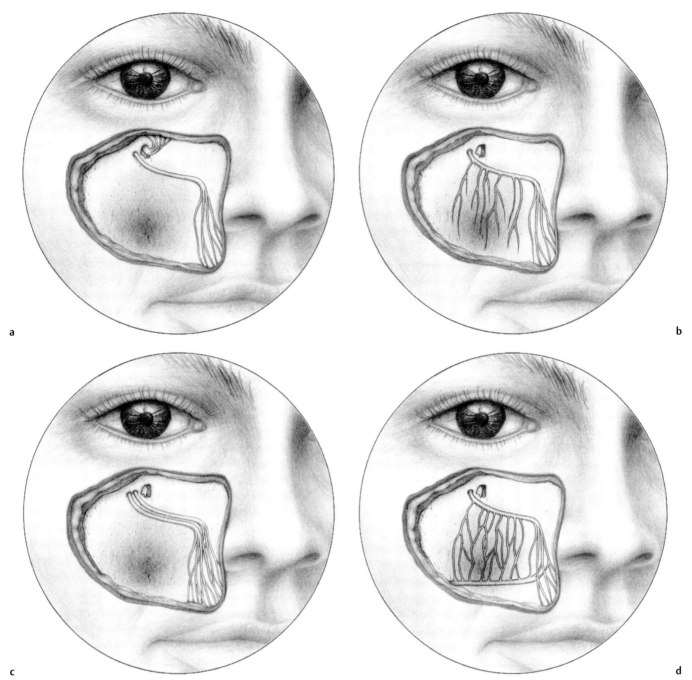

a

b

c

d

Fig. 5.26 The most common nerve patterns are single trunk (75%) as seen in (**a**) (type 1) and (**b**) (type 2). (**c**) A double trunk is uncommon (10%) (type 4). The middle superior alveolar nerve is seen in 23% of patients and may have no branches (10%) or multiple branches (13%; type 7) as seen in (**d**).

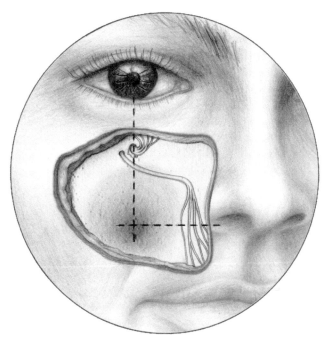

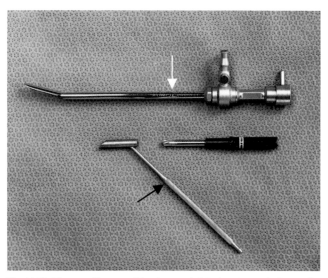

Fig. 5.28 The maxillary trephination set* (Medtronic ENT) shows the endoscope sheath for holding the soft tissue away from the end of the endoscope (*white arrow*), the drill guide (*black arrow*), and the drill bit which fits into the end of the microdebrider.

Fig. 5.27 The landmarks for canine fossa puncture/trephine are the intersection between a vertical line through the pupil and a horizontal line drawn through the floor of the nose.

drilled through the anterior face of the maxilla (**Fig. 5.29b**). A Frasier suction is used to remove any bone dust from the hole and surrounding soft tissues and the 4-mm straight microdebrider blade is placed through the trephine into the maxillary sinus. Using a 70-degree endoscope placed transnasally at the maxillary antrostomy, the debrider blade can be opened and then visualized in the sinus. Activating the blade before it is visualized could result in damage if the blade had inadvertently been placed into the orbit or soft tissues (**Fig. 5.30**). The blade is then used to enlarge the max-

illary sinus antrostomy. Any residual uncinate is removed and the posterior fontanelle is removed up to the posterior wall of the maxillary sinus. Polypoid tissue and residual uncinate are removed from the anterior lip of the antrostomy. The widest possible view is now able to be obtained through the antrostomy and the surgeon can remove the polyps and thick mucin from the maxillary sinus. Angled microdebrider blades are used for the lateral regions and anterior face of the maxillary sinus. The endoscope can also be placed through the trephine and the interior of the maxillary sinus inspected to ensure complete removal of polyps and mucus. Note that only the polypoid tissue and mucus are removed. The basement membrane of the maxillary sinus is retained. This al-

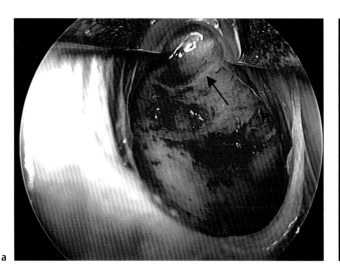

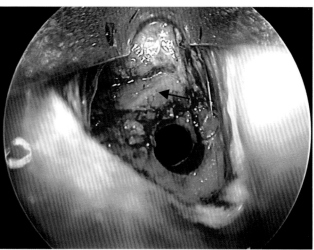

a   b

Fig. 5.29 (**a**) The left anterior superior alveolar nerve (*black arrow*) is exposed and therefore can be avoided during placement of the canine fossa trephine (**b**).

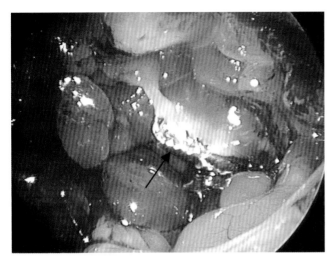

Fig. 5.30 The microdebrider blade has been placed through a canine fossa trephine access port and can be seen emerging from amongst the massive polyposis filling the left maxillary sinus.

lows speedy re-epithelialization in the postoperative period with re-ciliation and restoration of the maxillary sinus function (**Fig. 5.25**).

Clinical Study of Complications with New Technique of Canine Fossa Puncture or Trephine[25]

In order to assess whether these new landmarks and technique reduced the incidence and severity of complications, a clinical study of 63 patients was performed.[25] Thirty-six patients had bilateral procedures resulting in 99 canine fossa punctures or trephines. Initial postoperative complication rates reduced from 75% to 44% with only 3.3% of patients having a persisting neurological complication after 6 months compared to 28.8% with the old CFP technique. In addition, the number of patients suffering from more than one side effect decreased from 70% to 31%. If the 99 sides were separated into patients who underwent canine fossa trephine (n = 67) as apposed to puncture (n = 32) with the new guidelines, a further reduction in complications is seen. In patients who had CFT and in whom the anterior face of the maxillary sinus was inspected for a visible ASAN or MSAN, the complication rate was 40%. This was significantly less than the 53% seen in patients who had a CFP and in whom the trocar was introduced in a blind manner. Also, the CFT patients recovered from their symptoms faster with an 83.3% full recovery in 1 month compared to 62.5% a full recovery in CFP patients. Although both techniques utilized the described landmarks to place the trephine/puncture, it is thought that the additional visualization provided by the trephine technique allowed the ASAN and its branches to be seen and avoided.[25] In addition, the trephine technique creates a neat hole through which the debrider blade is passed whereas the puncture technique potentially creates fracture lines in the anterior face of the maxilla which may disrupt the nerves running in the bone and cause injury to these nerves.

◆ Postoperative Care

Patients who have undergone either CFT or CFP are advised to rinse their mouth after eating with saline for the first few days until the gingivobuccal incision seals. This incision is usually not stitched. All patients are advised to perform saline douches starting the day after surgery and all patients receive 5 days of broad-spectrum antibiotics. Toilet of the nasal cavity and maxillary sinuses is performed at 2 weeks.

Managing the Persisting Discharging Maxillary Sinus Cavity

In a small percentage of patients who have had adequate sinus surgery and have enlarged maxillary sinus ostia, the maxillary sinus continuous to discharge. Such recalcitrant infections are first treated by adequate courses of culture directed antibiotics and in some cases topical antibiotics and topical steroids. If medical therapy fails then a further surgical option is to try to achieve gravity-dependant drainage by creating a mega-antrostomy.[26]

Mega-antrostomy

The principle for this surgery is to lower the posterior part of the antrostomy to the floor of the nose while preserving the nasolacrimal duct. After enlarging the maxillary antrostomy to the posterior wall of the maxillary sinus, an artery forceps is used to crush the inferior turbinate about 2 cm behind the anterior end angling the forceps toward the posterosuperior wall of the maxillary sinus (**Fig. 5.31**). A curved endoscopic scissors is used to cut the turbinate flush with the lateral nasal wall. Next a scalpel blade is used to make a horizontal incision about 5 mm above the floor of the nose on the lateral nasal wall under the

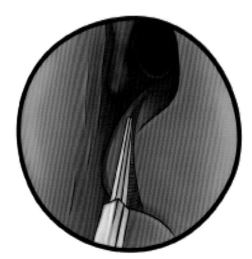

Fig. 5.31 The inferior turbinate is crushed with a curved artery forceps about 2.5 cm behind the head of the turbinate and then cut with an endoscopic scissors up to lateral nasal wall.

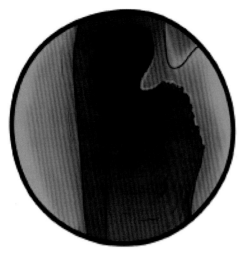

Fig. 5.32 The scalpel blade is used to make mucosal incisions as outlined by the *dotted lines* to create mucosal flaps to cover the exposed bone after enlargement of the maxillary ostium.

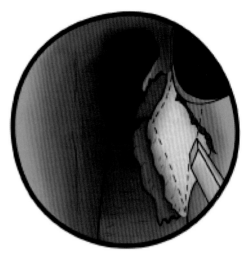

Fig. 5.33 An osteotome is used to remove the bone of the lateral wall the nose, enlarging the maxillary antrostomy to the floor of the nose.

inferior turbinate with a posterior and anterior cut onto the floor of the nose. A vertical mucosal incision is placed 5 mm anterior to the lateral wall and posterior wall junction of the lateral nasal wall (**Fig. 5.32**). A malleable suction Freer is used to mobilize this nasal floor flap medially exposing the bone of the lateral nasal wall and mobilizing the vertical posteriorly based flap posteriorly thereby exposing the bone of the posterior portion of the lateral nasal wall. An osteotome is used to remove the bone over the posterior half of the maxillary sinus leaving the anterior half intact (**Fig. 5.33**). If necessary, a drill can be used to lower the remaining bone between the floor of the nose and the maxillary sinus. In addition, if needed, the antrostomy can be enlarged anteriorly using a backbiter under the nasolacrimal duct and under the remaining inferior

turbinate (**Fig. 5.34**). The flap is then repositioned over the exposed bone along the floor of the nose and the posterior wall (**Fig. 5.35**).

◆ Conclusion

The severely diseased maxillary sinus should be dealt with in the same way as any other severely diseased sinus by removal of all polyps and mucus or pus. A large middle meatal antrostomy combined with canine fossa trephine or puncture utilizing the landmarks described allows access to all regions of the maxillary sinus with the microdebrider blade. This in turn allows polyps and mucus to be removed with the

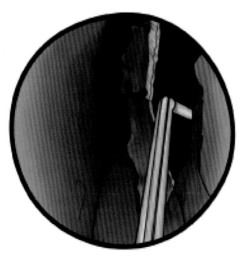

Fig. 5.34 A backbiter is used to further enlarge the antrostomy under the residual inferior turbinate and under the opening of the lacrimal duct.

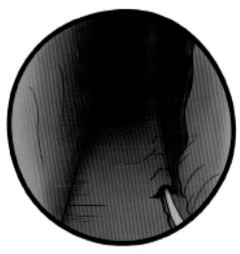

Fig. 5.35 The mucosal flaps are replaced over the exposed bone to improve the postoperative healing and reduce granulation tissue and crusting.

retention of the basement membrane of the sinus and rapid postoperative healing with restoration of the function of the maxillary sinus.

◆ Anterior Approach to the Maxillary Sinus

The anterior approach to the maxillary sinus follows similar steps to those presented in the description for an inferior turbinate shoulder osteotomy in Chapter 4. Its primary use is to provide access to the anterior wall of the maxillary sinus for patients who have a tumor attached to the anterior wall. It is not used for inflammatory disease of the maxillary sinus. The technique is presented in Chapter 16 where surgical techniques for tumors involving the maxillary sinus are presented.

◆ Key Points

Uncinectomy

Uncinectomy is the first and often the most important step of ESS.[1–4] If it is poorly performed there is a significant likelihood that the ESS will fail.[1–4] Critical evaluation of the CT scan before uncinectomy is important so that an atelectatic uncinate can be identified before surgery is undertaken. In our hands the swing-door technique of uncinectomy has few complications and a higher incidence of identification of the natural ostium.[4]

Enlargement of the Natural Maxillary Sinus Ostium

In revision ESS the surgeon should specifically look for a posterior fontanelle ostium during both the clinical examination and the CT evaluation. It is critical that the natural ostium of the maxillary sinus is identified and if there is a posterior fontanelle or accessory ostium that the two ostia are joined to form a single ostium. The natural ostium should be enlarged posteriorly if there is evidence of significant disease within the maxillary sinus that needs to be addressed through the natural ostium.

Canine Fossa Puncture or Trephine

A canine fossa puncture or trephine can be used to access anterior, medial, and inferior disease within the maxillary sinus. The patient should always be warned about the possibility of lip and teeth numbness after the surgery with a small risk of permanent numbness.

Mega-antrostomy

In patients who have persistent chronic maxillary sinus infections and in cystic fibrosis patients, the antrostomy can be lowered to the floor of the nose thereby facilitating gravity-dependant drainage and better sinus irrigation.

References

1. Owen R, Kuhn F. The maxillary sinus ostium: Demystifying the middle meatal antrostomy. Am J Rhinol 1995;9(6):313–320
2. Richtsmeier WJ. Top 10 reasons for endoscopic maxillary sinus surgery failure. Laryngoscope 2001;111(11 Pt 1):1952–1956
3. Parsons DS, Stivers FE, Talbot AR. The missed ostium sequence and the surgical approach to revision functional endoscopic sinus surgery. Otolaryngol Clin North Am 1996;29(1):169–183
4. Wormald PJ, McDonogh M. The 'swing-door' technique for uncinectomy in endoscopic sinus surgery. J Laryngol Otol 1998;112(6):547–551
5. Levine HL. Functional endoscopic sinus surgery: evaluation, surgery, and follow-up of 250 patients. Laryngoscope 1990;100(1):79–84
6. Yoon JH, Kim KS, Jung DH, et al. Fontanelle and uncinate process in the lateral wall of the human nasal cavity. Laryngoscope 2000;110(2 Pt 1):281–285
7. Stammberger H. Endoscopic endonasal surgery--concepts in treatment of recurring rhinosinusitis. Part I. Anatomic and pathophysiologic considerations. Otolaryngol Head Neck Surg 1986;94(2):143–147
8. Joe JK, Ho SY, Yanagisawa E. Documentation of variations in sinonasal anatomy by intraoperative nasal endoscopy. Laryngoscope 2000;110(2 Pt 1):229–235
9. Jog M, McGarry GW. How frequent are accessory sinus ostia? J Laryngol Otol 2003;117(4):270–272
10. Kirihene RK, Rees G, Wormald PJ. The influence of the size of the maxillary sinus ostium on the nasal and sinus nitric oxide levels. Am J Rhinol 2002;16(5):261–264
11. Moncada S, Palmer RMJ, Higgs EA. Nitric oxide: physiology, pathophysiology, and pharmacology. Pharmacol Rev 1991;43(2):109–142
12. Nathan CF, Hibbs JB Jr. Role of nitric oxide synthesis in macrophage antimicrobial activity. Curr Opin Immunol 1991;3(1):65–70
13. Bentz BG, Simmons RL, Haines GK III, Radosevich JA. The yin and yang of nitric oxide: reflections on the physiology and pathophysiology of NO. Head Neck 2000;22(1):71–83
14. Nakane M, Schmidt HHHW, Pollock JS, Förstermann U, Murad F. Cloned human brain nitric oxide synthase is highly expressed in skeletal muscle. FEBS Lett 1993;316(2):175–180
15. Arnal J-F, Flores P, Rami J, et al. Nasal nitric oxide concentration in paranasal sinus inflammatory diseases. Eur Respir J 1999;13(2):307–312
16. Lundberg JON. Airborne nitric oxide: inflammatory marker and aerocrine messenger in man. Acta Physiol Scand Suppl 1996;633:1–27
17. Schlosser RJ, Spotnitz WD, Peters EJ, Fang K, Gaston B, Gross CW. Elevated nitric oxide metabolite levels in chronic sinusitis. Otolaryngol Head Neck Surg 2000;123(4):357–362
18. Sathananthar S, Nagaonkar S, Paleri V, Le T, Robinson S, Wormald PJ. Canine fossa puncture and clearance of the maxillary sinus for the severely diseased maxillary sinus. Laryngoscope 2005;115(6):1026–1029
19. Desrosiers M. Refractory chronic rhinosinusitis: pathophysiology and management of chronic rhinosinusitis persisting after endoscopic sinus surgery. Curr Allergy Asthma Rep 2004;4(3):200–207
20. Seiberling K, Ooi E, MiinYip J, Wormald PJ. Canine fossa trephine for the severely diseased maxillary sinus. Am J Rhinol Allergy 2009;23(6):615–618
21. Seiberling KA, Church CA, Tewfik M, et al. Canine fossa trephine is a beneficial procedure in patients with Samter's triad. Rhinology 2012;50(1):104–108
22. Robinson SR, Baird R, Le T, Wormald PJ. The incidence of complications after canine fossa puncture performed during endoscopic sinus surgery. Am J Rhinol 2005;19(2):203–206
23. Bernal-Sprekelsen M, Kalweit H, Welkoborsky HJ. Discomforts after endoscopy of the maxillary sinus via canine fossa. Rhinology 1991;29(1):69–75
24. Robinson S, Wormald PJ. Patterns of innervation of the anterior maxilla: a cadaver study with relevance to canine fossa puncture of the maxillary sinus. Laryngoscope 2005;115(10):1785–1788
25. Singhal D, Douglas R, Robinson S, Wormald PJ. The incidence of complications using new landmarks and a modified technique of canine fossa puncture. Am J Rhinol 2007;21(3):316–319
26. Costa ML, Psaltis AJ, Nayak JV, Hwang PH. Long-term outcomes of endoscopic maxillary mega-antrostomy for refractory chronic maxillary sinusitis. Int Forum Allergy Rhinol 2015;5(1):60–65

6 The Anatomy of the Frontal Recess and Frontal Sinus with Three-Dimensional Reconstruction

◆ Introduction

In recent years, ESS has become accepted as the treatment of choice for chronic sinusitis that is resistant to medical management.[1] As ESS has become more widely adopted, the understanding of the complex and varied anatomy of the sinuses has improved.[2,3] However, the frontal recess and frontal sinus remain a challenge for surgeons. The anatomy is complex, varied, and can be confusing.[4,5] To better understand the anatomy of the paranasal sinuses, it is important to be aware of the embryology of the turbinates and sinuses. There are six embryological lamellae or "ridges" that form from the lateral nasal wall and give rise to important structures in the nose. Early in the fetal development, these lamellae fuse to form four lamellae. Persistence of the fifth lamella will result in the presence of a supreme turbinate. This is rare and only present in 15% of population. The first lamella forms the uncinate process, the second the bulla ethmoidalis, the third the middle turbinate, the fourth the superior turbinate, and the fifth (if present) the supreme turbinate (**Fig. 6.1**). The frontal, anterior ethmoid, and maxillary sinuses pneumatize from the furrow between the uncinate and bulla ethmoidalis. The posterior ethmoids pneumatize from the furrow between the middle and superior turbinates and the sphenoid sinus from the furrow above the superior turbinate.

The key to safe surgery in the frontal recess is a clear understanding of the anatomy. This chapter explains how computed tomography (CT) software can view cells in the coronal, parasagittal, and axial planes and, using building blocks, how a three-dimensional (3D) picture of the anatomy of the frontal recess can be created. Such a 3D picture allows the surgeon to plan a surgical approach to the frontal recess so that each cell in the frontal recess can be entered in a predetermined sequential manner and then removed. This allows the surgeon to be able to turn to the CT scan at any point during the dissection and identify the cell that is currently being dissected. This mental picture gives the surgeon greater confidence that the complex anatomy of the frontal recess and frontal sinus is fully understood and removal of obstructing cells can be safely achieved. Insecurity during dissection in the frontal recess may result in either inadequate surgery with ESS failure or may increase the risk of injury to the skull base, orbit, and the anterior ethmoid artery.[4,6]

◆ Basic Anatomy of the Frontal Recess and Frontal Sinus

A common reason for ESS failure is inadequate removal of cells obstructing the outflow of the frontal sinus.[4,6] The location of the frontal recess creates anxiety for the surgeon as operating in this region places the lateral wall of the olfactory fossa (the thinnest part of the skull base), the anterior skull base (fovea ethmoidalis), the anterior ethmoidal artery, and the orbit at risk. The anterior wall of the frontal recess is formed by the thick bone of the frontal process of the maxilla, the so-called "beak" of the frontal process (**Fig. 6.2**). The size of this beak will vary according to the degree of pneumatization of the agger nasi cell. If there is a large agger nasi cell then the beak will be small. If, however, the agger nasi cell is absent or under-pneumatized, then the beak will extend significantly into the frontal recess and create a narrow frontal ostium as the beak approaches the forward projecting anterior skull base. Thus the anteroposterior distance from the skull base to the frontal beak is largely determined by the pneumatization of the agger nasi cell (**Fig. 6.3**).

The medial wall of the frontal recess is formed by the lateral wall of the olfactory fossa. The height of this wall is determined by the level of the cribriform plate. Keros[7] classified the depth of the olfactory fossa as a Keros type 1 (less than 3 mm), type 2 (3–7 mm), and a type 3 (>7 mm). Depending on the Keros type, a variable amount of the lateral wall of the olfactory fossa will be exposed during dissection in this

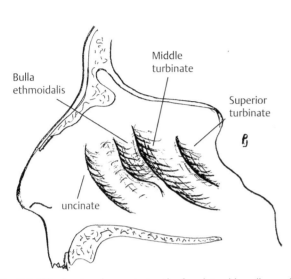

Fig. 6.1 This drawing demonstrates the four lateral lamellae and the corresponding structures into which they develop.

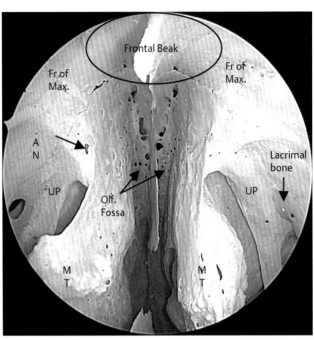

Fig. 6.2 Endoscopic image of dry skull demonstrating the dry bone anatomy of the frontal recess and frontal beak. Both frontal process of the maxilla (*Fr of Max*) join in the midline to form the frontal beak. The olfactory fossa (*olf. fossa*) are bounded by the middle turbinates (*MT*) and the nasal septum, and roofed by the cribriform plate. The location of the agger nasi cell (*ANC*) is shown, and the extent of pneumatization of this cell will determine the size of the frontal beak. *UP*, uncinate process.

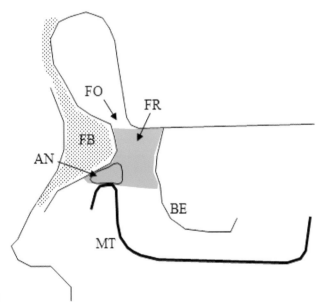

a

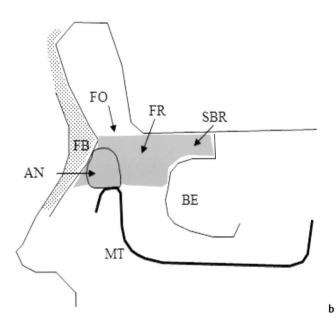

b

Fig. 6.3 (**a**) The effect of a small under pneumatized agger nasi cell (*ANC*). The frontal beak (*FB*) is large and the AP diameter of the frontal ostium (*FO*) small. The frontal recess (*FR*) is shaded and extends from the beak to the bulla lamella (*BE*). (**b**) The effect of a well pneumatized agger nasi cell (*AN*) cell with a small frontal beak (*FB*) and large frontal ostium. If the bulla lamella does not reach the skull base, a supraullar recess (*SBR*) is formed. *MT*, middle turbinate.

region. The bone of the lateral wall of the olfactory fossa varies in thickness between 0.05 mm and 0.2 mm and provides little resistance to penetration.[8]

The lateral wall of the frontal recess is formed by the lamina papyracea and the posterior wall by the upward continuation of the anterior face of the bulla ethmoidalis. On occasion, this anterior wall of the bulla ethmoidalis may not reach the skull base and a suprabullar recess is formed (**Fig. 6.3**). The frontal recess is then continuous with this recess.

The roof of the frontal recess is formed by the fovea ethmoidalis. This bone is relatively thick and normally provides significant resistance to penetration. In a study conducted in our department we found that the right fovea ethmoidalis was higher than the left in 59% of patients.[9] It should also be noted that the roof (fovea ethmoidalis) may slope, placing the medial aspect of the roof at a lower level than the lateral aspect. The anterior ethmoidal artery and nerve runs across the fovea ethmoidalis at a 45-degree angle from lateral to medial (**Fig. 6.4**). In most instances, it can be found behind the upward continuation of the bulla ethmoidalis. However, when this is absent and a suprabullar recess is present, the anterior ethmoidal artery will be in the frontal recess. The anterior ethmoidal artery may lie in a mesentery suspended from the skull base in 14 to 43% of patients (in our study the incidence was 34%).[9] It is important that the CT scan is reviewed carefully before surgery to establish if the anterior ethmoidal artery is against the skull base or in a mesentery and if a suprabullar recess is present or not (**Fig. 6.5**).

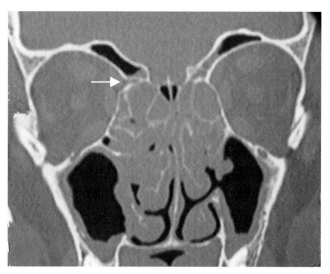

Fig. 6.5 The right anterior ethmoidal artery is on a mesentery (*white arrow*). Note the pinching of the lamella papyracea as the artery exits the orbit.

If the anterior ethmoidal artery is cut during surgery (this is only likely if it is on a mesentery), it may retract into the orbit and cause bleeding within the orbital tissues. This creates an increase in the intraorbital volume with resultant proptosis. Increasing pressure stretches the optic nerve and may result in decreased arterial blood flow to the retina and subsequent loss of vision.

◆ The Uncinate Process

The uncinate process has in the past been thought to be the key to the frontal recess.[8] This text adopts an alternate approach and suggests that the agger nasi cell is the key that unlocks the frontal recess.[10,11] The agger nasi cell is present in more than 90% of patients.[12] As the agger nasi cell is the key, it is important to understand the interaction between the uncinate and the agger nasi cell. The interaction between the upward continuation of the uncinate and the agger nasi cell is often poorly understood. The attachment of the root of the uncinate into either the lamina papyracea, skull base, or middle turbinate have been well described (**Fig. 6.6**)[5,8,13] but how this upward continuation of the uncinate interacts with the agger nasi cell and anterior ethmoidal cells in the frontal recess is sometimes poorly understood.

Attachment of the Uncinate to the Lamina Papyracea

In most cases, the uncinate forms the medial wall of agger nasi but only in the posterior half of the cell. The anterior half is embedded in the frontal process of the maxilla and does not interact with the uncinate. In 85% of patients the uncinate, after forming the posteromedial wall of the cell, implants on the lamina papyracea. In a large proportion of these patients, this upward extension will give off a leaflet of

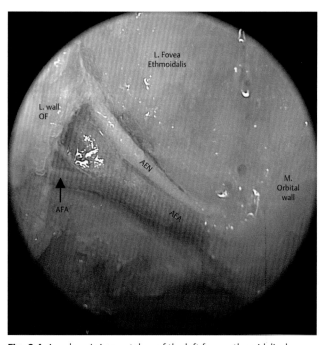

Fig. 6.4 A cadaveric image taken of the left fovea ethmoidalis demonstrating the anterior ethmoidal artery (*AEA*) and nerve (*AEN*) leaving the orbit and traveling in a 45-degree angle from lateral to medial along the skull base. This artery can be seen giving off the anterior falcine artery (*AFA*) as it approaches the lateral wall of the olfactory fossa (*L. wall OF*). *M.* Orbital wall, medial orb.

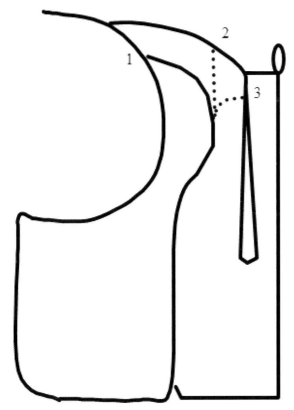

Fig. 6.6 The classical description of the insertions of the uncinate process.[8] 1, insertion into the lamina papyracea; 2, insertion into the skull base; 3, insertion into middle turbinate.

bone to the bulla lamella forming a plate of bone that divides the frontal recess vertically from posterior to anterior[14,15] as it extends from the bulla ethmoidalis to the medial wall of the agger nasi cell and onto the frontal beak. In this situation the frontal sinus will drain medial to this plate (**Fig. 6.7**).

The relationship of a single large agger nasi cell (AN) to the frontal sinus ostium (FS) is considered; it is better understood by viewing the coronal and parasagittal scans (see **Fig. 6.13**). This example shows the simplest anatomical configuration of the frontal recess. The next important step is to decide where the frontal sinus drains in relation to these cells.[16–18] Placement of the building blocks is illustrated in **Fig. 6.8**.

Attachment of the Uncinate to the Middle Turbinate

The second anatomical variation to consider is that of a larger agger nasi cell. A large cell may push the upward continuation of the uncinate medially so that it attaches to the middle turbinate (**Fig. 6.9**).

This configuration alters the drainage of the frontal sinus as the agger nasi cell pushes the frontal drainage pathway posteriorly. Therefore, the surgeon can no longer access the frontal recess medial to the uncinate. Access is obtained by passing the curette along the frontal sinus drainage pathway behind the posterior wall of the agger nasi cell and fracturing

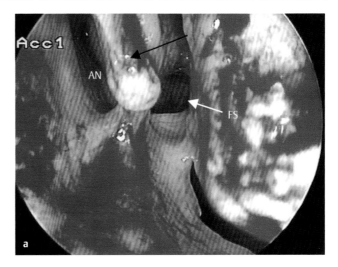

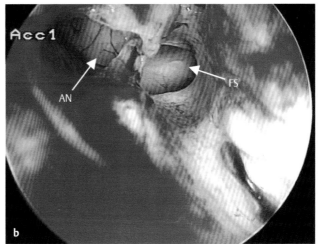

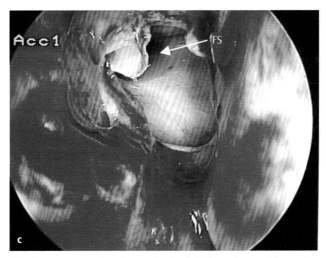

Fig. 6.7 Intraoperative pictures in the right frontal recess illustrating (**a**) the upward continuation of the uncinate (*black arrow*) forming the medial wall of the agger nasi cell (*ANC*). In (**b**) the further removal of the medial wall/uncinate superiorly reveals the roof of the agger nasi cell (*ANC*) and frontal ostium (*FS*). (**c**) A small residual part of the roof of the agger nasi cell remains. The frontal sinus ostium (*FS*) can be seen.

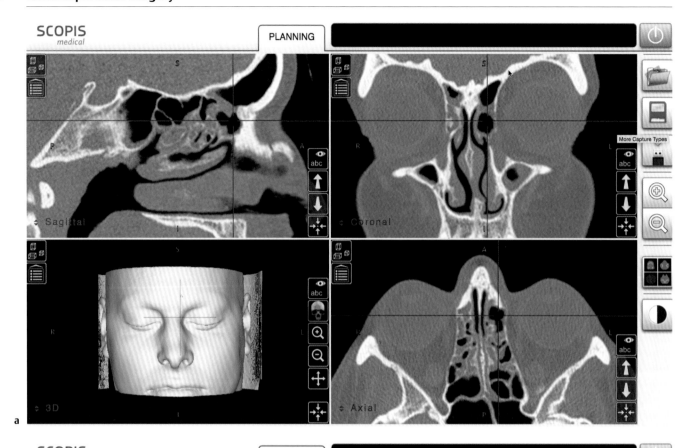

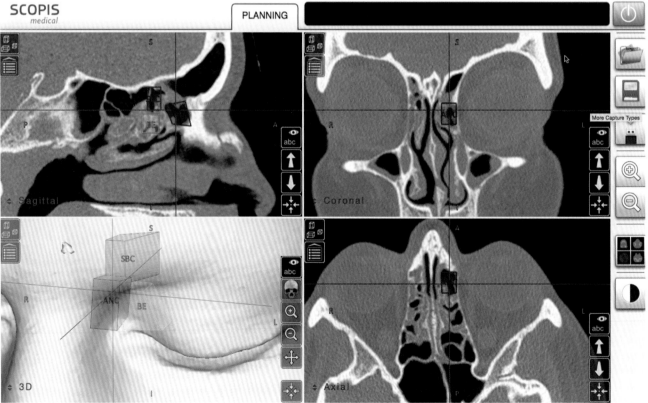

Fig. 6.8 (**a**) Coronal, axial, and parasagittal scans illustrating a single agger cell (*crosshairs*) on the left side. (**b**) Three-dimensional building block reconstructions have been placed over the agger nasi cell (*ANC*), bulla ethmoidalis (*BE*), and supra bulla cell (*SBC*).

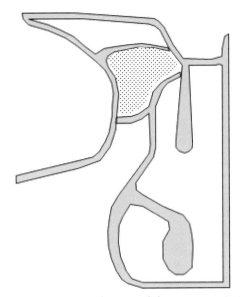

Fig. 6.9 A diagram illustrating how a single large agger nasi cell pushes the insertion of the uncinate onto the middle turbinate.

the posterior wall and roof of the agger nasi cell forward to fully expose the frontal ostium.

The following series of CT scans and operative dissection pictures illustrates the upward continuation of the uncinate, which forms the medial wall of the agger nasi cell and has been pushed by this cell to insert on the middle turbinate before progressing superiorly, forming the roof of the agger nasi and then implanting on the lamina papyracea (**Fig. 6.10** and **Fig. 6.11**).

Attachment of the Uncinate to the Skull Base

The third scenario involves the further upward continuation of the uncinate onto the skull base. In a small percentage of patients, the uncinate may have no relationship with the agger nasi cell. Usually in this configuration the uncinate will progress superiorly to implant on the skull base. The following series of CT scans and anatomical dissections illustrates this variation (**Fig. 6.12**).

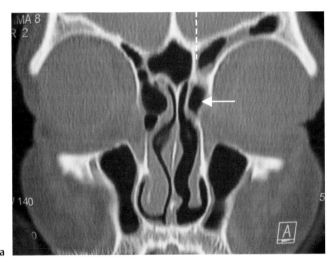

a

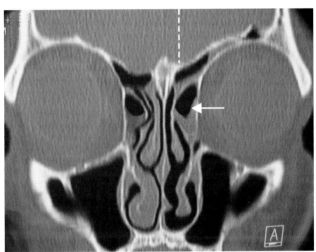

b

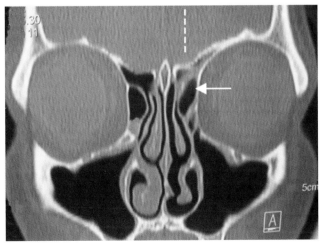

c

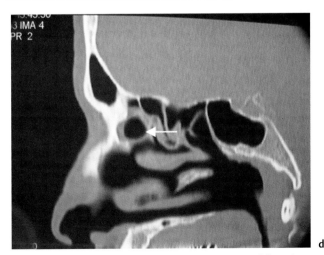

d

Fig. 6.10 The agger nasi cell is indicated by the *white arrow*. The *broken line* indicates the position of the parasagittal scan. The scans follow the sequence (**a**), (**b**), (**c**), and (**d**). The uncinate can be seen to be pushed medially by the agger nasi cell, touching the middle turbinate before turning more posteriorly to form the posterior wall and roof of the agger, and implanting on the lamina papyracea.

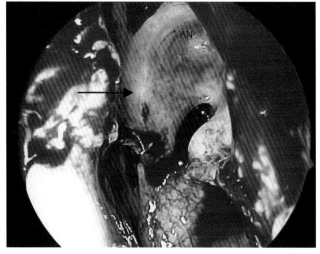

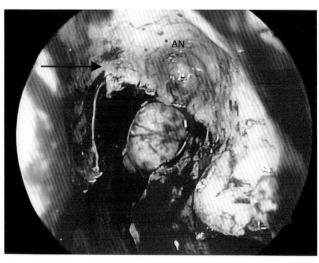

Fig. 6.11 These left-sided operative pictures are taken of the patient in the scans of **Fig. 6.10**. The *black arrow* indicates the uncinate process, which forms the medial wall of the agger nasi cell (*ANC*) and attaches to the middle turbinate before progressing superiorly to form the roof of the agger cell and implanting on the lamina papyracea.

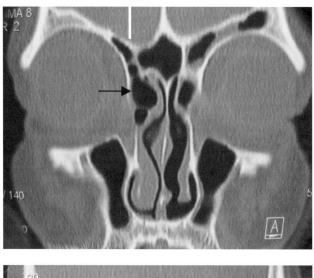

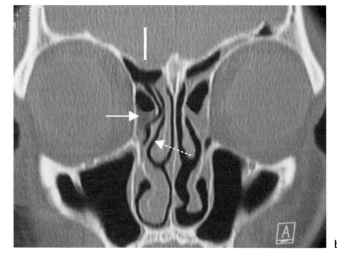

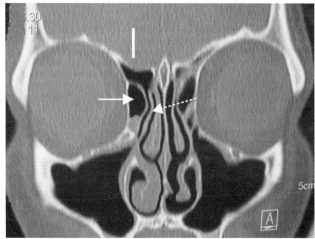

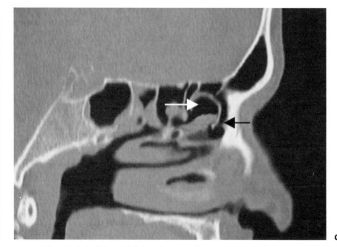

Fig. 6.12 (**a–d**) On the right side of the CT scans (**b**), (**c**), and (**d**), the *white arrow* indicates the agger nasi cell. The *black arrow* indicates the space anterior to the agger nasi cell in scans (**a**) and (**d**). The *solid white vertical line* in (**a**), (**b**), and (**c**) indicates the position of the parasagittal scan (**d**). The *broken white arrow* indicates the uncinate process separate from the agger nasi cell in scans (**b**) and (**c**). (*continued*)

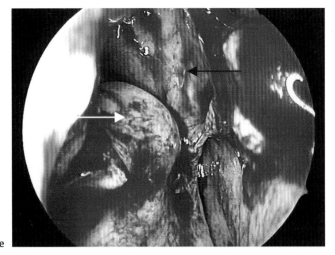

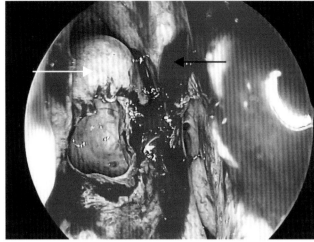

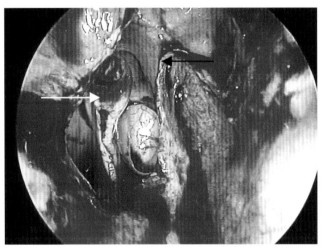

Fig. 6.12 (*continued*) (**e–g**) These are the right-sided operative pictures of the CT scans shown in (**a–d**). (**e**) Corresponds to CT scan in (**a**) and shows the agger nasi cell intact (*white arrow*); the *black arrow* indicates the uncinate process as it progresses upward to implant on the junction of the middle turbinate and the skull base. (**f**) The anterior face of the agger nasi cell opened with the uncinate process (*black arrow*) seen to be separate from the agger nasi cell. (**g**) The uncinate (*black arrow*) implanting onto the skull base. The *white arrow* indicates the remaining roof of the agger nasi cell.

The uncinate can be seen passing medial to the agger nasi cell and implanting at the junction of the middle turbinate and skull base. The broken line indicates the position of the parasagittal scan.

Alternatively the uncinate process may form the medial wall of a frontoethmoidal cell that is sitting above the agger nasi cell. This frontoethmoidal cell may push the upward continuation of the uncinate superiorly to attach onto the skull base (**Fig. 6.13**). The variations associated with the frontoethmoidal cells will be considered below with the discussion on the classification of the frontal ethmoidal cells. The following cadaver dissection and CT scan illustrate a cell on the right side pushing the insertion of the uncinate onto the skull base.

The Agger Nasi Cell[10]

There are a large number of possible variations in the anatomy of the frontal recess. To gain a functional understanding of the anatomy of the frontal recess the simplest configurations should be understood first before more complex variations are tackled. The simplest anatomical configuration is the single agger nasi cell without frontal ethmoidal cells.

The agger nasi cell is the most anterior ethmoidal cell and is present in 93% of people.[12] The agger nasi cell forms a bulge on the lateral nasal wall anterior to the middle turbinate (**Fig. 6.14**). If sequential coronal CT scans are evaluated in an anterior to posterior direction, the agger nasi cell can be seen before the middle turbinate comes into view (**Fig. 6.15**).[5,12]

Note that the uncinate only has a relationship with the posterior half of the agger nasi cell and not the anterior half, which is why the uncinate cannot be seen on the coronal CT scans taken through the anterior half of the agger nasi cell as seen in **Fig. 6.15**. This relationship can be viewed in **Fig. 6.16** and **Fig. 6.17**.

The Transition from Frontal Sinus to Frontal Recess on the Coronal CT Scans

The surgeon reviewing a patient's CT scans before surgery needs to understand how the anterior coronal CT scan through the agger nasi cell relates to the frontal beak and frontal sinus and to be able to tell when on sequential coronal CT scans the frontal sinus transitions to the frontal recess. **Fig. 6.16** is a diagrammatic illustration of how a coronal CT scan through the anterior half of the agger nasi

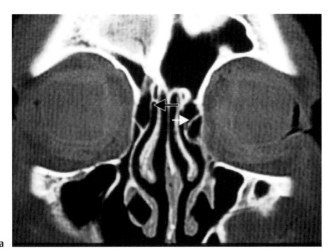

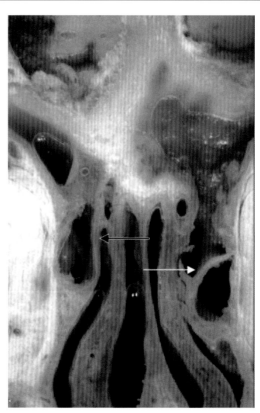

a   b

Fig. 6.13 (a,b) The CT scan is taken of the cadaver dissection speci-men pictured along with it. On the right side the uncinate process (*white arrow*) is pushed up toward the skull base and onto the middle turbinate by a small cell sitting above and medial to the agger nasi cell. On the left the upward continuation of the uncinate can be seen forming the roof of the agger nasi cell (*gray arrow*). Note the frontal sinus draining directly above the agger nasi cell.

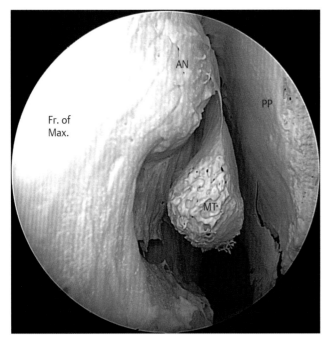

Fig. 6.14 Endoscopic image of a dry skull taken within the right nasal cavity. The bulge on the lateral nasal wall created by the agger nasi cell (*ANC*) can clearly be seen above and anterior to the middle turbinate (*MT*). *Fr. of Max*, frontal process of maxilla; *PP*, perpendicular plate.

cell and through the frontal sinus can be identified on a coronal CT scan.

If line 1 is drawn in the coronal plane, the frontal beak can be seen as continuous ridge of bone with the frontal sinus above it (*diagonally shaded area* in **Fig. 6.16** and **Fig. 6.17**). This line (line 1) is anterior to the uncinate with no uncinate visible on the coronal diagram (**Fig. 6.16**). This makes it simple

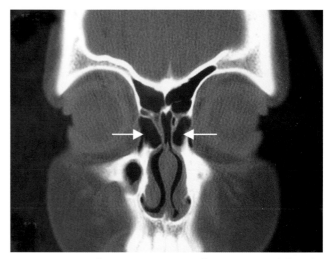

Fig. 6.15 CT scan illustrating agger nasi cells anterior to middle turbi-nate insertion (*white arrows*).

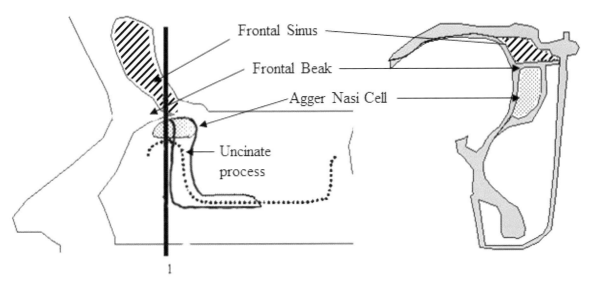

Fig. 6.16 A diagrammatic illustration of a parasagittal view of the agger nasi cell with line 1 representing a coronal cut through the anterior aspect of the agger nasi cell anterior to the middle turbinate. The diagonally striped shaded area represents the area of the frontal sinus above the frontal beak.

to differentiate the frontal sinus (above the beak) from the frontal recess. Line 2 in **Fig. 6.17** shows a coronal cut through the uncinate process and posterior half of the agger nasi cell behind the beak. This illustrates the transition from the frontal sinus to the frontal recess with loss of the continuity of bone (illustrated as the "frontal beak" in **Fig. 6.16**) and by the presence of the uncinate. This coronal cut illustrates the posterior part of the agger nasi cell's relationship to the superior extension of the uncinate process. This part of the uncinate forms the medial and posterior medial wall of the agger nasi cell and represents the relationship between the anterior agger nasi cell (*shaded with dots*) and the frontal beak and the floor of the frontal sinus (*diagonally shaded area*).

The *diagonally shaded area* in **Fig. 6.16** and **Fig. 6.17** is the frontal sinus above the frontal beak. The frontal beak forms

the floor of the frontal sinus (**Fig. 6.2**). From these diagrams it can be seen that most of the agger nasi cell is anterior to the uncinate but the posterior half of the agger nasi cell has an intimate relationship with the upward extension of the uncinate process[10] (**Fig. 6.18**).

Transition from Frontal Sinus to Frontal Recess on the Axial Scans

Understanding the axial CT scans is crucial for the surgeon to be able to determine how the frontal sinus drains into the frontal recess. To determine exactly where the frontal sinus drains the surgeon sequentially scans through the axial scans from cranial to caudal following the frontal sinus

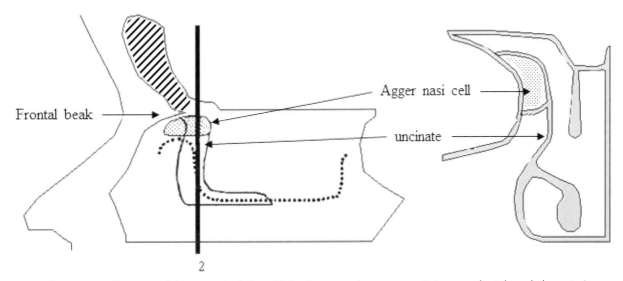

Fig. 6.17 A diagrammatic illustration of the parasagittal view with line 2 representing a more posterior coronal cut through the posterior aspect of the agger nasi cell.

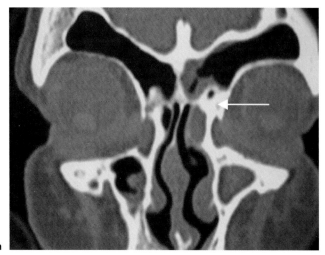
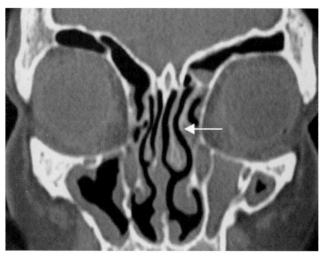

a   b

Fig. 6.18 (**a**) Coronal CT anterior to uncinate with the floor of the frontal sinus ("beak") illustrated by *white arrow* on the left. (**b**) Coronal CT through the uncinate process (*white arrow*) with the uncinate forming medial wall and roof of agger nasi cell on the left.

outflow tract. Understanding the transition from the frontal sinus to the frontal recess on these scans is important. The frontal sinus scans should be viewed from the top down (cranial to caudal). The frontal sinus is easy to identify. As the frontal sinus approaches the frontal recess (**Fig. 6.19a**) it narrows and forms a square (**Fig. 6.19b**). At this level, the posterior wall of the two frontal sinuses forms a straight line (**Fig. 6.19b**). As the skull base turns posteriorly, these squares elongate posteriorly but still maintain a roughly rectangular shape. This is the transition stage from frontal sinus to frontal recess (**Fig. 6.19d,f**). As the posterior ends of these boxes become pointed, so the scans reach the frontal recess. Note how the bone of the anterior wall changes at each of these levels. At **Fig. 6.19b,d**, the bone of the anterior wall of the frontal sinus is even and relatively flat and not very thick. The anterior wall bone becomes much thicker as the upper region of the frontal beak is reached (**Fig. 6.19f**). At **Fig. 6.19f,h** the anterior wall is curved indicating that the nasion has been reached. In **Fig. 6.19h**, the nasion is fully developed and the frontal beak bone is thick, whereas in **Fig. 6.19j**, the beak disappears with only the nasal bones present anteriorly. Also note how the supra bulla frontal cell (SBFC) is seen early on the posterior wall of the frontal sinus (**Fig. 6.19d**, *white arrow*).

Frontal Ethmoidal Cells

Classification

A single agger nasi cell in the frontal recess is only one of the many anatomical variations. In 1995, Fred Kuhn classified the cells[14] seen in the frontal recess and frontal sinus but a recent consensus statement published in 2016 presented a more user-friendly and easier to understand classification as seen in **Table 6.1**.[14]

The classification of the cells is important as it lends structure to our 3D understanding of the anatomy of the frontal recess. However, the drainage pathway is the most important feature to determine during review of the anatomy on the CT scans. The new International Frontal Sinus Anatomy Classification (IFAC)[15] groups the cells into the frontal sinus into three main groups: cells that push the drainage pathway medially, posteromedially, or posteriorly (agger nasi cell, supra agger cells, supra agger frontal cells—these cells are usually associated with the frontal process of the maxilla); cells that push the drainage pathway of the frontal sinus anteriorly (bulla ethmoidalis, supra bulla cells, supra bulla frontal cells, supraorbital ethmoid cells—cells usually associated with the skull base); and cells that push the frontal sinus drainage pathway laterally—cells usually associated with the frontal sinus intersinus septum (frontal septal cell). The IFAC is a consensus document from some of the leading rhinologists in the world in which the previous frontal recess and frontal sinus cell classification (Modified Kuhn Classification)[16,17] has been simplified and improved with the emphasis on both cell position as well as how these cells affect the frontal sinus drainage pathway. The frontal process of the maxilla is the bone forming the anterior wall of the frontal recess (**Fig. 6.20**).

This bone goes on to form the frontal beak. The frontal ethmoidal cells are further divided depending on how many there are and how far these cells extend into the frontal sinus through the frontal ostium.[15] The IFAC defines these cells as supra agger cells and those that extend through the frontal ostium as supra agger frontal cells.

◆ The Building Block Concept for the Reconstruction of the Anatomy of the Frontal Recess

To reconstruct in three dimensions the cells in the frontal recess, building blocks are arranged, one block for each cell.[10,16,17] When operating in this area the surgeon needs to know exactly which cell is being dissected and in what sequence each cell will be opened so that the frontal recess can be safely and competently cleared. In order to build a mental picture of the cells in the frontal recess, the cursor

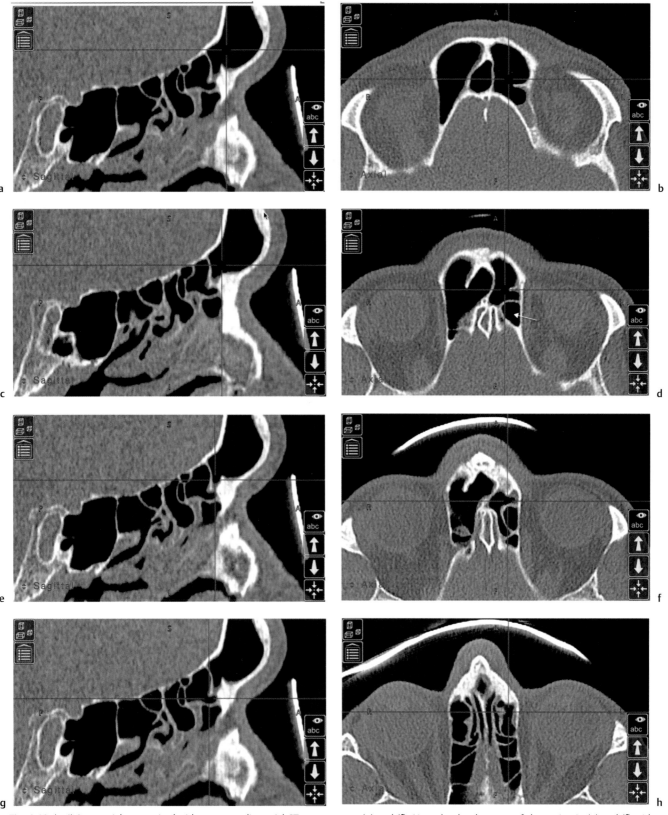

Fig. 6.19 (**a–j**) Sequential parasagittal with corresponding axial CT scans with the *crosshairs* on the parasagittal indicating the level at which the axial cut is taken. The transition from frontal sinus to frontal recess is from cuts (**e**) and (**f**). Note the development of the nasion in (**e**) and (**f**) with thick bony beak visible. The *crosshairs* are on the frontal sinus (**a**) and (**b**), frontal ostium (**c**), supra agger cell (**g**), and agger nasi cell (**i**). (*continued*)

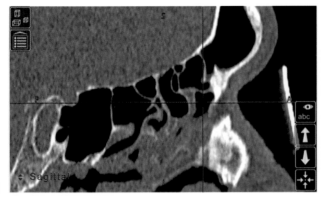
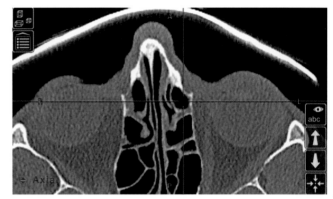

Fig. 6.19 (continued)

is placed on the axial CT on the nasal bones and then the coronal CTs are slowly scrolled through from anterior to posterior. This gives an overview of the cells in the frontal recess in the coronal plane. The cursor is now moved from side to side in the axial CT while the parasagittal CTs are viewed again, confirming the overview obtained when the coronal CTs were viewed. In conjunction with Scopis, software has been developed to draw building blocks and the frontal sinus drainage pathway directly on the CT scans. The software also allows for the blocks to be manipulated in one of the three planes. The cursor is placed in the first cell seen on the coronal CT (this is usually the agger nasi cell but in this example the supra agger frontal cell is used as the first cell) (**Fig. 6.21a**). This cell should now be identified on the parasagittal and axial CT scans (**Fig. 6.21a**). A building block is now placed over this cell on the coronal CT scan (**Fig. 6.21a**). The block when first placed on the CT scan is white. After placement of the block, the surgeon reviews the block in the coronal, parasagittal, and axial planes

and then decides in which of these planes it is best to manipulate the block to get the best possible fit of the block to the cell. In the example (**Fig. 6.21a**) the block is placed over the SAFC and is a poor fit on the parasagittal scan. The choice is made to manipulate the block in the parasagittal plane and the corners of the block are moved until the best fit is achieved (**Fig. 6.21b**). Once the circles on the corners of the block have been grabbed by the mouse and manipulated, it will no longer be possible to manipulate the block in the other planes (coronal and axial). If you decide that you wish to manipulate the block in one of the other planes, the block will need to be deleted and a new block placed; the new block can now be manipulated in any of the planes. The block can be named according to the IFAC by clicking on the "IFAC" button on the screen (**Fig. 6.21c,d**). The other cells that make up the frontal recess are identified and blocks placed and manipulated for each cell (**Fig. 6.21e**). Note that there are two supra agger cells (SACs) and these have been named SAC1 and SAC2. The blocks that make up the frontal

Table 6.1 International Frontal Sinus Anatomical Classification (IFAC)[15]

Name	Definition	Abbreviation
Anterior cells (push the drainage pathway of the frontal sinus medial, posterior, or posteromedially)		
Agger nasi cell	Cell that sits either anterior to the origin of the middle turbinate or sits directly above the most anterior insertion of the middle turbinate into the lateral nasal wall.	ANC
Supra agger cell	Anterolateral ethmoidal cell, located above the Agger nasi cell (not pneumatizing into the frontal sinus).	SAC
Supra agger frontal cell	Anterolateral ethmoidal cell that extends into the frontal sinus. A small SAFC will only extend into the floor of the frontal sinus, whereas a large SAFC may extend significantly into the frontal sinus and may even reach the roof of the frontal sinus.	SAFC
Posterior cells (push the drainage pathway anteriorly)		
Bulla ethmoidalis	Cell above the maxillary ostium	BE
Supra bulla cell	Cell above the bulla ethmoidalis that does not enter the frontal sinus.	SBC
Supra bulla frontal cell	Cell that originates in the supra-bulla region and pneumatizes along the skull base into the posterior region of the frontal sinus. The skull base forms the posterior wall of the cell.	SBFC
Supra orbital ethmoid cell	An anterior ethmoid cell that pneumatizes around, anterior, or posterior to the anterior ethmoidal artery over the roof of the orbit. It often forms part of the posterior wall of an extensively pneumatized frontal sinus and may only be separated from the frontal sinus by a bony septation.	SOEC
Medial cells (push the drainage pathway laterally)		
Frontal septal cell	Medially based cell of the anterior ethmoid or the inferior frontal sinus, attached to or located in the interfrontal sinus septum, associated with the medial aspect of the frontal sinus outflow tract pushing the drainage pathway laterally and frequently posteriorly.	FSC

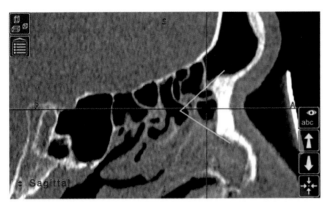

Fig. 6.20 The region between the divergent *solid green arrows* is the frontal process of the maxilla. In this example we have a large agger nasi cell (*crosshairs*) and a supra agger cell above ANC.

recess and frontal sinus anatomy can now be viewed, enlarged, and rotated; look at the 3D reconstructed image in **Fig. 6.21e**. This naming of each cell can be hidden by clicking the ABC button with the image of an eye on the button (**Fig. 6.21f**) and the cells remain but each acronym for each cell has been removed. Re-clicking on this icon restores the names to the cells. Next, the software is used to place the frontal sinus drainage pathway amongst the cells (building blocks). The easiest way to identify where best to draw in the drainage pathway is to use the arrow buttons on the

parasagittal CT to move back and forth through these parasagittal scans until a scan is identified that is most likely to allow the drainage pathway to be seen and drawn onto the scan (**Fig. 6.21g**). Once the drainage pathway has been drawn onto a CT scan a slider appears on each of the views. This slider is used to scroll through the images in that plane. To identify whether the frontal drainage pathway has been correctly placed the slider in the axial CT scan is used to follow the drainage pathway from the frontal sinus through the frontal ostium and frontal recess. If adjustment to the placement of the pathway is necessary while following the drainage pathway, the mouse is placed on the pathway and the mouse icon becomes a hand symbol, which is used to grab the pathway and simply pull it into the correct position. Note in **Fig. 6.21h** the pathway runs through the SAFC and not medial to it as it should be. This is grabbed and moved in the axial plane until it is in the correct position (**Fig. 6.21i**). This can also be done on the other CT scans in the coronal and parasagittal planes. Once the surgeon is happy that the pathway has been correctly placed they can review the anatomy of both the cells and the drainage pathway and plan the surgery; note how the pathway runs anterior then medial to the SAFC, medial to the SACs, and medial to the ANC (**Fig. 6.21j**). In **Fig. 6.21k** the names have been replaced in the cells to give the surgeon a complete 3D understanding of the cells and the drainage pathway.

So far we have concentrated on the ANC, SAC, and SAFC. As we move further posterior in the anterior ethmoid cells

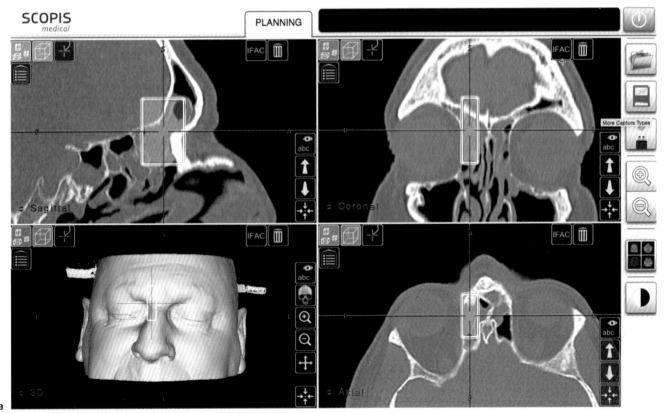

Fig. 6.21 In this series of screen shots (**a**) to (**k**), the basics of the Scopis planning software are illustrated. (**a**) A building block is placed over the supra agger frontal cell. (*continued*)

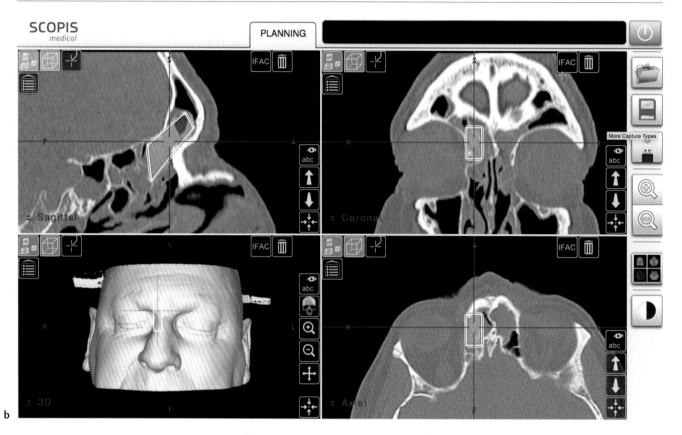

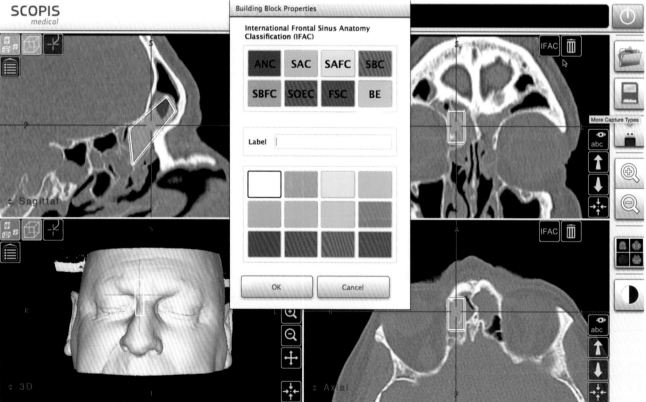

Fig. 6.21 (*continued*) (**b**) The corners of the block are manipulated in the parasagittal plane. (**c**) The IFAC classification drop menu is opened and the cell type selected and this is demonstrated in (**d**).

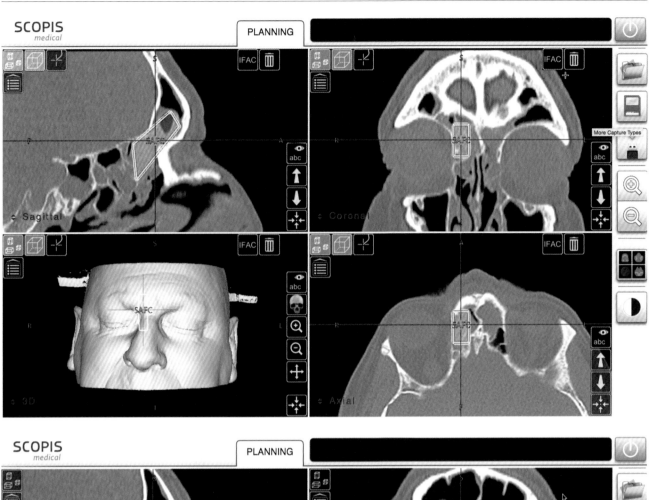

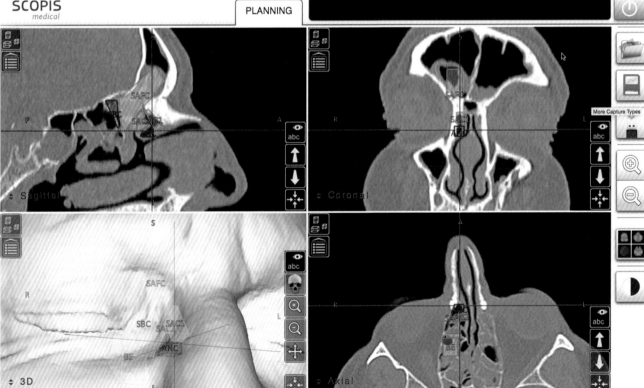

Fig. 6.21 (*continued*) (**e**) All the other cells have building blocks placed over them the cells identified using the IFAC.

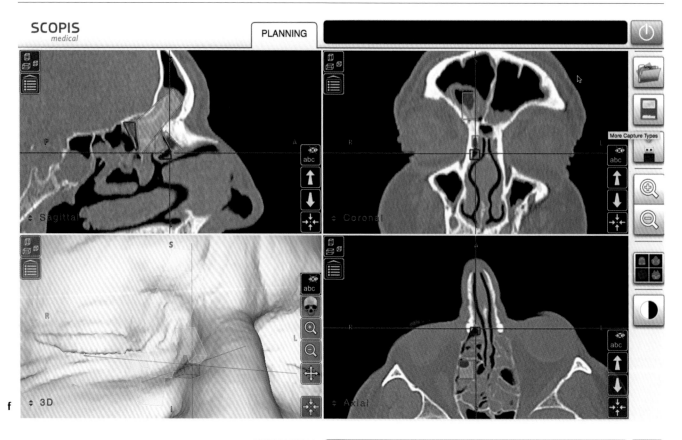

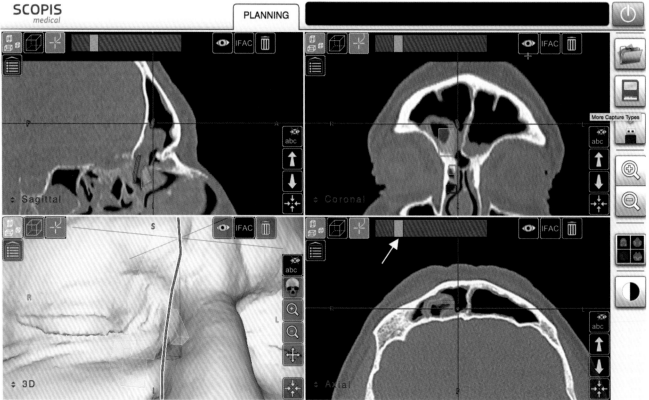

Fig. 6.21 (*continued*) The acronyms can be hidden by clicking on the "eye" icon as shown in (**f**). The frontal sinus drainage pathway is drawn onto the scans in (**g**).

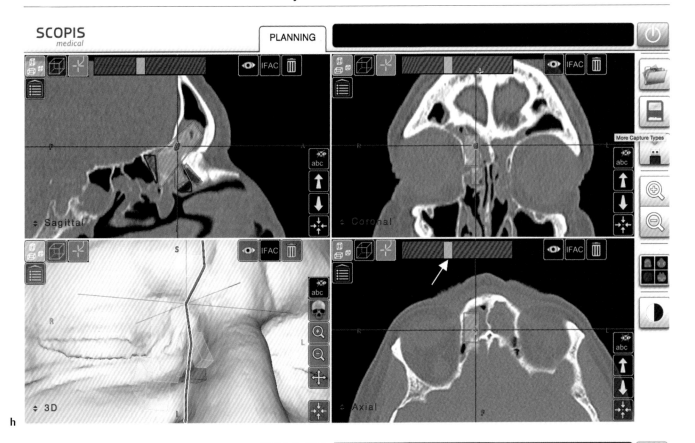

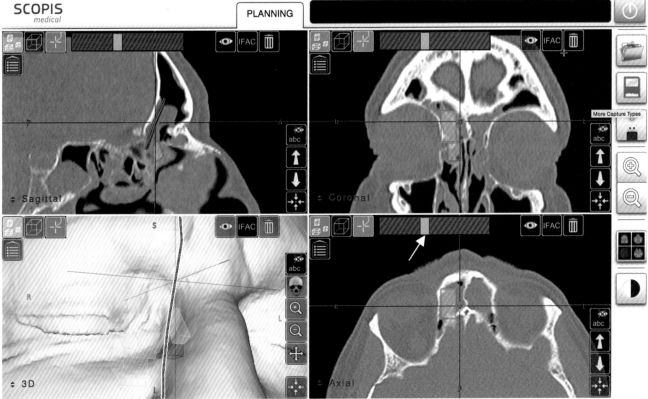

Fig. 6.21 (*continued*) In order to manipulate the position of the frontal drainage pathway, the slider (*white arrow*) is used to scroll through the sequential axial slices (**h**). The mouse icon changes to a hand as it passes over the frontal drainage pathway and by clicking on the pathway it can be dragged into a new position on the scan. This changes in all three planes (**i**).

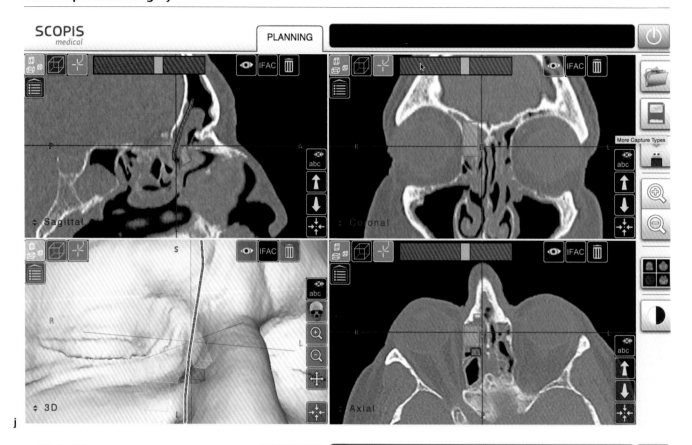

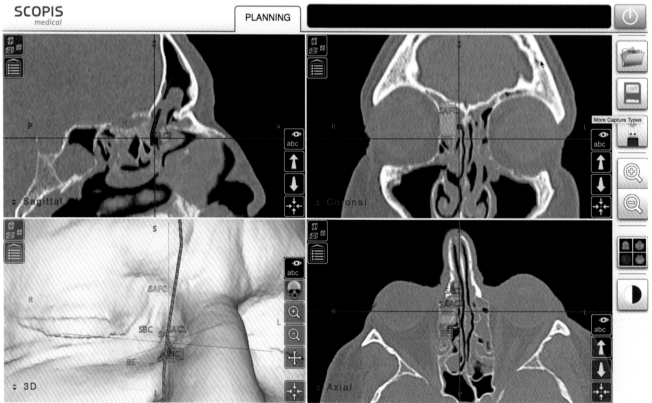

Fig. 6.21 (*continued*) The final 3D reconstruction is presented in (**j**) with the blocks representing the cells and the line the frontal drainage pathway.

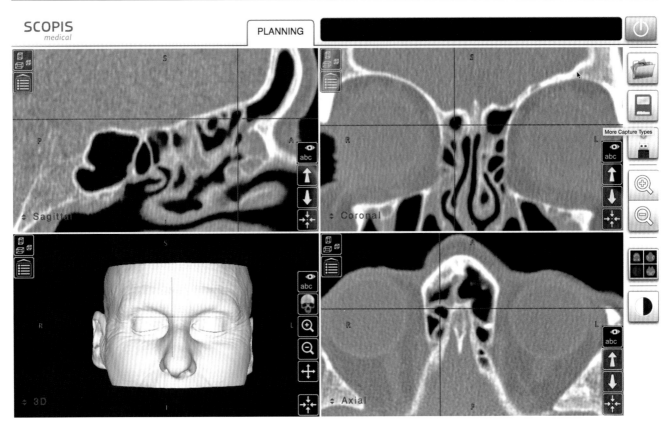

Fig. 6.22 The cell directly above the bulla ethmoidalis is identified as a suprabulla cell (*crosshairs*) and visualized in all three planes. Note its anterior wall encroaches on the frontal sinus drainage pathway.

the bulla ethmoidalis and supra bulla cells become important. In most patients a supra bulla cell is present. This cell can be difficult to identify on the coronal scan if the septation between it and the frontal drainage pathway is not actively sought in the parasagittal and axial planes (**Fig. 6.22**). This cell lies against the skull base so the skull base forms its roof (**Fig. 6.22**). It may be confused with the frontal sinus drainage pathway especially if it projects forward toward the frontal ostium.

Drainage Pathways: A Critical Concept in Frontal Recess Dissection[16–18]

The most important concept that the surgeon needs to establish is how the frontal sinus drains through the cells of the frontal recess. Once the cellular construction and their relationship with one another has been established the surgeon needs to identify the frontal sinus drainage pathway.[16–18] Once this drainage pathway has been identified and drawn in on the CT scans, this pathway can be placed in the 3D reconstruction of the anatomy of the frontal recess. The best scans to check that the pathway is correctly placed is to sequentially view the pathway using the slider above the axial CT scan (**Fig. 6.21g**). The surgeon starts in the frontal sinus (**Fig. 6.21g**) and then follows the drainage pathway down through the frontal ostium and then through the cells of the frontal recess (**Fig. 6.21g–j**). Should the pathway not

be correctly placed, the cursor is placed over the pathway and it is simply grabbed with the cursor and dragged into the correct position on the CT scans. This manipulation of the position of the pathway is best done in the axial plane but can be done in the parasagittal and coronal planes as well. During the dissection of the frontal recess, instruments (probes or curettes) are passed along this pathway and the identified cells fractured to clear the pathway.[17] Usually the pathway is medial (as in this example) or posterior to the cell(s) and the cell(s) can be fractured laterally or anteriorly quite safely. However, when the pathway is anterior, care needs to be taken when fracturing the cell wall posteriorly against the skull base. When the drainage pathway is lateral, the cell wall should be removed by a very gentle fracture if the bone is thin or by placing the instrument as far posterior to the cell wall as possible and fracturing the cell wall anteriorly. For removing residual bony fragments, a through-cutting giraffe forceps can be used. Instruments should not be passed through the roof of a cell as occasionally the surgeon may be confident that he or she is in a cell with space between the roof of the cell and the skull base. But, if mistaken and they are in the space above the cell, pushing the instrument through the "roof" of the cell will result in the instrument entering into anterior cranial fossa. If instruments are passed along pathways, and this can be done very gently without undue force or pressure, cell walls can be fractured safely clearing the drainage pathway of the frontal sinus without endangering the anterior cranial fossa or the orbit.[16–19]

◆ The Anatomical Variations of the Frontal Recess and Frontal Sinus

The Supra Agger Cellular Configuration[15]

An SAC configuration is one or more anterior ethmoidal cell(s) above the ANC (**Fig. 6.23**). This configuration of a single or multiple cells associated with the ANC is common but also may induce significant variability into the frontal recess. The 3D conceptualization of this arrangement is either one or two building blocks sitting one on top of the ANC (**Fig. 6.23**).

The CT scan (**Fig. 6.23**) illustrates the supra agger configuration on the left side with ANC representing the agger nasi cell and cells SAC1 and SAC2, the supra agger cells above it. Review of the parasagittal scan and 3D reconstruction would confirm the position and placement of these cells. Note how the two SACs sit above the ANC and each other but don't project into the frontal sinus. The frontal sinus drains medial to these cells (**Fig. 6.23**).

Supra Agger Frontal Cell[15]

Further pneumatization of these frontal ethmoidal cells into the floor (inferior part) of the frontal sinus above the frontal beak (into the *diagonally shaded area* in **Fig. 6.8**) are classified as SAFCs (**Fig. 6.24**). If the section where the frontal sinus becomes the frontal recess is reviewed (**Fig. 6.16** and

Fig. 6.17), the transition from the frontal sinus to the frontal recess occurs when the continuous bony line that forms the floor of the frontal sinus disappears. For the cell to be pushing into the floor of the frontal sinus, the cell needs to be visualized above this bony line in the floor of the frontal sinus (**Fig. 6.16** and **Fig. 6.17**). Supra agger frontal cells (**Fig. 6.24**, *crosshairs*) are usually found in the lateral aspect of the frontal sinus ostium and push the drainage pathway medially and narrow (obstruct) the drainage pathway of the frontal sinus (**Fig. 6.24**, *pink dot*). The bony beak can be visualized forming the floor of the frontal sinus on the left side of **Fig. 6.25** (*red crosshairs*). These cells will often significantly narrow the frontal sinus outflow (**Fig. 6.24** and **Fig. 6.25**).

Supra Agger Frontal Cells: Small or Large

Small SAFCs pneumatize into the floor of the frontal sinus, whereas large SAFCs pneumatize extensively into the frontal sinus. In example **Fig. 6.26**, a large SAFC is seen to pneumatize into the frontal sinus and therefore narrows the frontal sinus drainage pathway (**Fig. 6.26**). In a recent article[17] we suggested that it is worthwhile to discriminate between very large SAFCs and a small SAFC.[17] Most small SAFCs that push into the floor of the frontal sinus can be removed from below through the frontal ostium. In patients with a narrow anteroposterior frontal ostial dimension, removal of large SAFC may not be possible through a purely transnasal

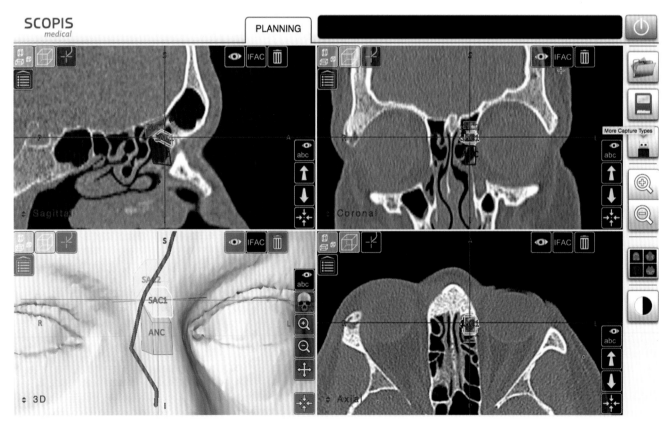

Fig. 6.23 This 3D reconstruction of the frontal recess reflects a combination of an ANC with two supra bulla cells (SAC1 and SAC2) which sit above the ANC and partially obstruct the drainage pathway of the frontal ostium (*pink line/dots*).

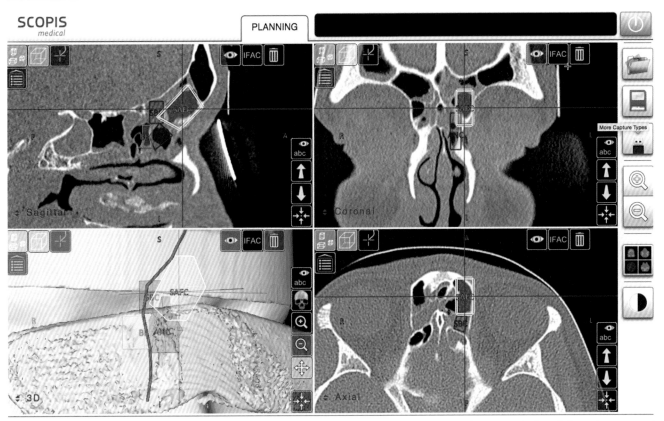

Fig. 6.24 The large SAFC (*crosshairs*) is demonstrated in all three planes. The frontal sinus drainage pathway is pushed medially and compressed between the cell and the skull base (*pink dot* axial CT).

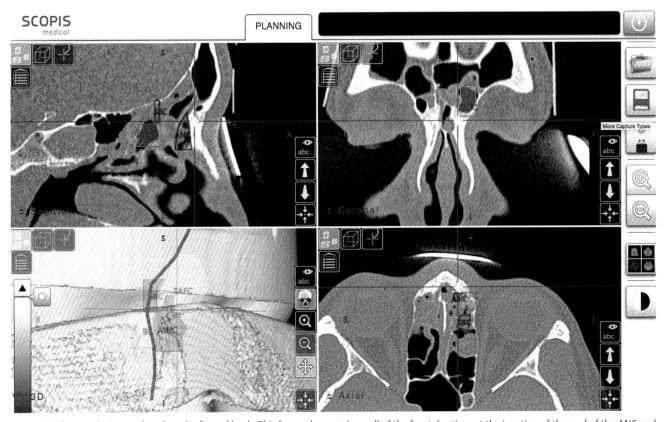

Fig. 6.25 The *crosshairs* are placed on the frontal beak. This forms the anterior wall of the frontal ostium at the junction of the roof of the ANC and SAFC (see parasagittal CT).

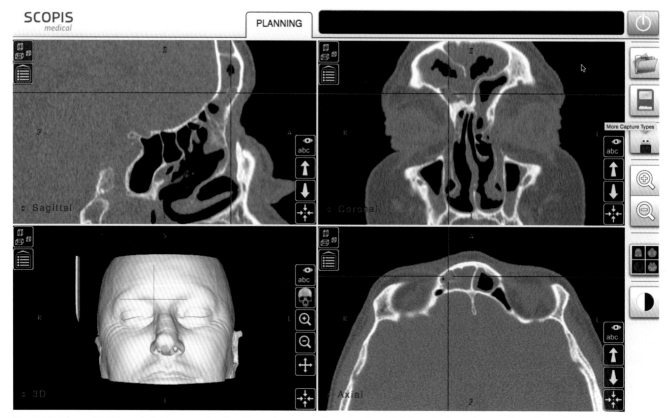

Fig. 6.26 A large SAFC (*crosshairs*) is seen migrating through a narrow frontal ostium high into the frontal sinus. This cell may be difficult to remove completely from below.

endoscopic approach and may well require a frontal drill-out procedure or trans eyebrow frontal trephine for instrument access and subsequent removal of the cell.

Supra Bulla Cells

Supra bulla cells (SBCs) are cells that sit above the bulla ethmoidalis. Often the SBC's anterior face is continuous with that of the bulla ethmoidalis (**Fig. 6.27**) unless there is a

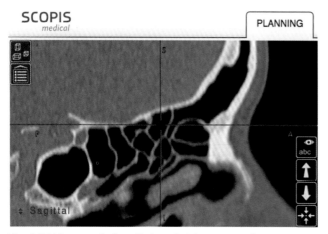

Fig. 6.27 The supra bulla cell's (*crosshairs*) anterior wall is continuous with the anterior face of the bulla ethmoidalis below.

supra bulla recess. A supra bulla recess is space above the bulla ethmoidalis (**Fig. 6.28**) that is continuous with the outflow tract of the frontal sinus and frontal recess. If a medial frontal sinus drainage pathway is followed with the bulla ethmoidalis intact, again the medial wall of the bulla ethmoidalis may not be distinguishable from the medial wall of the SBC. However, SBCs will usually migrate toward the frontal ostium and often play an important part in the obstruction of the frontal ostium. **Fig. 6.29** shows how the anterior face of a large SBC (*crosshairs*) impedes the outflow of the frontal sinus and influences the size and position of the frontal sinus drainage pathway (**Fig. 6.29**).

Supra Bulla Frontal Cells

SBFCs are SBCs that originate in the supra bulla region and because they migrate through the frontal ostium into the frontal sinus become SBFCs. The skull base always forms the roof of these cells and they are seen on the parasagittal to hug the skull base as they migrate into the frontal sinus (**Fig. 6.30**, *crosshairs*). On the axial CT they can be clearly seen on the posterior wall of the frontal sinus. If these cells protrude off the skull base in an anterior manner, they will often appear as an isolated cell in the frontal sinus (**Fig. 6.31**, *crosshairs*). The clinical importance of these cells is that they push the drainage pathway of the frontal sinus anteriorly and to be removed the curette or probe needs to be passed anterior to their wall and the cell wall carefully fractured in a posterior direction.

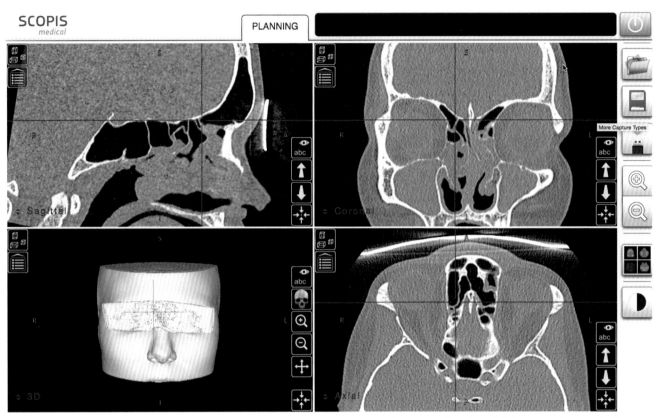

Fig. 6.28 If there is no cell above the bulla ethmoidalis or the cell is small, the space above the bulla ethmoidalis becomes the supra bulla recess (*crosshairs*).

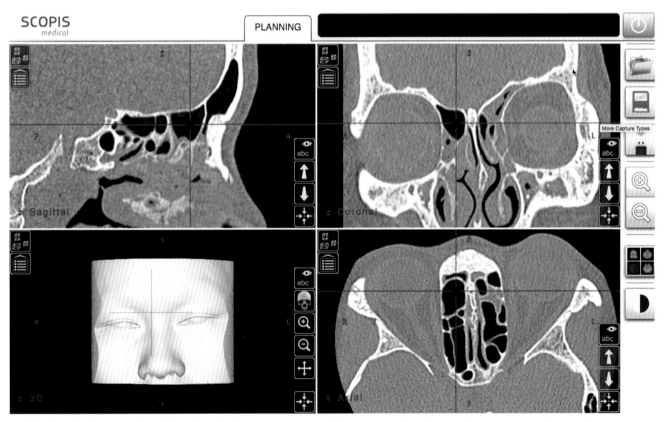

Fig. 6.29 The large supra bulla cell (*crosshairs*) migrates along the skull base into the frontal sinus and encroaches on the frontal sinus drainage pathway, pushing it anteriorly.[17]

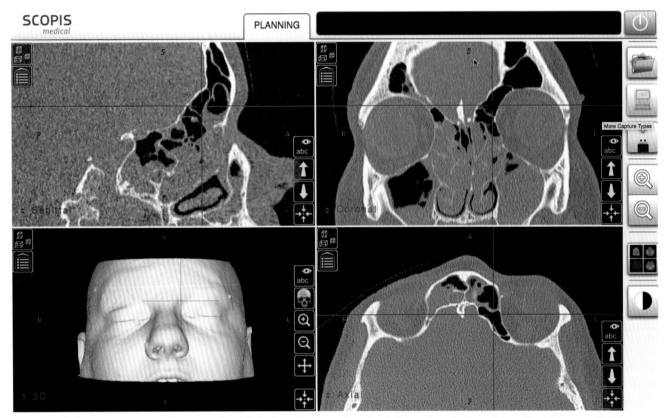

Fig. 6.30 The large SBFC (*crosshairs*) migrates through the frontal ostium along the skull base into the frontal sinus. It pushes up against the supra agger frontal cell and the two cells almost completely obstruct the frontal ostium.

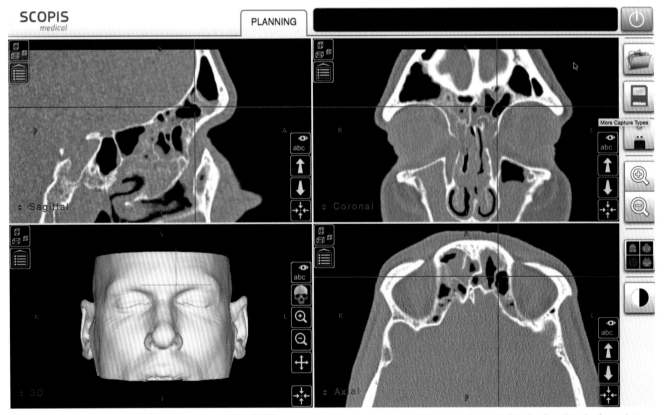

Fig. 6.31 This large SBFC (*crosshairs*) protrudes off the skull base and can appear on a coronal CT scan to be an isolated cell within the frontal sinus. However, when all three planes are visualized, it is quite clear that the cell is a SBFC pneumatizing from the supra bulla region into the frontal sinus.

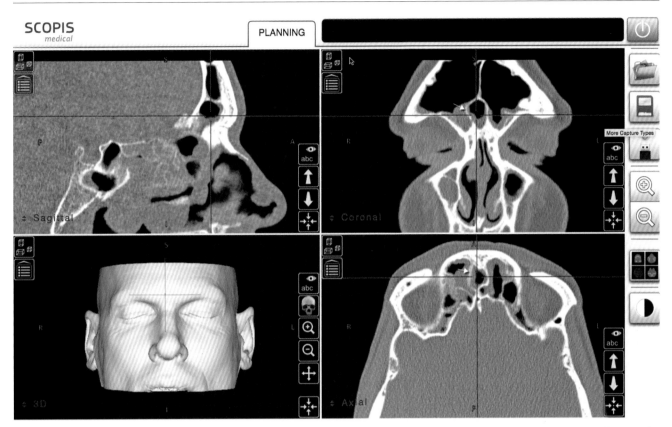

Fig. 6.32 A large frontal septal cell (*crosshairs*) partially obstructs the right frontal drainage pathway and pushes this pathway laterally. Note the thick lateral wall of this cell (*white arrows* in coronal and axial CTs) may not be able to be fractured during surgery.

Frontal Septal Cells

These are cells associated with the intersinus septum of the frontal sinus. This cell pneumatizes from the frontal recess through the frontal ostium and its medial wall is the intersinus septum of the frontal sinus. This cell may vary in size but it always pushes the frontal sinus drainage pathway laterally. If this cell is large it may significantly compromise the drainage of the frontal sinus (**Fig. 6.32**, *crosshairs*) and if the lateral wall of the cell is thick (**Fig. 6.32**, *white arrow*) it may not be possible to fracture this wall, making removal with normal handheld instruments difficult. In these patients we do not advocate drilling this septum as the drill always creates significant mucosal trauma often leading to a scarred or stenosed frontal ostium as healing takes place.

◆ Identifying the Frontal Sinus Drainage Pathways in the Different Anatomical Variations

Cellular Configurations and Associated Drainage Pathways

In the preceding pages the various cellular configurations have been detailed. Although it is vital to determine the number of cells in the frontal recess and their relationship to

the frontal ostium, it is equally important to understand how these cells interact with the drainage pathway of the frontal sinus.[15–18] One of the most difficult tasks is to determine with each cellular variation where the particular drainage pathway is. In the following examples the cellular configuration is first established and then for each configuration the drainage pathway is determined. Once the drainage pathway has been identified, the surgeon can work out where to slide the frontal sinus probe or curette so that the cells can each be removed sequentially, clearing the drainage pathway and exposing the frontal sinus ostium.

Supra Agger Cell Variations

Supra Agger Cell Configuration with a Posterior Drainage Pathway

Once the ANC is identified, the large SAC is seen (**Fig. 6.33**, *crosshairs*). In the coronal plane the frontal sinus drainage pathway is pushed above the SAC and in the axial scan the drainage pathway can be seen to be posterior (*pink dot* indicates pathway). Note how the large SAC contacts the middle turbinate and lamina so that the only possible drainage pathway is posterior (**Fig. 6.33**).

The surgeon should now be able to visualize the anatomy prior to surgery being performed. If the ANC is opened via an axillary flap approach,[20] the roof of the agger nasi will be seen.

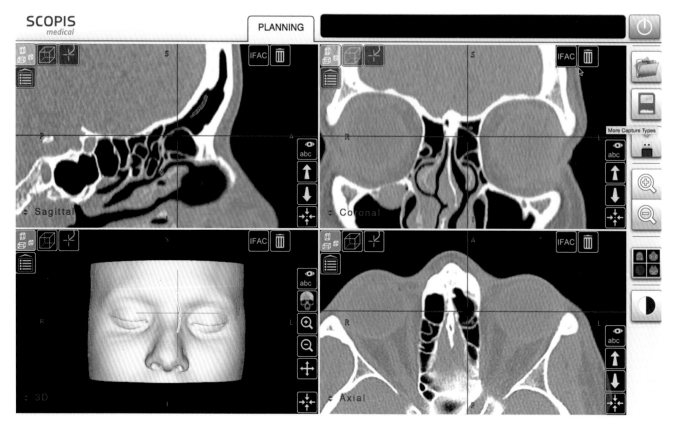

Fig. 6.33 A large SAC (*crosshairs*) completely occupies the anterior region of the frontal recess and pushes the drainage pathway (*pink dots/line*) posteriorly.

The malleable suction curette is placed up the drainage pathway posterior to the roof of the cell. The roof of the agger nasi is removed and the large SAC visualized. The posterior drainage pathway as seen in **Fig. 6.33** should be identified and the suction curette gently slid up the pathway and the roof of the SAC removed with exposure of the frontal ostium. If not clearly visible, the posterior wall of the SAC should be gently manipulated until the drainage pathway of the frontal sinus is clearly identified. This allows safe removal of the cell and exposure of the frontal ostium. Failure to correctly identify the frontal drainage pathway on the CT scan will cause indecision and may result in the probe being placed in the incorrect position and potentially, if force is used, may breach the skull base.

SAC Configuration with a Medial Drainage Pathway

This is one of the more common configurations where the SAC sits directly above the ANC and pushes the drainage pathway of the frontal sinus in a medial direction. This is caused by the upward continuation of the uncinate process forming the medial wall of not only the agger cell but also of the SAC before finally implanting on the lamina papyracea. In this example, the ANC and SAC (**Fig. 6.34**, *crosshairs*) is seen and is identified on the parasagittal CT scan.

The next step is to identify the drainage pathway in this example. The scans are scrolled in the parasagittal plane to establish which scan shows the best example of

the frontal drainage pathway and once that's decided the frontal sinus drainage pathway is drawn on the CT scan (**Fig. 6.34**, *pink dots and lines*). The pathway is viewed by manipulating the slider above the axial CT scan until the best possible route of frontal sinus access is decided and the pathway has been dragged into this pathway. The frontal sinus drainage pathway is best identified by starting high up in the frontal sinus and then by following the drainage pathway by scrolling through the axial CT scans inferiorly. Once this has been done a few times, the frontal sinus drainage pathway can be drawn onto the parasagittal CT scan and then, using the slider (*white arrow*) in the axial CT scan, can be followed inferiorly into the frontal recess (**Fig. 6.35**). The pathway can be manipulated by using the hand to grab the pathway in any of the slices in the CT scan and pull it into the correct position. It is best adjusted in sequential axial CTs but can also be adjusted on the coronal and parasagittal scans.

SAC with an Anterior Drainage Pathway

If the SAC expands so that it touches the supra bulla cell and the frontal process of the maxilla in the lateral region, it will push the drainage pathway of the frontal sinus anteromedially. This SAC configuration is illustrated by the following example on the right side (*pink dot* on **Fig. 6.36**). The SAC is identified by the crosshairs. The patient also has a very large

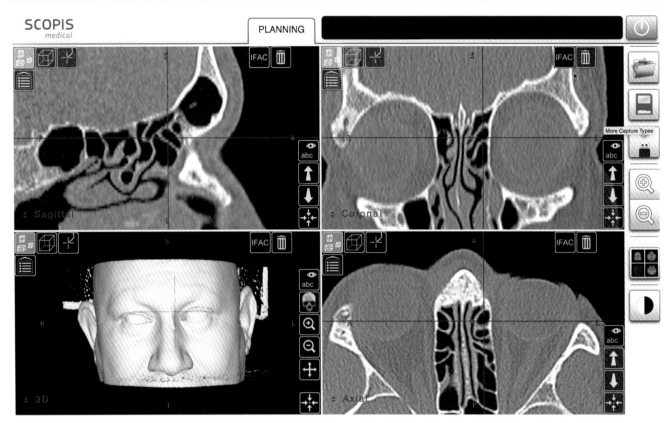

Fig. 6.34 The SAC (*crosshairs*) pushes the drainage pathway medially. This is the most common configuration within the frontal recess.

SBFC (*white arrow*) pushing anteriorly into the frontal sinus, which contributes to the drainage pathway being pushed anteriorly.

It is important to be able to pick the drainage pathway of the frontal sinus around these cells. In this patient the frontal sinus drains anteriorly adjacent to the SAC and anterior to the SBFC (**Fig. 6.36**). Again, if we follow the drainage pathway of the frontal sinus from the frontal sinus inferiorly into the

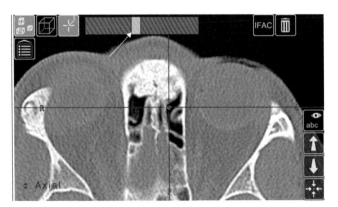

Fig. 6.35 In this axial CT the frontal drainage pathway is indicated by a *pink circle*. The slider (*white arrow*) is slid up and down while the axial CT scans are examined to ensure that the drainage pathway is correctly placed. The cursor can be passed over the pathway at any stage and changes to a hand by which the pathway can be grabbed and manipulated into position.

frontal recess on the axial CT scans, the relationship between the pathway and the SAC is clearly seen (**Fig. 6.36**).

To add a clinical perspective, the following intraoperative pictures of this example are shown (**Fig. 6.37** and **Fig. 6.38**). In **Fig. 6.37a**, the SAC is seen (*white arrow*) with a tight anterior pathway (*black arrow*). In **Fig. 6.37b**, the SAC (*white arrow*) is opened and the SBFC (*orange arrow*) is identified. The tight anterior frontal drainage pathway is still seen (*black arrow*). In **Fig. 6.38a**, the SAC has been removed and the SBFC (*white arrow*) opened with the further opening of the anterior drainage pathway (*black arrow*). In **Fig. 6.38b**, the anterior face of the SBFC (*white arrow*) has been partially removed to expose the frontal sinus (*black arrow*). The surgeon should be able to visualize the configuration of the frontal recess cells and drainage pathway and should be able to picture this in their mind before surgery is commenced. When the surgeon looks up into the frontal recess, the SAC should be seen anteriorly with the drainage pathway anteromedially.

Once the ANC is removed and the SAC identified, the surgeon should know where to look for the frontal sinus drainage pathway. In this patient if attempts were made to push probes posterior to the cell, injury and penetration of the skull base would be possible. However, if the pathway is recognized, a small probe can be slid up between the SAC and the medial wall of the olfactory fossa and the cell fractured laterally thereby clearing the frontal recess. Review the Chapter 6 tutorials and videos to see how this configuration was dissected and how it compares to your mental 3D reconstruction of the anatomy.

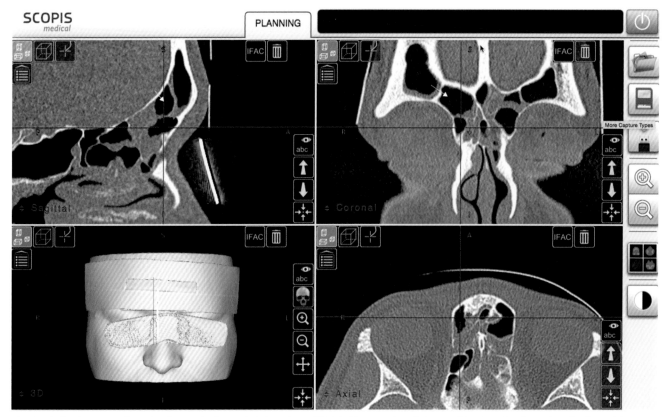

Fig. 6.36 The large SAC (*crosshairs*) is pushed anteriorly by a large SBFC (*white arrow*) and the combination of cells pushes the frontal drainage pathway anteriorly up against the frontal beak (*pink dot*).

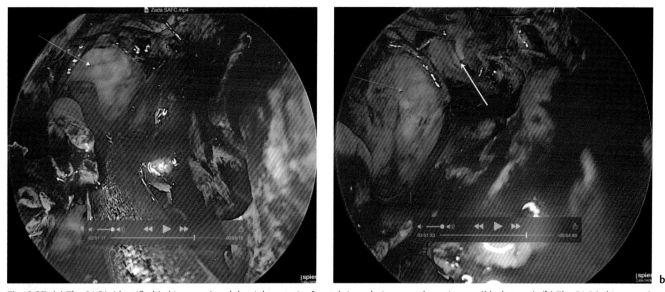

Fig. 6.37 (**a**) The SAC is identified (*white arrow*) and the tight anterior frontal sinus drainage pathway is seen (*black arrow*). (**b**) The SAC (*white arrow*) is partially removed exposing the SBFC (*orange arrow*) with the tight anterior frontal drainage pathway indicated by the *black arrow*.

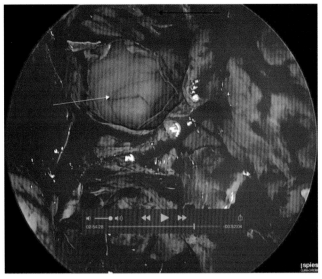 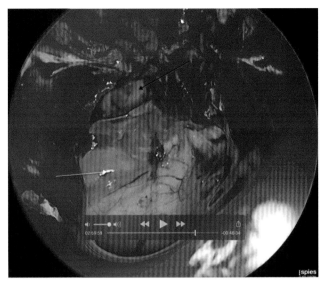

a   b

Fig. 6.38 (**a**) The SAC has been removed and the SBFC (*white arrow*) further exposed. The tight anterior frontal drainage pathway is indicated by the *black arrow*. (**b**) The anterior wall of the SBFC (*white arrow*) has been partially removed to show the frontal sinus (*black arrow*).

SAC with a Lateral Drainage Pathway

If an SAC abuts the insertion of the middle turbinate as it inserts to the skull base, the frontal sinus drainage pathway may be pushed laterally. This is relatively uncommon but is important to recognize when it occurs. It is more common for a medially based cell to be situated much higher and for it to be in contact with the frontal sinus septum and is termed a frontal septal cell (see below). Recognition of an SAC situated medially in the frontal recess will allow the frontal sinus drainage pathway to be sought laterally and allow this cell to be safely removed and the frontal ostium to be fully exposed. The following example shows the medially placed SAC (*crosshairs*) with the lateral drainage pathway (*pink dot/lines*) (**Fig. 6.39**).

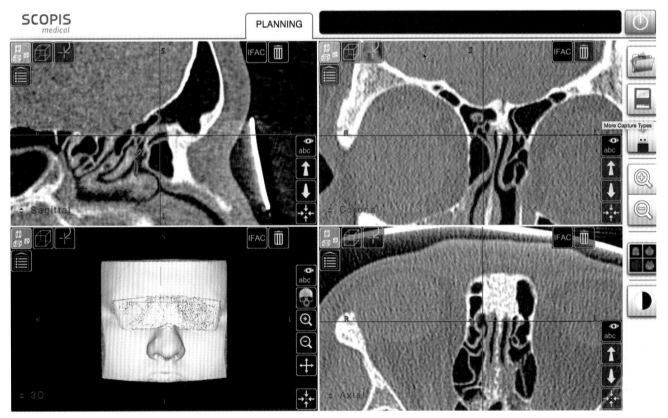

Fig. 6.39 In this example, a medially based SAC (*crosshairs*) pushes the frontal sinus drainage pathway laterally (*pink dots* on coronal and axial scans).

Although the axial CT scans are the primary scan we use to follow the frontal sinus drainage pathway, it is also important to view the coronal and parasagittal CT scans. In this example the frontal drainage pathway can be clearly seen in the coronal CTs as well as the axials.

If the surgeon had a clear 3D picture of the anatomy, then he or she would be able to visualize the SAC in the medial region of the frontal recess and the frontal sinus drainage pathway draining lateral to it. Make sure that your intraoperative visualization corresponds to how you thought the frontal recess would look prior to doing the surgery and if not redo the planning on the scans until the planning and clinical pictures correlate. In **Fig. 6.40a,b** the clinical image that the surgeon should imagine when looking at the CT scans is displayed. In **Fig. 6.40a** the ANC is opened and the roof of the agger identified (*white arrow*). In **Fig. 6.40b** the medial supra agger cell is seen (*black arrow*) and the lateral drainage pathway identified (*white arrow*). The drainage pathway (*white arrow*) is further opened in **Fig. 6.40c** to clearly illustrate the lateral drainage pathway. This clinical correlation to the CT scan is important and as each case is planned so should how each frontal recess will look at the time of surgery be imagined.

Supra Agger Frontal Cell Variations

SAFC with a Medial Drainage Pathway

In most cases, an SAFC will enter the frontal ostium laterally, pushing the frontal sinus drainage pathway medially (**Fig. 6.41**). In this example on the left side the SAFC occupies most of the frontal ostium as it pushes through the ostium into the floor of the frontal sinus. In this case the ANC then the SAFC are identified, followed by two SBCs and a large bulla ethmoidalis (**Fig. 6.42**). The SAFC is large and pushes backward onto the anterior wall of the SBC.

The drainage pathway of the frontal sinus (*white arrow*) is seen to run anteromedial to these cells. This is best appreciated in the axial CT scans and drawings. If we look at the intraoperative images taken from the dissection, we can correlate this complex anatomy with what was seen during surgery (**Fig. 6.43**).

In some patients with very large SAFCs, only the medial wall that occupies the frontal ostium may need to be removed and the roof of the cell may be left if this no longer obstructs the frontal sinus drainage pathway. This is usually only done if there is technical difficulty in reaching the

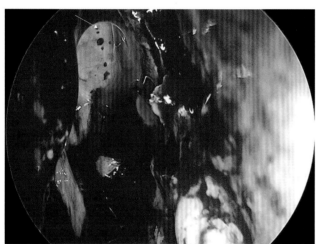

a

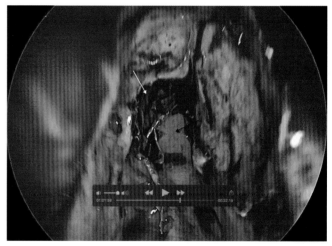

b

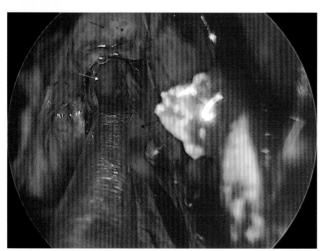

c

Fig. 6.40 (**a–c**) Intraoperative pictures display the cells seen on the CT scan in **Fig. 6.39**. (**a**) The ANC is opened and the roof of the ANC seen (*white arrow*). (**b**) The medial SAC is indicated with the *black arrow* and the frontal sinus drainage pathway is indicated with the *white arrow*. (**c**) The roof of the ANC has been further resected displaying the laterally based frontal sinus drainage pathway (*white arrow*).

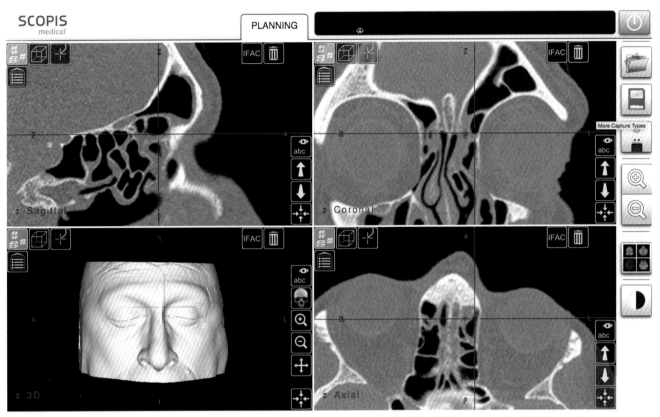

Fig. 6.41 A large SAFC (*crosshairs*) pushes the frontal sinus drainage pathway anteromedially (*pink dots* on coronal and axial scans).

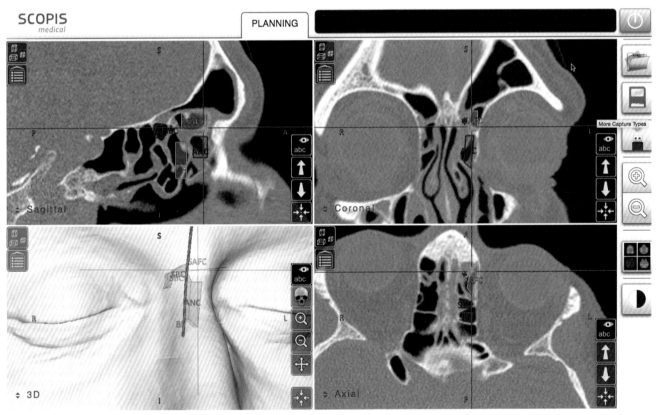

Fig. 6.42 To plan the surgery a full 3D reconstruction of the anatomy in **Fig. 6.41** is presented with building blocks placed over all the cells. Note how the SAFC pushes posteriorly within the frontal recess (coronal scan) and again how the drainage pathway is pushed anteromedially (*pink dot*).

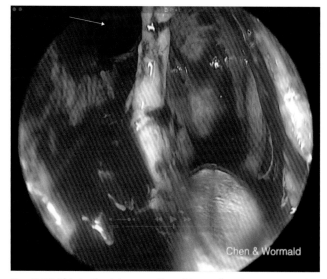

Fig. 6.43 This is the intraoperative picture of patient presented in **Fig. 6.41** and **Fig. 6.42** illustrating the large SAFC (instrument tip in cell) and the anteromedial frontal drainage pathway (*white arrow*).

roof or dome of the cell or if the roof is too thick to fracture easily with a probe or a curette. A large SAFC is a cell that usually enters the frontal sinus along the lateral wall of the frontal ostium pushing the drainage pathway medially. However, in the coronal plane, it can be seen that the

cell extends significantly into the frontal sinus on the scan (**Fig. 6.44**, *crosshairs*). The decision as to whether it would be possible to remove this is based on the anteroposterior dimension of the frontal ostium best evaluated on the parasagittal scan. In this case the frontal ostium is widely patent and the SAFC was able to be removed from below. If this is not felt to be the case then a modified Lothrop/frontal drill-out is performed for access and in all cases this provides more than adequate access to be able to remove large SAFCs.

SAFC with a Posterior Drainage Pathway

This situation occurs when a SAFC (*crosshairs*) pneumatizes through the frontal ostium and occupies the entire anterior region of the frontal ostium pushing the frontal sinus drainage pathway posteriorly (**Fig. 6.45**, *pink dot and lines*). In some instances this pathway can be very narrow and there may be significant risk when trying to manipulate a probe or curette through this narrow space due to the proximity of the skull base. In most patients this portion of the skull base (fovea ethmoidalis) is quite thick and there should be resistance to penetration. This should be checked on the CT scan prior to the probe being placed. Once the 3D picture has been created, the drainage pathway of the frontal sinus around these cells needs to be established. In the example (**Fig. 6.46**), the SAFC (*black arrow*) can be

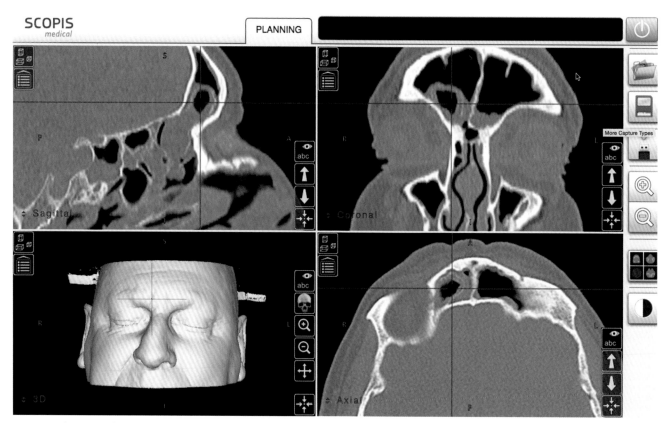

Fig. 6.44 This patient has a very large SAFC which extends significantly into the frontal sinus (*crosshairs*). The decision as to whether this can be removed endoscopically is largely based on the anteroposterior dimensions of the frontal ostium.

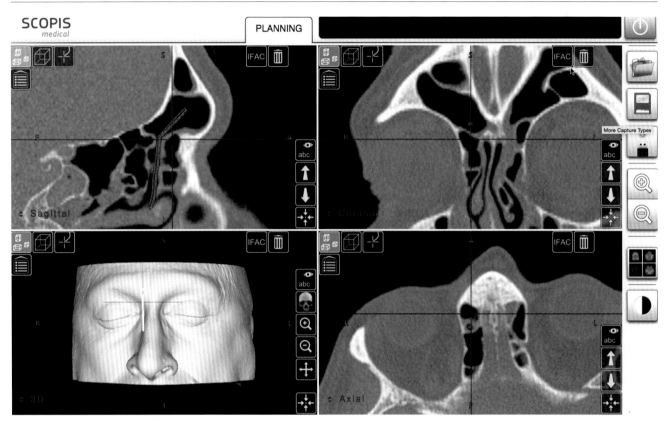

Fig. 6.45 This patient has a SAFC (*crosshairs*) that occupies the entire anterior portion of the frontal ostium and pushes the frontal sinus drainage pathway posteriorly (*pink dot/line*).

seen occupying most of the frontal ostium and pushing the drainage pathway (*white arrow*) of the frontal sinus posteriorly. Again, this picture should be able to be visualized at the time of viewing the CT scan and planning the anatomy and the surgery.

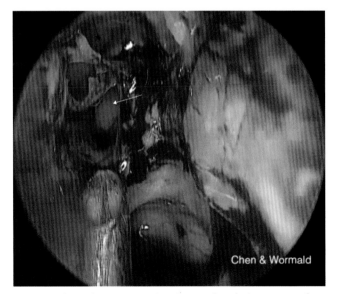

Fig. 6.46 This is the intraoperative picture taken during surgery of patient in **Fig. 6.45**. Note the anteriorly based SAFC with the posterior frontal sinus drainage pathway (*white arrow*).

SAFC, SBFC, and Frontal Septal Cell with an Anterior Drainage Pathway

If the SAFC is large and fills the frontal ostium it will push the drainage pathway medially, posteriorly, or anteriorly. The direction it pushes the drainage pathway is primarily dependent upon where the cell is based (anteriorly, laterally, or posteriorly) and what other cells are present in the frontal ostium/recess. If, for example, a frontal septal cell (FSC) is present, this will further narrow the frontal sinus drainage pathway and this cell will tend to push the pathway laterally. In such a case the pathway will be squeezed between these two cells. If there is also an SBFC this results in a very tight frontal sinus outflow tract. An example of this anatomical variation is presented in **Fig. 6.47**. The SAFC (*crosshairs*) extends significantly through the frontal ostium, and pushes the drainage pathway anteriorly (*pink dots*) so that it is squeezed between the SAFC and the FSC (*white arrow*). The large SBFC (*black arrow*) extends above the SAFC and additionally squeezes the pathway between itself and the other cells. If a building block is placed for each of these cells seen and for the bulla ethmoidalis and supra bulla cell, a 3D picture of this complex cellular configuration is established (**Fig. 6.48**). In order to work out the frontal sinus drainage pathway, the axial scans are viewed from cranial to caudal. As the frontal sinus is followed into the frontal recess its pathway is initially pushed anteriorly by the SAFC and laterally but the FSC then as the pathway reaches the SBFC, it is squeezed against the frontal beak. In **Fig. 6.49**, a frontal sinus

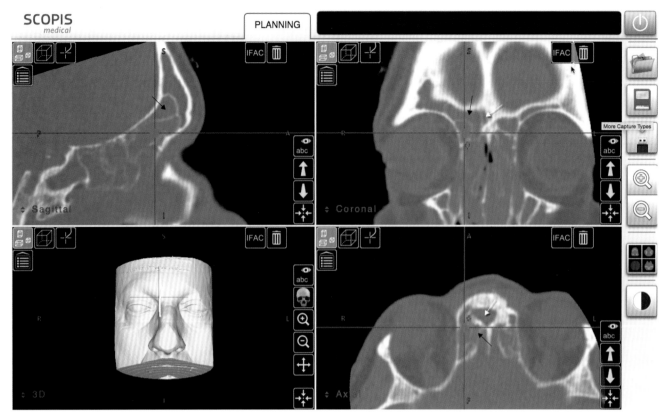

Fig. 6.47 This patient has extensive sinus disease with a large SAFC (*crosshairs*), a large SBFC (*black arrow*), and an FSC (*white arrow*) all combining to obstructing the frontal sinus drainage pathway (*pink dot*). Note how the FSC pushes the drainage pathway lateral and squeezes it between it and the SAFC. The SBFC occupies the posterior aspect of the frontal ostium (*black arrow*).

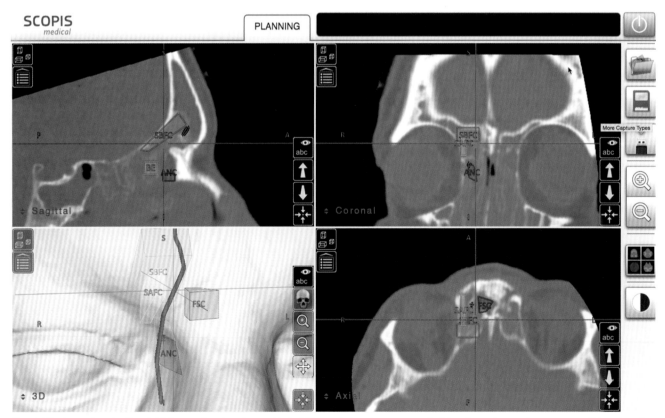

Fig. 6.48 The patient in **Fig. 6.47** has a planning done with building blocks placed for all cells illustrating the 3D configuration of the anatomy of this very difficult frontal recess. This aids with the surgery and helps the surgeon decide where the suction curette will be placed to allow each cell to be fractured and removed from the frontal ostium.

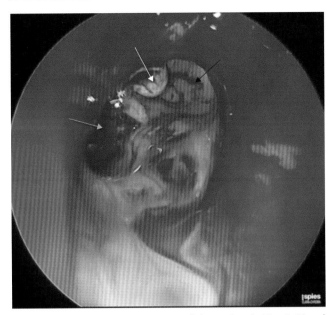

Fig. 6.49 This intraoperative picture of the patient in **Fig. 6.47** and **Fig. 6.48** shows the FSC (*black arrow*) and the SAFC (*green arrow*) with fluorescein having been placed into the frontal sinus through a frontal sinus mini-trephine and draining through the frontal sinus drainage pathway (*white arrow* indicates opening of pathway).

mini-trephine has been placed and fluorescein can be seen draining through the anteriorly based frontal drainage pathway (*white arrow*) with the medial FSC (*black arrow*) and the SAFC (*green arrow*) seen at the frontal ostium (**Fig. 6.49**). This allows the surgeon to decide exactly where the probe or curette should be placed so that it can be slid up the drainage pathway and the cells that are obstructing the frontal ostium can be removed.

Supra Bulla Frontal Cell with Anterior Drainage Pathway

This cell has been commonly confused with the type 4 cell of the original Kuhn classification in which a type 4 cell was defined as an isolated cell within the frontal sinus. In **Fig. 6.50**, the SBFC appears to be an isolated cell in the frontal sinus (*crosshairs*). However, when this cell is followed posteriorly and viewed on the parasagittal scan, it is quite clear that this is a frontal bulla cell that originated in the suprabullar space and pneumatizes forward along the skull base into the frontal sinus.

The frontal sinus drainage pathway can be followed from the frontal sinus into the frontal recess and is pushed anteriorly by the SBFC. Note the FSC which also impacts on the drainage pathway by pushing it laterally (*white arrow*).

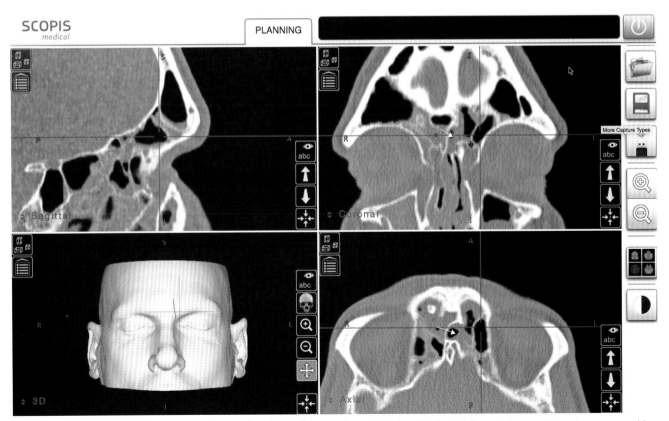

Fig. 6.50 This patient has what appears to be an isolated frontal sinus cell on the coronal scan (*crosshairs*) but when the other scans are viewed it is obvious that this is a large SBFC projecting anteriorly off the skull base. Note how the frontal sinus drainage pathway is compressed between the SBFC and the FSC (*pink dot*).

◆ Conclusion

The anatomy and common variations that occur in the frontal recess are poorly understood by a large number of endoscopic sinus surgeons. The ANC is proposed as the key to the understanding this complex area. Fine cut coronal and parasagittal reconstructed CT scans aid the identification of each individual cell and allow the surgeon to formulate a clear and precise surgical plan. Axial scans are useful for the identification of the frontal sinus drainage pathway. New software allows each cell to be visualized in all three planes simultaneously and with some software programs the building blocks can be placed directly onto the cells creating the 3D picture of the anatomy of the frontal recess. In addition, in this software, the frontal sinus drainage pathway can be drawn onto the CT scans and the pathway reviewed in all three planes as well as allowing the pathway to be adjusted so that the correct pathway is identified. Before surgery is performed in the frontal recess, the surgeon needs to fully review all the CT scans in the three planes and assume that they are in a surgical simulator. The surgeon should be able to mentally create an image of the cellular structure in the frontal recess with frontal sinus drainage pathway in this 3D picture. The surgeon should then go through the surgical steps to be performed. For example: create an axillary flap, raise the flap, remove the anterior wall of the ANC, place the suction curette medial or behind the ANC, and remove this cell (medial wall and roof). Identify the residual cells and the frontal sinus drainage pathway around these cells. Place the suction curette along the frontal sinus drainage pathway without force and fracture the cell and remove the cell(s) exposing the frontal ostium. Such a surgical plan formulated from a thorough understanding of the anatomy allows a confident dissection of a complex and difficult area.

Videos

There are a large number of videos accompanying this book illustrating all of the variations described above. All of these videos start with series of CT scans. Please review the CT scans carefully and try to build a mental picture of the anatomy of the frontal recess before watching the video. Repeat this often until the CT scans can be accurately correlated to the anatomy seen in the surgery.

References

1. Kaliner MA, Osguthorpe JD, Fireman P, et al. Sinusitis: bench to bedside. Current findings, future directions. J Allergy Clin Immunol 1997;99 (6 Pt 3):S829–S848
2. Davis WE, Templer J, Parsons DS. Anatomy of the paranasal sinuses. Otolaryngol Clin North Am 1996;29(1):57–74
3. Schaefer SD, Manning S, Close LG. Endoscopic paranasal sinus surgery: indications and considerations. Laryngoscope 1989;99(1):1–5
4. Kennedy DW, Senior BA. Endoscopic sinus surgery. A review. Otolaryngol Clin North Am 1997;30(3):313–330
5. Stammberger HR, Kennedy DW; Anatomic Terminology Group. Paranasal sinuses: anatomic terminology and nomenclature. Ann Otol Rhinol Laryngol Suppl 1995;167(supplement 167):7–16
6. Thawley SE, Deddens AE. Transfrontal Endoscopic Management of Frontal Recess Disease. Am J Rhinol 1995;9(6):307–311
7. Keros P. Über die praktische Bedeutung der Niveauunterschiede de Lamina cribrosa des Ethmoids. Laryngol Rhinol Otol (Stuttg) 1965;41: 808–813
8. Stammberger H, Hawke M, eds. Functional Endoscopic Sinus Surgery - The Messerklinger Technique. Chapter Special Endoscopic Anatomy. Philadelphia, PA: B.C. Decker Publishers; 1991:61–90
9. Floreani SR, Nair SB, Switajewski MC, Wormald PJ. Endoscopic anterior ethmoidal artery ligation: a cadaver study. Laryngoscope 2006;116: 1263–1267
10. Wormald PJ. The agger nasi cell: the key to understanding the anatomy of the frontal recess. Otolaryngol Head Neck Surg 2003;129(5): 497–507
11. Kew J, Rees G, Close D, Sdralis T, Sebben R, Wormald PJ. Multiplanar reconstructed CT images improves depiction and understanding of the anatomy of the frontal sinus and recess. Am J Rhinol 2002;16(2): 119–123
12. Bolger WE, Butzin CA, Parsons DS. Paranasal sinus bony anatomic variations and mucosal abnormalities: CT analysis for endoscopic sinus surgery. Laryngoscope 1991;101(1 Pt 1):56–64
13. Wake M, Takeno S, Hawke M. The uncinate process: a histological and morphological study. Laryngoscope 1994;104(3 Pt 1):364–369
14. Kuhn FA. Chronic frontal sinusitis: the endoscopic frontal recess approach. Operative techniques. Otolaryngol Head Neck Surg 1996;7(3): 222–229
15. Wormald PJ, Hoseman W, Callejas C, et al. The International Frontal Sinus Anatomy Classification (IFAC) and Classification of the Extent of Endoscopic Frontal Sinus Surgery (EFSS). Int Forum Allergy Rhinol 2016;6(7):677–696
16. Wormald PJ. Three Dimensional building block approach to understanding the anatomy of the frontal recess and frontal sinus. Op Tech in OL&HNS 2006;17(1):2–5
17. Wormald PJ. Surgery of the frontal recess and frontal sinus. Rhinology 2005;43(2):82–85
18. Kim KS, Kim HU, Chung IH, Lee JG, Park IY, Yoon JH. Surgical anatomy of the nasofrontal duct: anatomical and computed tomographic analysis. Laryngoscope 2001;111(4 Pt 1):603–608
19. Wormald PJ. The axillary flap approach to the frontal recess. Laryngoscope 2002;112(3):494–499
20. Wormald PJ, Chan SZX. Surgical techniques for the removal of frontal recess cells obstructing the frontal ostium. Am J Rhinol 2003;17(4): 221–226

7 Surgical Approach to the Frontal Sinus and Frontal Recess

◆ Introduction

The frontal recess has always been considered to be the most difficult area to dissect.[1–4] This is largely due to its location behind the beak of the frontal bone.[5] There are three major philosophies regarding the management of disease of the frontal recess and sinus. The minimal invasive sinus technique, or MIST, advocates management of the maxillary sinus and associated transitional spaces (hiatus semilunaris and ethmoidal infundibulum) without performing surgery in the frontal recess.[6–8] This philosophy states that treatment of the maxillary sinus and associated transitional spaces will result in clearance of the frontal recess and sinus disease. There are few published papers supporting this theory and all publications come from the same group of investigators.[6–8] Until there is substantial evidence that this approach works for a broad spectrum of frontal sinus and frontal recess disease, we do not advocate this approach. The second philosophy is that the frontal recess and frontal sinus should only be operated upon if there are symptoms that can be directly ascribed to the frontal sinus such as frontal headache and pain. Although we agree that surgery on a diseased frontal sinus or recess that is symptomatic is appropriate, we disagree that this is the only indication for surgery in this region. Patients who present with nasal obstruction, postnasal drip, purulent rhinorrhea, and anosmia and who have radiologic disease in the frontal sinus or recess need to have this region surgically addressed. These patients have their diseased maxillary sinuses, ethmoid, and sphenoid sinuses addressed and it makes no sense that just because they do not have localized frontal pain or tenderness, that the frontal sinus should not be addressed as well. It has been well recognized that retained or residual cells in the frontal recess/sinus is one of the most common causes of endoscopic sinus surgery failure.[1,2]

In this chapter we present our graduated approach to surgery of the frontal recess and sinus. In the easy frontal recess and sinus, simple maneuvers in terms of endoscopy and surgical access (axillary flap) are advocated and are, in most cases, sufficient to allow clearance of the frontal recess and frontal ostium. In the difficult frontal recess or sinus, the additional technique of frontal sinus mini-trephination is presented. These difficult patients may also benefit from the surgeon having computer-aided surgical navigation available.

The mainstay of our surgical technique is the axillary flap technique. This technique has similarities to the frontal sinus rescue procedure described by Kuhn et al[9] in that mucosal flaps are raised during the surgery on the frontal ostium. However, the major difference is that the frontal sinus rescue procedure is designed for the management of patients who have failed previous standard endoscopic sinus surgery and have a stenosed frontal ostium. The axillary flap technique is designed for all patients undergoing frontal recess or sinus procedures, including previously operated patients. The central concept of the axillary flap procedure is removal of the anterior wall of the agger nasi cell. This is not new and was described by May and Schaitken[10] as part of their nasofrontal approach (NFA I) to the frontal sinus. Schaefer and Close[11] have advocated a similar approach with removal of the bone above the insertion of the middle turbinate. The major difference between these approaches and the axillary flap approach is the elevation of a mucosal flap that can be replaced at the end of the procedure to cover the raw exposed bone that is seen after removal of the anterior wall of the agger nasi cell. This prevents granulation tissue from forming over the exposed bone with subsequent scarring and cicatrization of this area. Such scarring can pull the upper extension of the middle turbinate laterally and close off the anterior aspect of the frontal recess. This may in turn lead to blockage of the frontal outflow tract and result in recurrent frontal sinusitis.

May and Schaitkin advocated enlarging the frontal ostium in their NFA II and III approaches.[10] This is unnecessary and not advocated in the vast majority of patients as the removal of residual cells within the frontal recess with the exposure of the frontal ostium is usually sufficient to achieve resolution of frontal sinusitis. It is our philosophy that where patients have cells in the frontal recess or frontal ostium that obstruct the outflow of the frontal sinus, these should be removed without enlarging the frontal ostium. Even very small frontal ostia can function well if their outflow pathway is not obstructed and the patient should be given the opportunity to see if the natural size of their frontal ostium is sufficient. In some patients, especially those with severe mucosal disease, this ostium may become edematous and obstruct; if this causes symptoms, then enlargement of the ostium is indicated. However, this occurs in the minority of cases and it's not possible to predict which patients with a particular frontal ostium size will obstruct and become symptomatic. In most patients, the only way to enlarge a frontal ostium is with a drill. Drilling in the frontal ostium without creation of the largest possible ostium is likely to result in an intense fibrous reaction from the exposed raw bone and in most cases will increase the likelihood of postoperative scarring and stenosis. As can be seen in Chapter 9, enlargement of the frontal ostium is usually done with a frontal drillout, modified Lothrop procedure/Draf 3, and very rarely with a Draf type 2 (unilateral enlargement of the frontal ostium) procedure, due to the increased incidence of fibrosis and stenosis seen with unilateral drilling on the frontal ostium.[12] This is especially true for patients who have severe mucosal disease and in whom the inflammatory process continues in the postoperative period.[13]

◆ Patients Suitable for Frontal Recess and Frontal Sinus Surgery

Our philosophy is that a patient who has undergone appropriate medical therapy (including systemic steroids) and is then found to have mucosal thickening in the frontal recess or sinus, should have all cells cleared from the frontal recess and frontal ostium exposed (**Fig. 7.1**).[13–16] In patients without significant disease of the frontal recess (**Fig. 7.1**), only the diseased sinuses are addressed and the frontal recess is left untouched. Partial surgery of the frontal recess is never indicated. If only the roof of the agger nasi cell is removed or one of the frontal ethmoidal cells is removed, scarring is likely to result. The cells in the frontal recess are usually in close approximation and partial clearance of cells will very likely result in adhesions forming between these closely approximated surfaces with obstruction of the drainage pathway of the frontal sinus. Our philosophy is an all or nothing approach. The frontal recess is either left entirely alone or all the cells are removed from the recess with visualization of the frontal ostium.

◆ Assessing the Frontal Recess and Frontal Sinus Prior to Surgery

In a patient who is to undergo frontal recess clearance and sinus surgery, the computed tomography (CT) scans need to be carefully assessed and the three-dimensional (3D) reconstruction of the anatomy performed (see Chapter 6). Once the surgeon has a clear understanding of the anatomy, a surgical plan should be formulated. An example of such a plan is presented in **Fig. 7.2**. The Scopis planning software is used to scroll through the CT scans, first looking at the coronal CT scans, then scrolling from lateral to medial through the parasagittal scans. This should give the surgeon an idea of the size, number, and position of cells within the left frontal sinus (see **Fig. 7.2a**). The software can be used to place building blocks over the cells and to draw the frontal sinus drainage pathway on the CT scans (see **Fig. 7.2b**). The frontal drainage pathway is now reviewed by using the slider on the

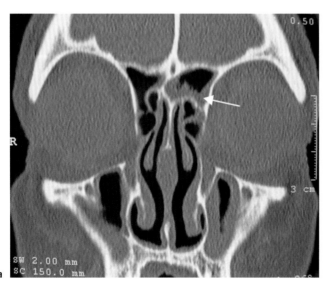
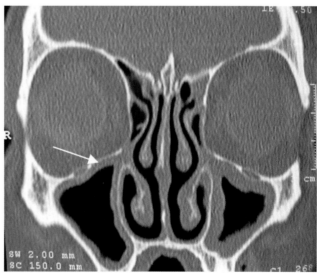

Fig. 7.1 (**a**) In coronal computed tomography, note the mucosal thickening in the left frontal sinus (*white arrow*) and recess with a normal right frontal sinus and recess. (**b**) In coronal computed tomography, note the mucosal thickening of the right maxillary sinus (*white arrow*). In this patient, the left frontal recess would be cleared of cells and the frontal ostium identified, whereas on the right side no surgery would be performed in the frontal recess. Both maxillary sinuses would be surgically addressed.

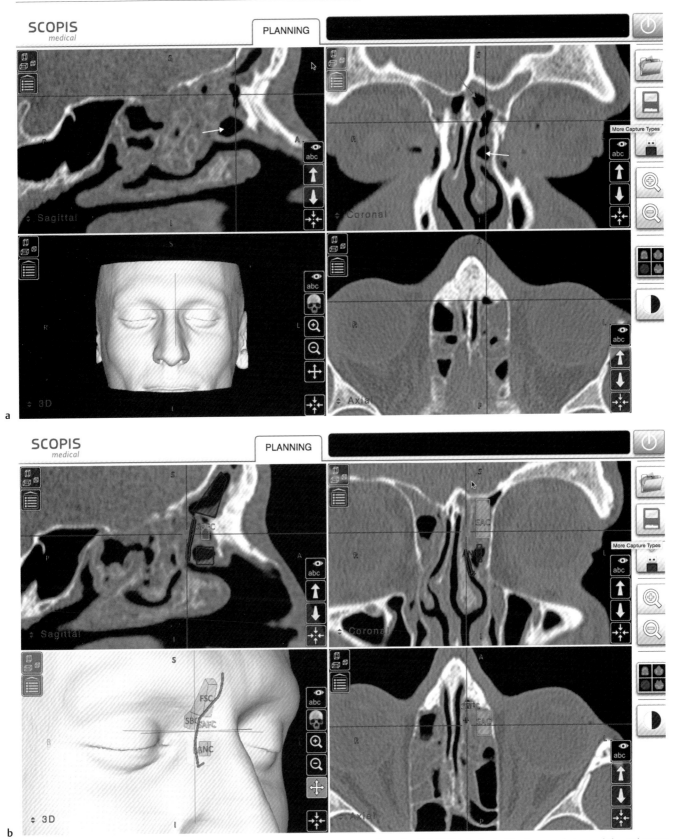

Fig. 7.2 (**a**) The agger nasi cell is indicated with a *white arrow*, the supra agger frontal cell (SAFC) is indicated by the *crosshairs*, and the *red arrow* indicates the frontal septal cell. (**b**) The building blocks have been placed over the cells. Note the green supra agger cell is posterior and inferior to the yellow SAFC which sits tight up against the frontal beak. The frontal septal cell is large and influences the drainage pathway in the frontal sinus but at the level of the crosshairs the drainage pathway (*pink circle*, axial scan) is medial to the supra agger cell and posterior to the SAFC. (*continued*)

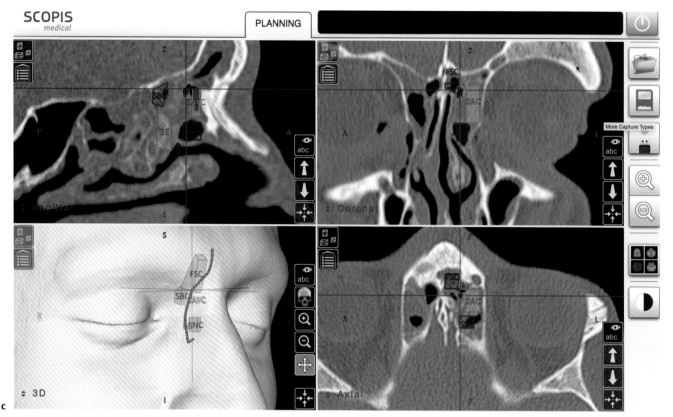

c

Fig. 7.2 (*continued*) (**c**) The influence of the FSC is seen pushing the drainage pathway (*crosshairs*) laterally but still posterior to the SAFC and medial to the SAC. This complex anatomy can now be understood and a surgical plan developed.

axial CT scan to scroll through the axial CTs from top to bottom starting in the frontal sinus and then moving progressively through the frontal ostium and frontal recess. If the frontal drainage pathway is not correctly positioned, then the pathway is simply grabbed with the cursor and repositioned on the CT scan until it is correctly positioned. Now a surgical plan can be made for this patient before surgery is actually performed. In this patient, after uncinectomy and middle meatal antrostomy, an axillary flap is performed to expose the anterior face of the agger nasi cell. This is removed with the Hajek Koeffler punch (Storz) and the agger nasi cell visualized. The malleable frontal sinus curette* (Integra) is placed posteromedially to the agger nasi cell's posterior wall and roof, and the cell removed by fracturing it forward. The resultant debris is removed with a microdebrider. The residual roof of the agger nasi cell (ANC) is cleared and the supra agger frontal cell (SAFC) and supra agger cell (SAC) are visualized. The SAFC is a small cell that will be sitting tight up against the anterior wall of the frontal beak whereas the SAC is a larger more posteriorly based cell sitting above the ANC. After careful assessment of the axial scans, we know that the frontal sinus drains medially around this cell and the suction curette is slid along this drainage pathway into the frontal sinus and the cell fractured laterally and removed. An angled microdebrider blade is used to clear debris, and small residual bony fragments are cleared with giraffe forceps and the malleable frontal sinus hooked probe* (Integra). The frontal ostium is visualized but all mucosa around the frontal ostium is preserved.

Identifying the Easy from the Difficult Frontal Recess and Sinus

Surgeons should recognize potentially difficult frontal recesses by studying the CT scans at the time the patient is listed for surgery.[13-16] Recognition of potential difficulties can aid the surgeon when discussing the likelihood of success of the procedure and the probable need for further surgery such as enlargement of a very narrow frontal ostium. In addition, the likelihood of possible ancillary procedures, such as a mini-trephine of the frontal sinuses, can be assessed and discussed with the patient. The need for computer-aided surgical navigation is assessed at the same time. The surgeon should assess the degree of difficulty of the surgery and if the case is too difficult for their level of expertise, the patient should be referred to a specialist rhinologist.

In order to aid the preoperative assessment of the complexity of surgery, we recently published a study looking at the various options for a classification system.[17] The degree of complexity classification system is present in **Table 7.1**.

This classification was found to be easy and quick to use but suited more toward patients who had not undergone prior surgery. It was equally accurate whether the ostium was measured or estimated which makes it easy to apply to all CTs preoperatively. It had a good inter- and intraobserver reliability. The classification allows grades 1 to 4 to be used to assess patient's surgical complexity prior to the surgery and if the surgeon is not comfortable in the higher degrees of

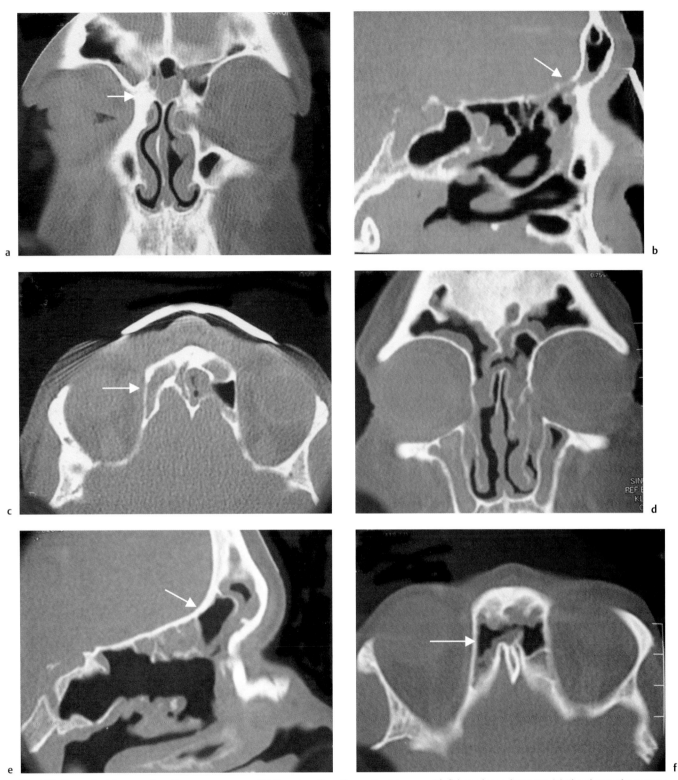

Fig. 7.3 The patient in scans (**a–c**) has a very narrow AP diameter; the other patient in scans (**d–f**) has a large diameter. (**a**) The clue to the narrow AP diameter is the thick bone (*white arrow*) on either side of the frontal ostia which is not present in equivalent coronal CT of the patient with a wide AP diameter (**d**). In the parasagittal scans, the difference between (**b**), with a narrow AP, and (**e**), with a wide AP is apparent (*white arrows*). On the axial CT scans (**c**) and (**f**), the difference in the AP diameter is again apparent (*white arrows*).

Table 7.1   Degree of complexity classification[17]

	Wide AP diameter ≥ 10 mm	Narrow AP diameter 5–9 mm	Narrowest AP diameter < 5 mm
Cells below ostium (Agger nasi, SAC, SBC)	Less complex (grade 1)	Moderate complexity (grade 2)	High complexity (grade 3)
Cells encroaching into the ostium (SAFC, SBFC, SOEC, FSC)	Moderate complexity (grade 2)	High complexity (grade 3)	Highest complexity (grade 4)
Cells extending significantly into frontal sinus (SAFC, SBFC, SOEC, FSC)	High complexity (grade 3)	Highest complexity (grade 4)	Highest complexity (grade 4)

Note: AP refers to the frontal ostium anteroposterior (AP) distance as measured from the frontal beak to the skull base on the parasagittal CT scan. Classification of the cells is from the International Frontal Sinus Classification (IFAC) published in IFAR in 2016.

Abbreviations: FSC, frontal septal cell; SAC, supra agger cell; SBC, supra bulla cell; SAFC, supra agger frontal cell; SBFC, supra bulla frontal cell; SOEC, supraorbital ethmoid cell.

complexity then the patient should be referred to an expert rhinologist.

Narrow versus Wide Anteroposterior Diameter of the Frontal Ostium

Patients who have a wide anteroposterior (AP) diameter (> 10 mm) will usually have a technically easier operation and will in most cases have a better prognosis for maintenance of health of the sinuses after surgery. This reflects the postoperative size of the frontal ostium that can be achieved without drilling on the ostium. **Fig. 7.3** illustrates a patient with a wide AP diameter compared with a patient with a narrow AP diameter. Note the space available to operate in the wide diameter patient.

Single Agger Nasi Cell or Simple SAC Configuration

A single ANC is the simplest configuration in the frontal recess and after removal of this cell, the frontal ostium can be identified (**Fig. 7.4**). A simple cell configuration of one or two associated SACs is also relatively easy to deal within the frontal recess.

SAFC Obstructing the Frontal Sinus Ostium

Even after an axillary flap approach these cells can be difficult to access and surgery often requires an angled endoscope thereby increasing the difficulty of the surgery. In addition, a high SAFC can be confused with the frontal sinus and the CT scans should be reviewed to ensure that the drainage pathway of the frontal sinus is identified and instrumented. These cells need to be removed to allow adequate ventilation and drainage of the frontal sinus. An example of this is given in **Fig. 7.5**.

Small Frontal Sinus with Poorly Pneumatized Agger Nasi Cells and Small Frontal Ostium

This can be problematic if the frontal sinus is completely opacified and the surgeon wishes to ensure the pus or inspissated mucus is cleared from the sinus. Failure to clear thick mucus or pus from the frontal sinus may allow the inflammatory process to continue in the postoperative period in the region of the frontal ostium. This delays the healing process and can increase the risk of scarring and adhesions in the frontal region. An example of a small frontal sinus ostium is presented in **Fig. 7.6**.

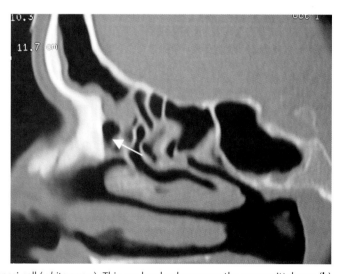

a   b

Fig. 7.4 In coronal CT scan (**a**) the left frontal recess has a single agger nasi cell (*white arrow*). This can be clearly seen on the parasagittal scan (**b**) (*white arrow*). This is the simplest configuration seen in the frontal recess.

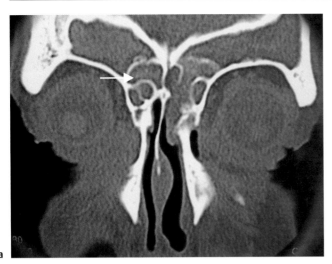
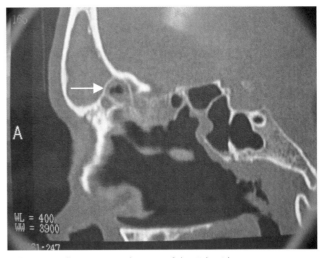

Fig. 7.5 (**a,b**) Bilateral supra agger frontal cells are seen obstructing the frontal ostium. The parasagittal view is of the right side.

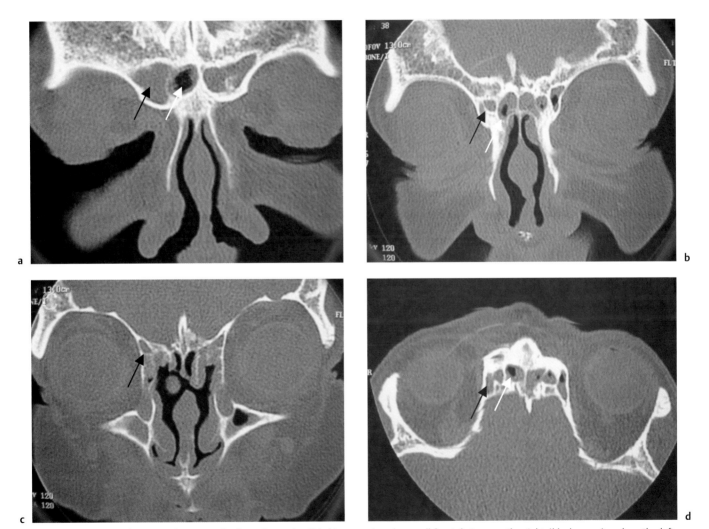

Fig. 7.6 This patient has a combination of a frontal septal cell (*white arrow*) and a small frontal sinus on the right (*black arrow*) and on the left. The small drainage pathway of the frontal sinus on the right is marked with a *black arrow* (**a–d**).

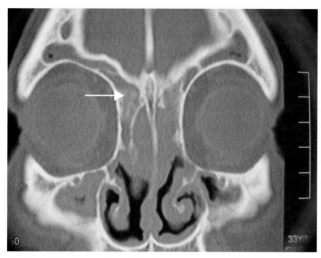

Fig. 7.7 New bone formation is seen in the right frontal recess (*white arrow*).

New Bone Formation in the Region of the Frontal Ostium

New bone formation in the region of the frontal ostium and recess often indicates osteitis of the surrounding bone. If the new bone obstructs the frontal ostium, removal will often leave vascular and inflamed exposed bone, which will usually produce significant fibrosis and scar tissue. Re-stenosis and obstruction of the frontal ostium will often result. An example of the CT scan appearance of new bone formation is shown in **Fig. 7.7**. There is considerable debate as to whether these bone changes are a result of infection or as a consequence of significant ongoing inflammation mediated through the eosinophils. Research has shown that eosinophils produce various toxic substances such a major basic protein (MBP), eosinophil peroxidase (EPX) and eosinophil cationic protein (ECP) which stimulate new bone growth.

Cultures with appropriate culture-directed antibiotics as well as topical and systemic steroids should be considered to suppress the inflammatory response during the healing period. This can be done by giving a 3-week course of oral steroids. Alternatively, or in combination with the oral steroids, the mini-trephine cannulas can be left in place for 3 to 4 days postoperatively and the frontal sinuses irrigated with prednisolone drops after saline douching. This serves two purposes as it keeps the frontal ostium clear of blood clot (which can contribute to fibrosis and scarring) and the prednisolone diminishes the inflammatory response in the immediate postoperative period.

Previous Surgery with Scarring of the Frontal Recess

Previous surgery, especially amputation of the middle turbinate with lateralization of the remnant with associated scar tissue formation, can make exposure of the frontal ostium difficult. Diagnosis is made both on the CT scan appearance and on endoscopy. The CT scan can show residual cells and new bone formation and endoscopy can confirm the presence of scar tissue in the frontal recess. An example is shown in **Fig. 7.8**.

Extensive Disease in the Frontal Recess

Some patients may have extensive and severe disease in the frontal recess (**Fig. 7.9**). In this example, the patient has allergic fungal sinusitis with expansion of the frontal recess and double densities visible on soft tissue settings (*white arrow*). The frontal recesses in this patient were filled with highly vascular polyps and inspissated fungal material. Not only were the normal anatomical landmarks distorted in this patient but there was extensive bleeding in the frontal recess as the polyps were removed. As previously stated such vascularity can significantly increase the degree of difficulty

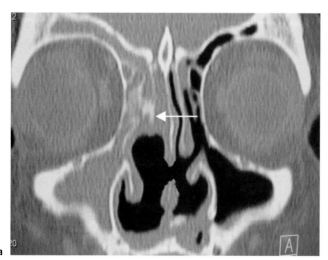

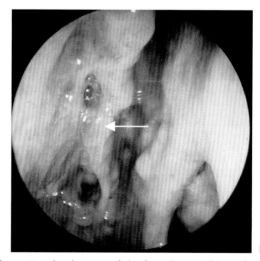

Fig. 7.8 (**a**) The amputated right middle turbinate is marked with a *white solid arrow* in both the CT scan and on the endoscopy picture. The uncinate remains and abuts the retained anterior ethmoid cells obstructing the drainage of the frontal sinus. (**b**) On the endoscopic view, significant scarring is seen between the lateralized residual middle turbinate and lateral nasal wall (uncinate).

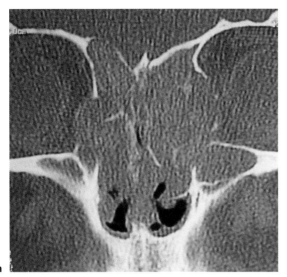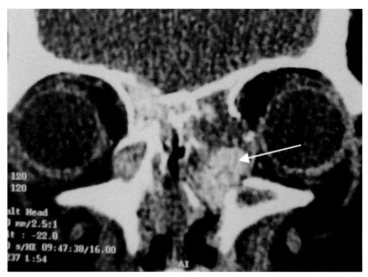

a   b

Fig. 7.9 (**a**) Expansile disease of the frontal recess. (**b**) Double densities marked with a *white arrow*.

for the surgeon during removal of the polyps and cells, and during identification of the frontal ostium.

Resected Middle Turbinates and Patients with Few or No Operative Landmarks

Patients who have previously had resection of their middle turbinates can be difficult to manage as the absence of the middle turbinate has removed the most important intraoperative landmark (**Fig. 7.10**).

If there are polyps present, identification of the residual middle turbinate can be difficult (**Fig. 7.11**). The first step is to identify the maxillary ostium and to clear the maxillary sinus of polyps using the maxillary trephination procedure if necessary (Chapter 5). This will allow positive

identification of the lamina papyracea, which is an important landmark in the further dissection of the frontal recess. The next step is to gently debride the polyps to reveal the underlying bony structures—the septum, olfactory recess, residual middle turbinate, and posterior bony choanae. If the anatomy is still unclear then the polyps in the region of the posterior bony choanae and the anterior face of the sphenoid should be removed. The natural ostium of the sphenoid is usually about 12 mm above the bony posterior choanae. The microdebrider blade is 4 mm and this can be used to measure 12 mm from the posterior bony choanae. A useful additional landmark is the roof of the maxillary sinus which can be used as a guide to enter the sphenoid. Harvey et al[18] have shown that a horizontal line taken from the maxillary sinus roof onto the anterior face of the sphenoid provides a safe point of entry into the sphenoid. Once

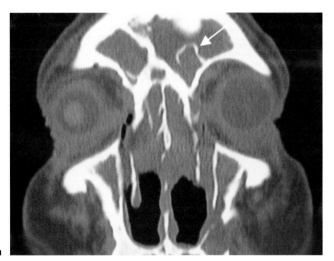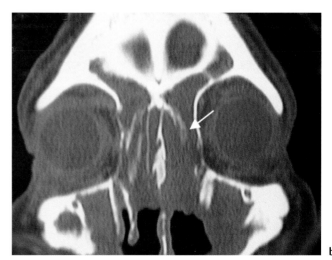

a   b

Fig. 7.10 (**a**) The *white arrow* indicates a residual supra bulla frontal cell in the frontal sinus. (**b,c**) The *white arrow* indicates the previously resected middle turbinate. Note the absence of the inferior turbinate on the left side from previous surgery. (**d,f**) The *white arrow* indicates the anterior wall of the supra bulla frontal cell. Note extensive polyps visible on all scans.

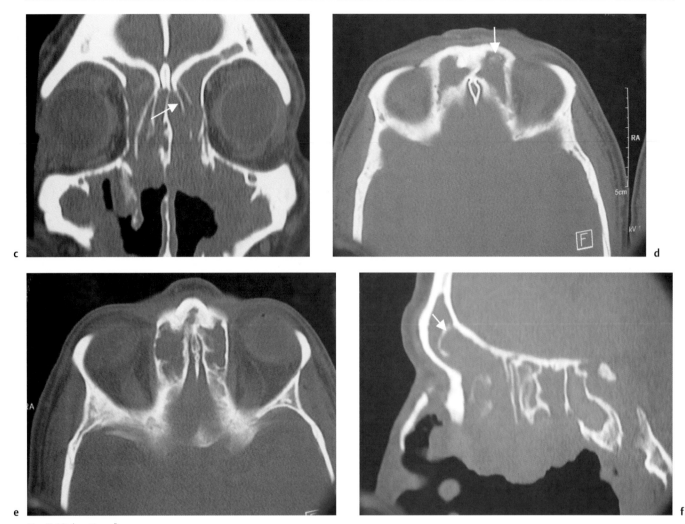

Fig. 7.10 (*continued*)

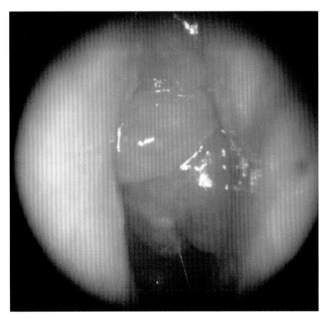

Fig. 7.11 Massive nasal polyps with no identifying landmarks visible.

the polyps in this region are cleared, the residual superior turbinate may come into view. If this has also been previously resected, then the polyps should be cleared from the skull base. The fovea ethmoidalis and olfactory fossa are normally in the same horizontal plane in this posterior region of the ethmoids and gentle removal of polyps (without bone removal) should safely expose the skull base and residual superior turbinate. The previously identified lamina papyracea is an important additional landmark. The next step is to identify the ostium of the sphenoid sinus (the method is described in Chapter 8) and enlarge the natural ostium of the sphenoid. This will allow the skull base to be positively identified and the dissection can then be brought along the skull base anteriorly. The surgeon needs to check the CT scan to identify the position of the anterior ethmoid artery and whether it is suspended within a mesentery. Using the lamina papyracea as the lateral landmark, the skull base as the superior landmark and the beak of the frontal process of the maxilla as the anterior landmark, the frontal recess can be identified. In most patients a small stump of residual middle turbinate can be seen and an axillary flap is performed and the axilla opened with a

Hajek Koeffler punch. Now that all the landmarks for the frontal recess are established, the clearance of the frontal recess can continue according to the 3D reconstruction of the anatomy of that recess with localization of the frontal sinus drainage pathway and stepwise removal of each remaining cell in the frontal recess.

Classification of the Extent of Surgery in the Frontal Recess and Frontal Sinus

In a recent publication, the extent of surgery was classified according to the presence of cells below, in, and above the frontal sinus ostium as well as whether bony enlargement of the frontal ostium was performed.[19] This is presented in **Table 7.2**.

This classification presents an accurate record of the surgery performed in the frontal recess and frontal sinus. It will allow comparison between surgeons on outcomes of frontal sinus surgery and, in combination with the Degree of Complexity Classification, allow comparisons of outcomes for different techniques, standard surgery, versus highly complex procedures. It will also allow better assessments of intraoperative interventions such as dissolvable nasal packing in the difficult highly complex patient versus the standard patient. Finally, it will allow trainees to be able to work their way through the degrees of complexity but also the grades of surgery of the frontal sinus so that their progress and competence can be adequately monitored and assessed.

◆ Surgical Techniques for Managing the Frontal Recess and Frontal Sinus

1. Endoscopy
2. Surgical approach—the axillary flap
3. Frontal sinus mini-trephine
4. Computer-aided surgery (CAS, or image guidance surgery)

Most frontal recesses and frontal sinuses will be managed by utilizing techniques for grades 1–3 in the International Classification of the Extent of Endoscopic Frontal Sinus Surgery (EFSS). These techniques are used in a graduated approach. The combination of endoscopy utilizing the least angled endoscope with the axillary flap technique is used for all frontal recess and sinus dissections (EFSS grades 1–3). Frontal sinus mini-trephination and CAS may be used in the more difficult frontal recess dissections such as EFSS grade 3.

Endoscopy

The classic description of the technique for dissection in the frontal recess and frontal sinus involves the use of 30-, 45-, and 70-degree endoscopes.[2–4] It is also recognized that the more angulated the endoscope the greater the degree of difficulty of the dissection because of surgeon disorientation and the manipulation of angled instruments. A recent paper[20] described increasing unwanted trauma within the nose and sinuses from the passage of angulated instruments during dissection.[20] **Fig. 7.12** shows the increasing angulation of instruments required to keep the tip of the instrument in the

Table 7.2 International Classification of the Extent of Endoscopic Frontal Sinus Surgery[19]

No tissue removal
Grade 0 Balloon sinus dilation (no tissue removal)
Frontal recess/sinus clearance procedures (cell[s] removed)
Grade 1: Below the frontal ostium. Clearance of cells below the frontal ostium. These are supra agger cells and supra bulla cells that do not encroach on or obstruct the frontal ostium.
Grade 2: Within the frontal ostium. Clearance of cell(s) within the frontal sinus ostium. These are supra agger cells or supra bulla cells that encroach on and obstruct the frontal sinus drainage.
Grade 3: Above the frontal ostium. Clearance of cell pneumatizing through the frontal ostium into the frontal sinus without enlargement of the frontal ostium. These are typically SAFCs, SBFCs, and FSCs
Frontal ostium enlargement procedures by removal of bone from the frontal beak
Grade 4: Enlargement of the frontal ostium. Clearance of cell(s) with (not just removal of cell walls) removal of bone of the frontal beak.
Grade 5: Unilateral frontal drillout. Enlargement of the frontal ostium from the lamina papyracea to the nasal septum (also previously also known as the Draf 2b) with unilateral removal of the floor of the frontal sinus.
Grade 6: Frontal drillout. Removal of the entire floor of the frontal sinus with joining of the left and right ostia into a common ostium with septal window—previously known as the modified Lothrop or Draf 3.

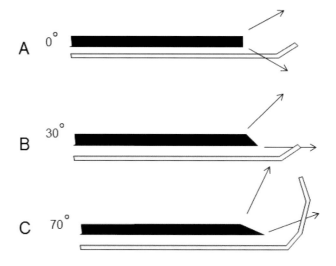

Fig. 7.12 When a zero-degree endoscope is used, the instrument passed beneath the scope will be in the center of the field of view as demonstrated in (**a**). If a 30-degree endoscope is used with a similar instrument passed below the scope, the instrument tip is on the extreme periphery of the visual field. If the tip of the instrument is brought into the center of the endoscope field of view, the endoscope is pushed upward by the instrument and the area of dissection may no longer be visible. If a 45- or 70-degree endoscope is used, the instrument needs to be sufficiently angled to be able to be placed in the center of the field of view of the endoscope as demonstrated in (**c**).

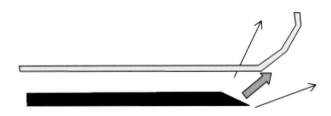

Fig. 7.13 If the instrument is positioned above the scope, the undersurface of the instrument is visualized (*block arrow*) and the working tip is not seen. This can be potentially dangerous if the working tip of the instrument is in a potentially vulnerable region of the frontal recess.

center of the field of dissection with increasing angulation of the endoscope.

As illustrated in Chapter 1 the vast majority of surgery is conducted with the endoscope placed above the instrument. If the endoscope is placed below the instrument, the working tip of the instrument cannot be visualized (**Fig. 7.13**).

The degree of difficulty is further increased if the surgical field is bloody. It can take longer for an angled endoscope (30 or 70 degrees) and a curved instrument to be positioned in the frontal recess before surgical dissection can take place. If bleeding in the surgical field is profuse, the surgical field may be covered in blood before the dissection begins. This situation may lead to frustration for the surgeon at the slow progress of surgery and the surgeon may be a tempted to proceed with dissection despite poor visibility. This can potentially lead to inadvertent injury to the skull base, lamina papyracea, or anterior ethmoidal artery. As with any surgical procedure, the wider the exposure, the easier the operation becomes. Most surgeons would recall a situation when they have needed the aid of a senior colleague during a procedure and that the first thing the senior surgeon did was to widen the incisions to

improve the surgical access. The axillary flap technique was designed to try to overcome some of the problems mentioned above by optimizing access to the frontal recess and allowing a large part of the dissection in the frontal sinus to be performed with a zero-degree telescope[13–16] (**Fig. 7.14**).

Surgical Technique for the Axillary Flap

The first step in the axillary flap approach is to make an incision about 8 mm above the axilla of the middle turbinate and to bring this forward by about 8 mm.[15] The incision is turned vertically down to the level of the axilla. It is then carried back under the axilla onto the root of the middle turbinate (**Fig. 7.15**). A number 15 scalpel blade on a number 7 BP scalpel blade holder is used to make these incisions.

The full thickness mucosal flap is then raised with a suction Freer elevator. It is important to ensure that the tip of the suction Freer is on bone when the flap is being raised and that the flap extends behind the root of the middle turbinate (**Fig. 7.16a**). The flap is connected at its inferior edge to tissue under the axilla of the middle turbinate. This needs to be separated from the flap with a sickle knife or scalpel (see videos) before the flap is tucked between the middle turbinate and the septum (**Fig. 7.16b**). Failure to expose the vertical bone of the middle turbinate just below where it attaches to the lateral nasal wall will often result in this bridge of tissue remaining. If this bridge of tissue is pulled by an instrument or suction then the flap will be pulled from between the turbinate and septum into the frontal recess. Here it may either be inadvertently removed by a microdebrider or instrument or irritate the surgeon by requiring it to be tucked away regularly before surgery can proceed. By exposing the vertical upper bony part of the middle turbinate, the surgeon ensures that the bridge of tissue is divided and once the flap is tucked between the middle turbinate and septum, it should not be

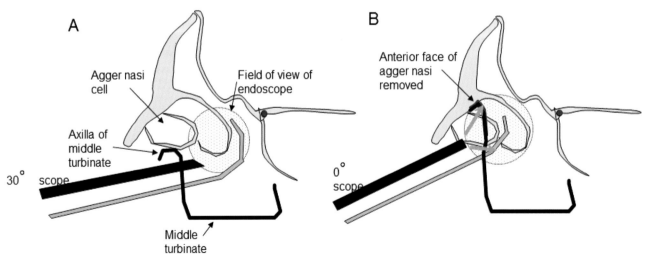

a

b

Fig. 7.14 (a) Illustration of the need to use an angled endoscope to view the frontal recess (visual field = *shaded circle*) with the axilla intact. After opening the anterior wall of the agger nasi cell (**b**), a zero-degree telescope can be used to view and operate in the frontal recess without having to use angled endoscopes and instruments.

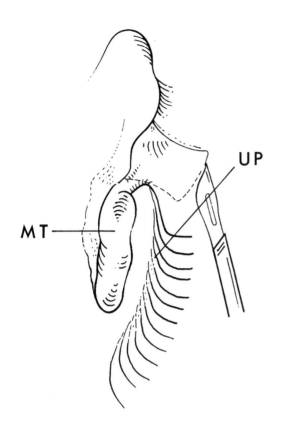

Fig. 7.15 The middle turbinate (*MT*) and uncinate process (*UP*) are marked in the left nasal cavity. The scalpel blade outlines the incisions for the axillary flap above the insertion of the middle turbinate on the left lateral nasal wall.

seen again until it is retrieved at the end of surgery to cover the raw bone of the newly created axilla.

A Hajek Koeffler punch is used to remove the anterior wall of the agger nasi cell. The thickness of the bone depends upon the extent of the pneumatization of the agger nasi cell. If it is well pneumatized this bone is thin and easy to remove and should be removed to the edge of the mucosal incisions (**Fig. 7.17**). If the agger nasi cell is small or absent, the bone can be thick and may only be able to be partially removed. If there are polyps in the agger nasi cell, these are removed with the microdebrider so that the extent of the cell can be clearly seen.

Now that the agger nasi cell has been entered and positively identified, the surgeon should review the 3D reconstruction of the anatomy of the frontal recess that has previously been performed (see Chapter 6). The location of the frontal drainage pathway should be sought with a probe or curette. The probe or curette should be gently slid up this drainage pathway and the obstructing cells removed by fracturing and removing the cell(s).

Once the frontal ostium has been visualized and is clear of any obstructing cells, the axillary flap is pulled forward and placed so that it partially rolls under the raw edge of bone of the residual anterior wall of the agger nasi cell (**Fig. 7.18**). This should provide cover for this area and prevent granulation tissue and subsequent adhesions from forming in this area.

Results of the Axillary Flap Technique[15]

In a recently published series,[15] the axillary flap approach in conjunction with the 3D building block concept provided visualization of 96% of the frontal sinus ostia in

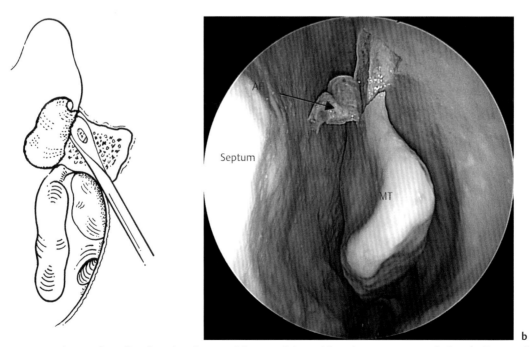

a   **b**

Fig. 7.16 (**a**) Suction Freer elevates the axillary flap. Identification of the root of the middle turbinate is necessary before the flap is tucked between the turbinate and septum. (**b**) Cadaveric image of a left sided axillary flap. *AF*, axillary flap; *MT*, middle turbinate.

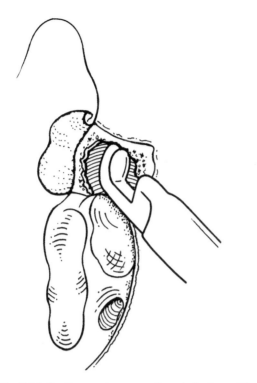

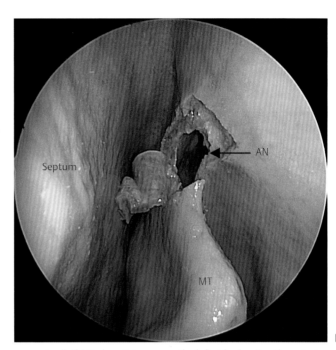

a

b

Fig. 7.17 (**a**) The Hajek-Koeffler punch removes the anterior face of the agger nasi cell. (**b**) Cadaveric image on the left side showing the anterior face of the agger nasi cell (*AN*) removed. *MT*, middle turbinate.

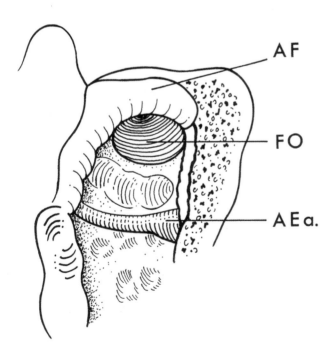

Fig. 7.18 The axillary flap (*AF*) is rolled over the raw edge of the newly formed axilla. The frontal ostium (*FO*) and anterior ethmoidal artery (*AEa*) are visible.

118 consecutive frontal recess procedures. The remaining frontal ostia were identified with the aid of the mini-trephine technique described below. Of the 118 cases, six had significant adhesions present that required outpatient treatment.[15] Therefore the axillary flap approach does not increase the risk of adhesion formation in the middle meatus.[13-16] **Fig. 7.19** shows the typical appearance of the region of the axillary flap after such an approach to the frontal recess.

Mini-Trephination of the Frontal Sinus

The mini-trephine of the frontal sinuses is a very helpful technique when the drainage pathway of the frontal sinus is not easily seen. Placement of a cannula in the frontal sinus allows the sinus to be flushed with fluorescein-stained saline and the pathway of this fluid in the frontal recess can be followed using a malleable frontal sinus probe* (Integra). As the probe is passed up the fluorescein-stained pathway, the probe is used to gently widen this pathway until a curette can be placed along the pathway. The cells in the frontal recess can then be fractured (usually anteriorly or laterally) and removed to expose the frontal ostium (see videos). In addition the trephine can be used to ensure clearance of pus, mucus, or fungal material from the frontal sinus where the surgeon does not wish to place an instrument through the frontal ostium and risk damage to the mucosa of the frontal ostium. If a frontal sinus suction is nearly as large as the frontal ostium (often the case with a standard 3- or 4-mm olive tip suction), it may cause circumferential damage to the mucosa of the frontal ostium if it is forced through the ostium

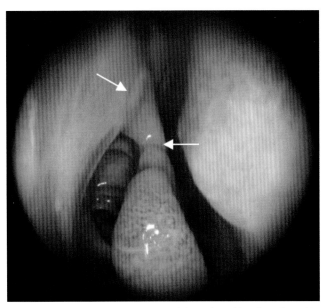

Fig. 7.19 Postoperative appearance of the right axillary flap. The *white arrows* mark the incision lines for the superior and inferior incisions.

into the frontal sinus. This may in turn lead to stenosis or obstruction of the ostium. Clearance of the frontal sinus by irrigating through the mini-trephine cannula can avoid such injury. The mini-trephine cannula can be removed at the end of surgery or may be left in place for a variable period of time after the surgery so that the frontal sinus and frontal ostium can be flushed with saline. This flushing process can remove blood clot from the frontal ostium which in turn may help maintain its patency as it heals. If the mucosa is significantly inflamed or polypoid, steroid drops may be placed into the frontal sinus for the period of time after surgery before the cannulae are removed. This in turn may help reduce the inflammation and potentially the formation of early scar tissue in the frontal ostia.

Technique of Placing the Mini-Trephines

The CT scans should be reviewed to establish the presence and size of the frontal sinus. **Fig. 7.20** shows absence of the right frontal sinus with a small left frontal sinus with a very narrow frontal ostium.

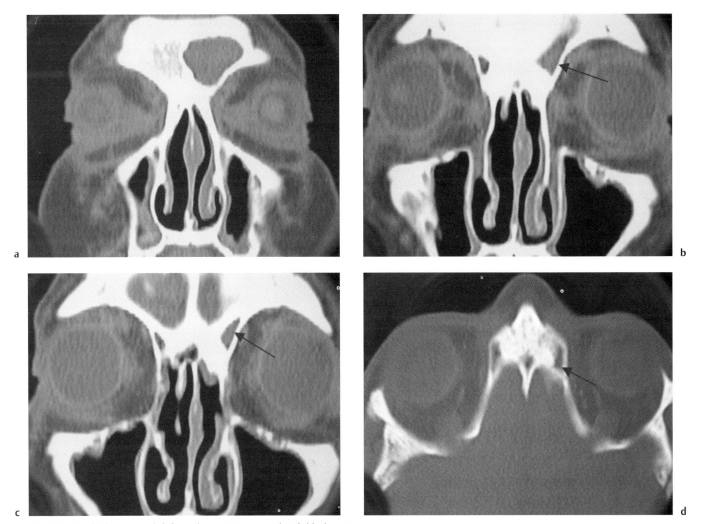

Fig. 7.20 (a–d) The narrow left frontal ostium is arrowed with *black arrows*.

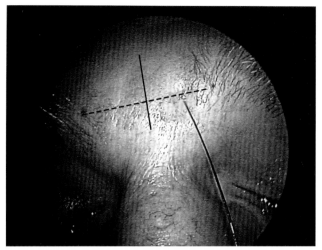
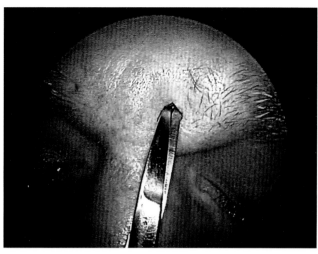

a

b

Fig. 7.21 (**a**) The *black line* marks the midline with the *asterisk* marking the medial aspect of the eyebrow. The *broken horizontal line* joins the ends of the eyebrows. The needle with local anesthetic is placed through a skin crease midway between these points. After a stab incision the wound is dilated with iris scissors (**b**).

Note that the left frontal sinus does not extend above the eyebrow (bony rim of the orbit). The extent of superior pneumatization of the frontal sinus needs to be assessed on the CT scan before the mini-trephine is placed.

The landmark for placement of the skin incision is the medial aspect of the eyebrow. In most patients the eyebrow is on the superior orbital rim and one should follow this medially on the CT scan to ensure that there is sufficient pneumatization of the frontal sinus above the superior orbital rim. Placement of the mini-trephine too high can result in intracranial penetration by the drill and a cerebrospinal fluid leak. If the frontal sinus is sufficiently pneumatized on CT, the skin landmarks for placement of the skin incision are as follows: Draw an imaginary horizontal line from the middle of the medial end of eyebrow to the medial end of the other eyebrow. Along this line, pick the midpoint between the eyebrows and then estimate 1 cm from the midline along this imaginary line (**Fig. 7.21**).

Infiltrate with 1 to 2 mL of local anaesthetic and adrenaline. A number 15 scalpel blade is used to make the stab incision through the skin onto bone. This incision can either be placed through a vertical frown line or, in the case of patients concerned about the possible aesthetic appearance of a scar, the incision can be placed through the medial hairs of the eyebrow. Although the latter two incisions may not be correctly placed between the medial aspect of the eyebrow and the midline, the skin over the frontal bone is mobile and after placement of the mini-trephine guide, this guide can be shifted by moving the skin until it is correctly placed on the bone as described above. If the bony trephine is placed too laterally it may either endanger the supratrochlear neurovascular bundle or be outside of the frontal sinus. The stab incision is gently dilated with a sharp-pointed scissors. A drill guide is placed through this incision by first laying the guide flat on the skin and then rotating it into the incision. This is done with the incision being held open by tension placed with fingers on either side of the wound (**Fig. 7.22**).

If the guide is pushed into the incision without opening the wound, a small ellipse of skin can be caught by the

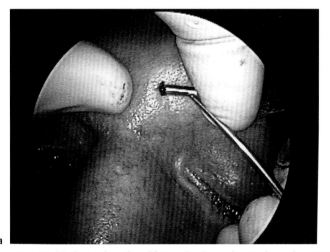
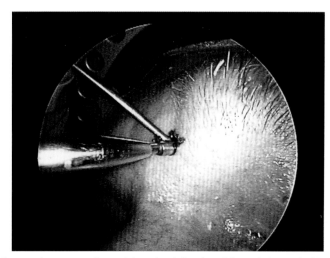

a

b

Fig. 7.22 (**a**) The guide is placed flat on the skin and rotated into the wound to avoid coring an ellipse of skin. The drill is placed through the guide (**b**).

teeth of the guide and the skin damaged as the guide is pushed into the wound. If the skin incision has been placed through the hairs of the eyebrow this point may be too lateral to perform the trephine. After placement of the drill guide, the skin is moved by pushing the guide to the point indicated by the above guidelines before the bone is trephined. The guide has teeth on the surface that come in contact with the bone and these should be securely engaged onto the bone so that the guide does not move during the trephination process. It is vitally important that the drill bit *not* be allowed to heat up. The drill bit should be removed almost immediately when it touches the bone. It should be completely withdrawn from the guide and the tip irrigated with saline or water to cool the drill bit down. Failure to do this results in significant heating of the drill tip and can lead to a burn of the bone and the skin around the trephine. On the skin this can result in a circular wound that leaves an unsightly scar and in the bone can predispose toward osteitis. The trephine bur is designed to extend 11 mm beyond the guide and should not be able to penetrate the posterior table of the frontal sinus. On rare occasions in patients with small (underpneumatized) frontal sinuses and a thick anterior table, the drill may not be long enough

to penetrate the anterior table of the frontal sinus. Should this occur, the surgeon can move the trephine guide inferiorly (the bone of the anterior table tends to thin as one moves inferiorly) and reattempt frontal sinus trephination. The skin over the frontal sinus is mobile and easily moved by the guide. Do not attempt to move the trephine site superiorly as this can risk trephination of the intracranial cavity. The trephine is removed while the guide is held firmly in place. A wire stylet is placed through the guide into the trephine hole. The guide is removed and the frontal cannula is placed over the stylet into the frontal sinus (**Fig. 7.23**). The cannula is placed in a rotatory fashion and is not pushed too firmly into skin as the barrel widens as this can put pressure on the skin around the shaft of the cannula.

A syringe half-filled with saline and fluorescein (500 mL saline and 0.5 mL of 5% fluorescein) is placed on the cannula and aspiration attempted. Aspiration of clear fluid indicates intracranial penetration and the cannula should be immediately removed and the wound sutured. Should fluorescein be inadvertently injected into the intracranial cavity, the concentration as described above should not cause meningeal irritation. Usually there is either air,

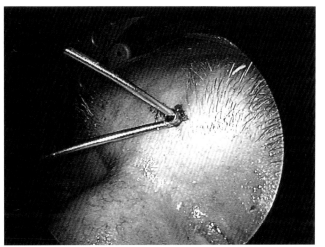

a

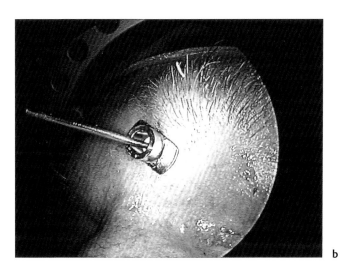

b

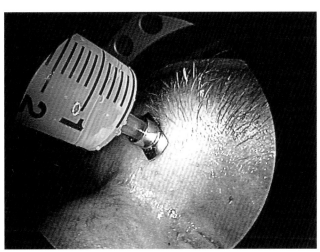

c

Fig. 7.23 (**a,b**) The frontal cannula is slid over the stylet into the trephine hole and into the frontal sinus. (**c**) A syringe half filled with fluorescein-stained saline is attached to the cannula and the frontal sinus aspirated before it is irrigated.

mucus, pus, or blood withdrawn into the syringe. When the frontal ostium is completely blocked, only a vacuum will be created in the syringe. In this situation, the frontal ostium is observed while gentle pressure is placed on the syringe. Pus or mucus followed by fluorescein-stained saline should be seen. This area of emergence of the fluorescein can then be probed to identify the drainage pathway of the frontal sinus. Before any significant pressure is placed on the syringe, check the CT scan to ensure that there are no dehiscences of the posterior table or floor of the frontal sinus.

Computer-Aided Surgery

Computer-aided surgery (CAS) utilizes new technology where the patient has undergone either a CT or MRI scan (or both) prior to surgery. These images are downloaded onto a computer in the CAS machine and the images presented to the surgeon in three planes (coronal, axial, and parasagittal). This is similar to the standard CT scans performed on our patients. There are a number of software programs that can be downloaded from the internet. For Apple Mac users, Scopis® planning or Osirix® can only be used—they all read DICOM files so any CT scan in DICOM format can be read in the same manner as is done on the CAS machines. Scopis® planning is also available for PCs and many radiology companies will supply a software program that can be copied onto the PC and used to view the images. The benefit of these software systems is that crosshairs can be placed on a cell and the crosshairs will appear in the same cell on the other two views (**Fig. 7.24**). The surgeon can identify a cell and see where that cell is in the other plane and, in the same way as described in Chapter 6, can build a 3D image of the anatomy of the patient. Surgical planning can also be effectively performed on the image guidance machine prior to surgery.

There are two systems: the first is optical system where a camera tracks light emitting diodes (LEDs) on the patient (headframe) and the instruments. The second system is electromagnetic where the computer tracks movement of electromagnetic markers on the patient (headframe) and on instruments. Recent CAS machines are able to perform either the LED or electromagnetic tracking, depending upon the surgeon's preference. Both systems work well and have different advantages and disadvantages. To register the patient on the computer, landmarks are identified on the scans on the computer and then on the patient or a laser tracer is run over the face. The headframe monitors the movement of the patient's head. The instruments are tracked either optically or electromagnetically. In patients without intranasal landmarks (absent middle turbinate, etc.), these systems allow important structures such as the skull base, orbit, optic nerve, and carotid to be identified. In addition they allow residual cells within the frontal recess and sinus to be identified and removed. If a frontal sinus drainage pathway cannot be found, they can track an instrument tip so that the pathway can be identified and the instrument slid up the pathway and remaining cells removed from the frontal recess or sinus.

◆ Difficult Surgical Situations in Frontal Recess and Frontal Sinus During Surgery

Narrow Frontal Ostium with Obstructive Cells with Thick Bony Walls

This situation is not uncommon but results in a difficult intraoperative situation. In this particular example, the patient has a thick beak with very under-pneumatized agger nasi cell and frontal septal cell (FSC) with thick bony walls that cannot be easily fractured with standard instruments to enlarge the frontal ostium (**Fig. 7.25**). The agger nasi cell is very small and narrow and the bulla ethmoidalis pushes forward into the frontal recess squashing the frontal sinus drainage pathway anterolaterally (best seen on the axial scans; **Fig. 7.25**). The beak of the frontal process is very thick and although there is an FSC, the wall of this cell is formed by thick bone that separates this cell from the frontal drainage pathway. It would be impossible to enlarge the frontal sinus drainage pathway without resorting to a drill. As discussed previously, drilling in this situation is more likely to result in postoperative scarring and obstruction of the frontal ostium with iatrogenic long-term frontal sinusitis that can be difficult to manage. The intraoperative management of this patient should include complete clearance of the opacified maxillary sinus with a canine fossa trephine and creation of a large middle meatal antrostomy followed by an axillary flap with removal of as much of the axilla of the middle turbinate as possible. This will expose the small thin agger nasi cell. Because the bulla pneumatizes anteriorly this should be opened as well as the supra bulla cell allowing identification of the skull base and anterior ethmoidal artery which should be seen adjacent to where the posterior wall of this cell touches the skull base. The curette can now be slid up the frontal sinus drainage pathway behind the agger nasi cell and this cell fractured forward and removed. Next the anterior wall of both the bulla and supra bulla cells should be removed up to the skull base. The FSC will be seen with the frontal ostium pushed laterally. Because the frontal ostium is narrow and could not be enlarged, and due to the inflamed state of the mucosa around the frontal ostium, a frontal sinus mini-trephine should be inserted and the frontal ostium irrigated for 3 days postoperatively with both saline flushes and prednisolone drops.

Postoperatively, the frontal ostium was edematous for some months before settling down. The patient remained asymptomatic and the ostium healed (**Fig. 7.26**). This emphasizes the importance of removing the obstructive cells from the frontal recess (agger nasi, bulla, and supra bulla cells) and clearing the drainage pathway. I believe that any attempt to enlarge this ostium with a drill would not have had such a positive outcome.

That is not to say that all patients will respond in this manner and some patients may develop chronic edema with obstruction of a narrow ostium (**Fig. 7.27**). Such patients should be treated with systemic and topical steroids, douches, and regular office toilet and if the symptoms persist, revision surgery is indicated (usually an endoscopic frontal drillout/modified Lothrop procedure/Draf 3 as described in Chapter 9).

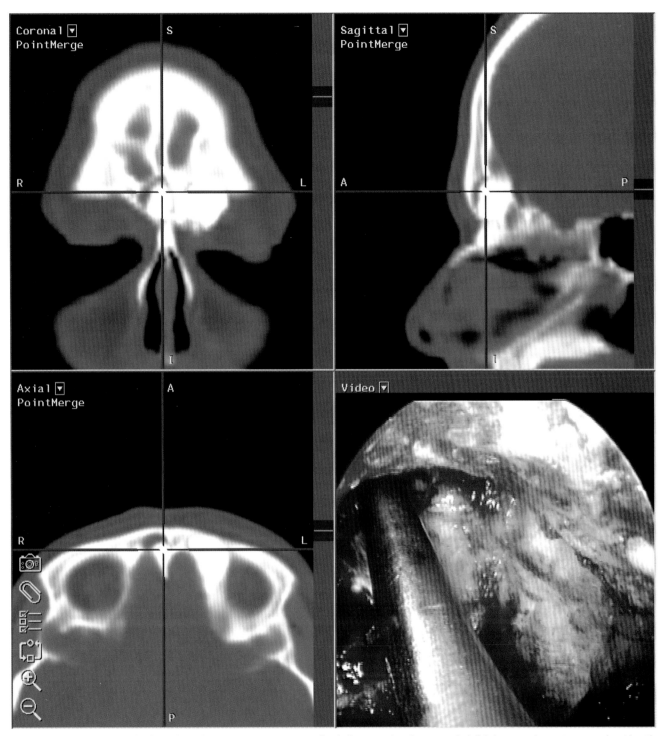

Fig. 7.24 In this patient with a large frontal sinus osteoma, computed-aided surgery (CAS) was very helpful during endoscopic removal to identify and prevent injury to the skull base. The *crosshairs* indicate the roof of the frontal sinus after removal of the osteoma.

Large SAFC Obstructing the Frontal Ostium

In some patients, there are cells that extend significantly into the frontal sinus through the frontal ostium and, in so doing, compromise the ostium and the drainage and ventilation of the frontal sinus. These cells can be very difficult to manage

and the approach depends on the size of the frontal ostium. If the patient has pneumatized sinuses then there is a reasonable chance the AP distance of the frontal ostium may be quite large as is the case in this example (*black arrow,* **Fig. 7.28**). In this case, the large SAFC is originating from the supra agger region and is anterior to the SBC and skull base

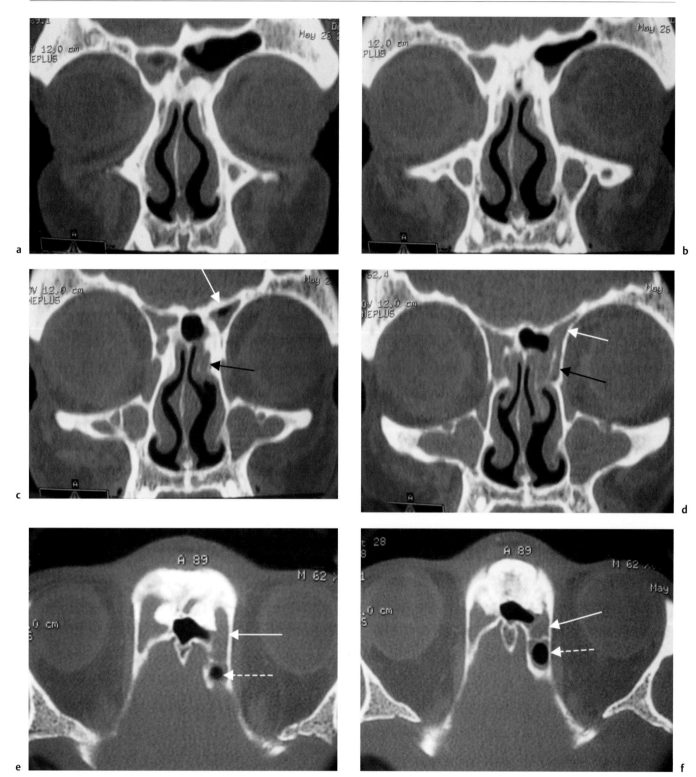

Fig. 7.25 The frontal ostium and frontal sinus drainage pathway are indicated with a *solid white arrow* on the left side (**c–g**). The small agger nasi cell can be seen in (**c,d**, *black arrow*). The suprabullar cell (*broken white arrow*) can be seen in (**e–h**). (*continued*)

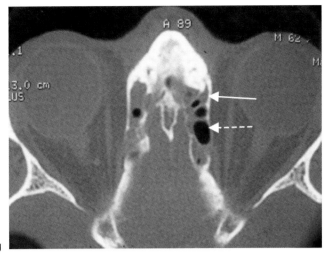
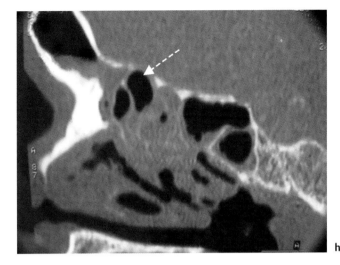

g   h

Fig. 7.25 (*continued*)

progressing almost to reach the roof of the frontal sinus. If the AP distance is large (*black arrow*), then the cell can be reached through the natural frontal ostium and removed. In this case it was possible to remove the entire cell from below without enlarging the frontal ostium. However, if the AP distance was small then the cell would need ancillary measures for removal. In our department this would usually be a frontal drillout/endoscopic modified Lothrop/Draf 3 procedure but removal may also be performed by a combined approach (trephine into the frontal sinus through the eyebrow big enough to admit either an endoscope or an instrument). The instrument is introduced through the frontal sinus trephine

and viewed through the frontal ostium or vice versa. Alternatively, an osteoplastic flap into frontal sinuses can be performed and the cell removed under direct visualization.

◆ Postoperative Frontal Sinus Irrigation Regimes

The frontal sinus cannulas are left in place during the following scenarios: if there has been inadvertent circumferential trauma to the frontal ostium mucosa, if the natural frontal

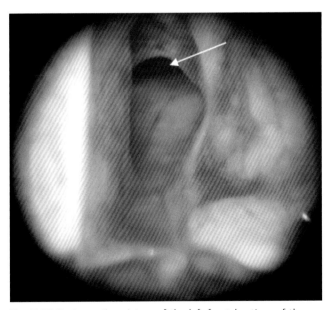

Fig. 7.26 Postoperative picture of the left frontal ostium of the patient presented in **Fig. 7.25**. Note the healthy left frontal ostium (*white arrow*).

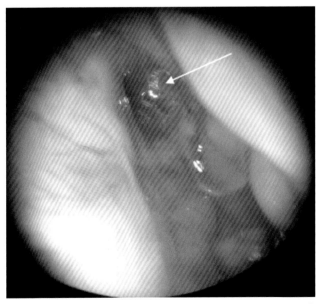

Fig. 7.27 A patient who had a very narrow left frontal ostium with edema obstructing the ostium (*white arrow*). A thin suction could still be passed through this ostium but, despite ongoing medical treatment, the edema in this region has remained. If the patient remains symptomatic further surgery is indicated.

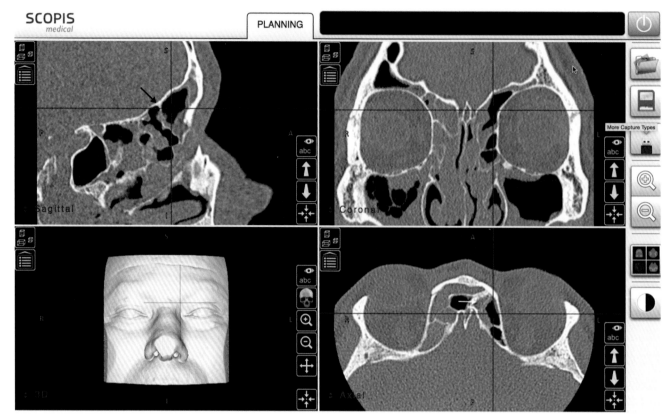

Fig. 7.28 The large SAFC is indicated by the *crosshairs* and on the parasagittal CT the large AP diameter is indicated by the *black arrow*. Note how the SAFC almost reaches the top of the frontal sinus. The drainage pathway (*white arrow*) can be seen on the axial CT scan medial to the SAFC (*crosshairs*).

sinus ostium is very narrow (< 3 mm), if there was evidence of osteitis with new bone formation in the frontal recess or ostium or if there were extensive polyposis resulting in significant traumatized mucosa after the polyp removal. The frontal cannulas are flushed with 5 mL of normal saline every 2 hours starting immediately after surgery. If prednisolone drops are to be used, 0.5 to 1 mL is instilled with a syringe into the frontal sinus after every second douche.

Sinus Packing after ESS

Over the past number of years our department has conducted a number of studies into Chitogel (Wellington, New Zealand) to assess its effect on hemostasis, development of adhesions, and maintenance of sinus ostial patency.[21–25] Chitogel on its own has been shown to have antibacterial properties, inhibit fibroblast migration, and have anti-inflammatory properties[21] which all lead to improved healing postoperatively.[22–25] In addition, Chitogel has been shown to be a very good hemostatic agent[22,25] and to prevent adhesion formation.[23] One of the more important features of Chitogel is the maintenance of sinus ostial patency[25] which is especially important in patients with narrow sinus ostia as it can improve the outcome for these patients. More recent studies have shown that the effect of Chitogel can be enhanced by the addition of budesonide to the gel as the gel slowly releases the steroid as the gel dissolves

over the 10–14 days after surgery. Note conflict of interest as I am an investor and on the board of the Chitogel company.

Postoperative Care and Debridement

All patients are placed on a 10-day course of broad spectrum antibiotics and requested to flush their nose and sinuses four to six times a day with saline after surgery. If significant polyps were found during surgery, patients are placed on a 3-week reducing course of oral prednisolone. Patients are reviewed in the office between 10 to 14 days after surgery. At this visit all residual blood clots are removed and the sinus ostia inspected. A thin curved suction is passed through the frontal sinus ostia and any secretions removed from the frontal sinus. All other sinus ostia are similarly checked. Any adhesions are divided. If these are significant an early return visit is scheduled but if all appears to be healing well the patient is reviewed 4 to 6 weeks later.

References

1. Levine HL. Endoscopic Sinus Surgery: Reasons For Failure. Oper Tech Otolaryngol–Head Neck Surg 1995;6(3):176–179
2. Kennedy DW, Senior BA. Endoscopic sinus surgery. A review. Otolaryngol Clin North Am 1997;30(3):313–330

3. Stammberger H, Kopp W, Dekornfeld TJ, Hawke M. Functional Endoscopic Sinus Surgery: The Messerklinger Technique. Special Endoscopic Anatomy. Philadelphia, PA: B.C. Decker Publishers; 1991:61–90

4. Stammberger H, Posawetz W. Functional endoscopic sinus surgery. Concept, indications and results of the Messerklinger technique. Eur Arch Otorhinolaryngol 1990;247(2):63–76

5. Thawley SE, Deddens AE. Transfrontal Endoscopic Management of Frontal Recess Disease. Am J Rhinol 1995;9(6):307–311

6. Setliff RC III. Minimally invasive sinus surgery: the rationale and the technique. Otolaryngol Clin North Am 1996;29(1):115–124

7. Catalano PJ, Setcliffe RC III, Catalano LA. Minimally invasive sinus surgery in the geriatric patient. Oper Tech Otolaryngol–Head Neck Surg 2001;12(2):85–90

8. Catalano P, Roffman E. Outcome in patients with chronic sinusitis after the minimally invasive sinus technique. Am J Rhinol 2003;17(1):17–22

9. Kuhn FA, Javer AR, Nagpal K, Citardi MJ. The frontal sinus rescue procedure: early experience and three-year follow-up. Am J Rhinol 2000;14(4):211–216

10. May M, Schaitkin B. Frontal Sinus Surgery: Endonasal Drainage Instead of an External Osteoplastic Approach. Oper Tech Otolaryngol–Head Neck Surg 1995;6(3):184–192

11. Schaefer SD, Close LG. Endoscopic management of frontal sinus disease. Laryngoscope 1990;100(2 Pt 1):155–160

12. Kuhn FA. Chronic frontal sinusitis: the endoscopic frontal recess approach. Operative techniques. Otolaryngol Head Neck Surg 1996;7(3):222–229

13. Wormald PJ. Three Dimensional building block approach to understanding the anatomy of the frontal recess and frontal sinus. Op Tech in OL&HNS 2006;17(1):2–5

14. Wormald PJ. Surgery of the frontal recess and frontal sinus. Rhinology 2005;43(2):82–85

15. Wormald PJ. The axillary flap approach to the frontal recess. Laryngoscope 2002;112(3):494–499

16. Wormald PJ. The agger nasi cell: the key to understanding the anatomy of the frontal recess. Otolaryngol Head Neck Surg 2003;129(5):497–507

17. Wormald PJ, Hoseman W, Callejas C, et al. The International Frontal Sinus Anatomy Classification (IFAC) and Classification of the Extent of Endoscopic Frontal Sinus Surgery (EFSS). Int Forum Allergy Rhinol 2016;6(7):677–696

18. Harvey RJ, Shelton W, Timperley D, et al. Using fixed anatomical landmarks in endoscopic skull base surgery. Am J Rhinol Allergy 2010;24(4):301–305

19. Wormald PJ, Hoseman W, Callejas C, et al. The International Frontal Sinus Anatomy Classification (IFAC) and Classification of the Extent of Endoscopic Frontal Sinus Surgery (EFSS). Int Forum Allergy Rhinol 2016;6(7):677–696

20. Kang SK, White PS, Lee MS, Ram B, Ogston S. A randomized control trial of surgical task performance in frontal recess surgery: zero degree versus angled telescopes. Am J Rhinol 2002;16(1):33–36

21. Paramasivan S, Jones D, Baker L, et al. The use of chitosan-dextran gel shows anti-inflammatory, antibiofilm, and antiproliferative properties in fibroblast cell culture. Am J Rhinol Allergy 2014;28(5):361–365

22. Valentine R, Athanasiadis T, Moratti S, Robinson S, Wormald PJ. The efficacy of a novel chitosan gel on hemostasis after endoscopic sinus surgery in a sheep model of chronic rhinosinusitis. Am J Rhinol Allergy 2009;23(1):71–75

23. Athanasiadis T, Beule AG, Robinson BH, Robinson SR, Shi Z, Wormald PJ. Effects of a novel chitosan gel on mucosal wound healing following endoscopic sinus surgery in a sheep model of chronic rhinosinusitis. Laryngoscope 2008;118(6):1088–1094

24. Valentine R, Athanasiadis T, Moratti S, Hanton L, Robinson S, Wormald PJ. The efficacy of a novel chitosan gel on hemostasis and wound healing after endoscopic sinus surgery. Am J Rhinol Allergy 2010;24(1):70–75

25. Ngoc Ha T, Valentine R, Moratti S, Robinson S, Hanton L, Wormald PJ. A blinded randomized controlled trial evaluating the efficacy of chitosan gel on ostial stenosis following endoscopic sinus surgery. Int Forum Allergy Rhinol 2013;3(7):573–580

8 Surgery of the Bulla Ethmoidalis, Middle Turbinate, Posterior Ethmoids, and Sphenoidotomy, Including Three-Dimensional Reconstruction of the Posterior Ethmoids

◆ Introduction

If the embryology of the sinuses is reviewed, the middle turbinate forms from the third lamella and the superior turbinate from the fourth lamella. The ground lamella of the middle turbinate divides the ethmoid sinuses into anterior ethmoid sinuses (anterior to the ground lamella) and posterior ethmoid sinuses (posterior to the ground lamella). Anterior ethmoid sinuses are further subdivided into those associated with the agger nasi and frontal process of the maxilla—the agger nasi cell (ANC) and supra agger cells, and cells associated with the bulla ethmoidalis. The bulla ethmoidalis forms from the second embryological lamella. It is a large ethmoid air cell directly anterior to the middle turbinate lamella. Cells directly above the bulla ethmoidalis are referred to as supra bulla cells. Posterior ethmoidal cells are found behind the middle turbinate ground lamella and anterior to the lamella of the superior turbinate.

◆ The Bulla Ethmoidalis and Supra Bulla Cells

The variations associated with the supra bulla cells are discussed in Chapter 6. The bulla ethmoidalis is either a single cell or group of cells that are visible directly behind the free edge of the middle and horizontal portions of uncinate process. The gap between the anterior face of the bulla ethmoidalis and the free edge of the uncinate process is known as the hiatus semilunaris which is the entrance to the ethmoidal infundibulum. The bulla ethmoidalis will usually have a posterior wall that is separate from the vertical portion of the ground lamella. The space between its posterior wall and the ground lamella is known as the retro-bulla recess. A supra bulla recess can also form from the retro-bulla recess as it pneumatizes over the top of the bulla. The bulla ethmoidalis, like all sinuses, drains via a natural ostium. This can usually be found on its posteromedial aspect in the retro-bulla recess.

To find the natural ostium, a double right-angled probe is passed medial to the bulla between the bulla and the middle turbinate. The tip of the probe is gently rotated laterally until it falls into the natural ostium (**Fig. 8.1**). As the probe is pulled forward, the medial and anterior walls are fractured. This fracture should be in continuity with the natural ostium.

To open the bulla ethmoidalis, a microdebrider is placed in this fractured area and the medial wall and anterior wall of the bulla removed. This allows the natural ostium to be enlarged and be a part of the opening created into the bulla. This follows the general philosophy of endoscopic sinus surgery of including the natural ostium in any opening made into a sinus. If only a mini-ESS is being performed (uncinectomy and opening of the bulla), then 3 or 4 mm of the anterior and inferior edge of the bulla is retained. This 3–4 mm of the anterior face of the bulla forms the posterosuperior part of the final common drainage pathway (see Chapter 5). This region is termed the "final common drainage pathway" as mucus from the frontal and anterior ethmoid cells and maxillary sinus is cleared to the nasopharynx along this pathway (**Fig. 8.2**).

If a posterior ethmoidectomy is to be performed in addition to opening the bulla, none of its anterior wall is retained. Removing the bulla in its entirety gives improved access to the posterior ethmoid complex but also allows the lamina papyracea to be identified. Identification of the lamina at this point is vitally important to understanding the position of the orbit during dissection of the posterior ethmoids. Failure to properly identify the lamina will often leave cells attached to the lamina and result in the surgery being driven medially and result in dissection being performed in a narrow corridor where identification of the other important landmarks becomes increasingly difficult. If the surgeon is confined to a narrow medial corridor, identification of the superior turbinate and anterior wall of the sphenoid becomes more difficult. Once the sphenoid is opened, identification of the skull base is also more difficult. The narrowness of the working corridor plus any blood in the field often will result in tentative surgery and incomplete removal of cells with a less than ideal postsurgery result. To accurately identify the lamina at this stage, the sur-

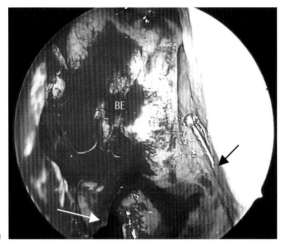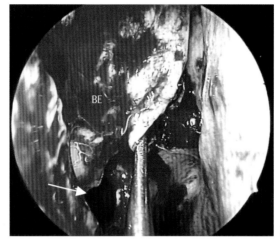

Fig. 8.1 (**a**) The ball-probe (*black arrow*) is slid medial to the anterior face of the bulla ethmoidalis (BE). (**b**) The anterior face of the bulla is fractured, creating an edge for the microdebrider. The maxillary sinus ostium marked by a *white arrow*.

geon should first identify the natural ostium of the maxillary sinus. Once this has been enlarged the roof of the maxillary sinus is identified and then followed to where the bulla attaches to the lamina, the lamina should be visible behind the anterior wall of the bulla with a zero- or 30-degree scope.

◆ The Three-Dimensional Reconstruction of the Posterior Ethmoids

As described in Chapter 6, three-dimensional (3D) anatomical reconstruction and planning of each surgical step is performed prior to dissection of the frontal recess. In a similar

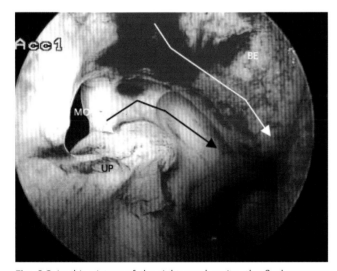

Fig. 8.2 In this picture of the right nasal cavity, the final common drainage pathway is indicated by the *black arrow*. This also indicates the drainage pathway of the maxillary sinus. The *white arrow* indicates the drainage pathway of the frontal and anterior ethmoidal cells along the anterior face of the bulla ethmoidalis (BE). This portion of the BE forms the posterosuperior part of the final common drainage pathway. The residual portion of the uncinate process (UP) after uncinectomy and the natural ostium of the maxillary sinus (MO) are marked.

manner as the agger nasi cell is used as the cornerstone of the dissection of the frontal recess dissection, a cell or space in the posterior ethmoids needs to be identified that can be accurately correlated to the CT scan. The space used in the 3D reconstruction of the posterior ethmoids is the superior meatus. To be able to accurately identify the superior meatus on sequential CT scans, the transition from the anterior to the posterior ethmoids must be established on the CT scans. If the coronal CT scans are evaluated, the first landmark that is sought is the superior turbinate. Each sequential coronal CT is evaluated until the superior turbinate is identified (**Fig. 8.3**).

Once the transition between the anterior and posterior ethmoids is established on the CT scans, the superior meatus (SM) should be sought. This is clearly marked in **Fig. 8.3b–d**, with the *crosshairs*. This space is directly above the horizontal part of the ground lamella and should be easily located on all CT scans. The ability of the surgeon to locate this space on both the CT scan and the patient is critical as it provides the starting point of the surgery. Once penetration of the posterior ethmoids has taken place through the ground lamella, the superior meatus and superior turbinate are identified (**Fig. 8.4**). The surgeon now has a landmark in the dissection that can be clearly placed on the CT scan. Each sequential cell in the posterior ethmoids is identified and using the building block principle, a 3D picture of the posterior ethmoids can be constructed. However, before a complete understanding of the anatomy of the posterior ethmoids is possible, a clear understanding of the transition between posterior ethmoids and sphenoid is necessary. This follows the theme of understanding the transition between the frontal sinus and anterior ethmoids, between the anterior and posterior ethmoids, and finally between the posterior ethmoids and sphenoid. The key to determining the transition from the posterior ethmoids to the sphenoid is identifying the first coronal CT scan in which the solid posterior bony choanae can be seen. In **Fig. 8.5a**, the crosshairs are just anterior to the anterior face of the sphenoid and both on the coronal and parasagittal images a clear space extending to the skull base is seen (*white arrows*). In **Fig. 8.5b**, the crosshairs are placed on the bone of the anterior wall of the sphenoid and on the coronal CT (crosshairs) the horizontal

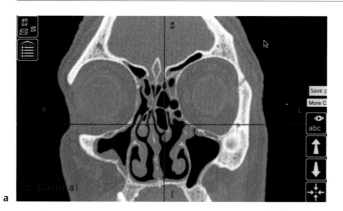

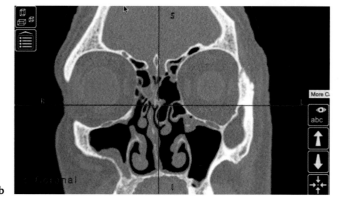

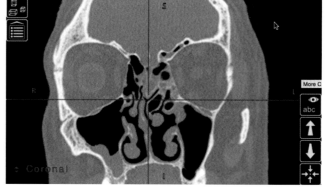

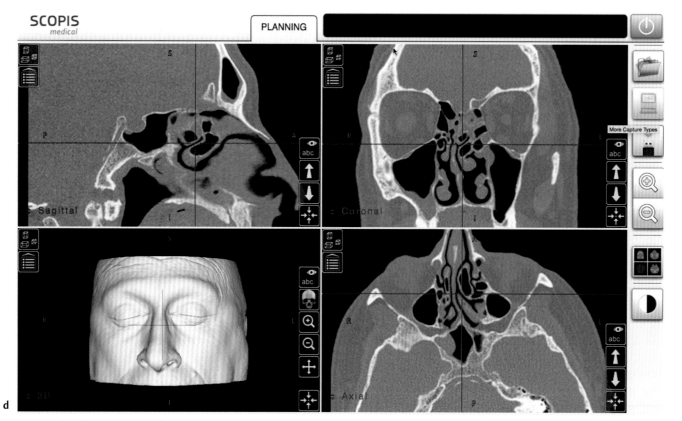

Fig. 8.3 The following sequential coronal CT scans show the transition of the anterior to the posterior ethmoids. (**a**) The *crosshairs* mark the middle turbinate. If the medial edge of the turbinate is followed superiorly, no superior turbinate can be seen. (**b**) The first indentation of the superior turbinate is seen (*crosshairs*). (**c**) The superior turbinate is well developed and (**d**) the position of the superior turbinate is clearly seen on both the parasagittal and axial CTs.

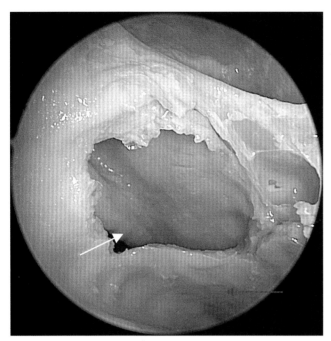

Fig. 8.4 This cadaveric image shows the horizontal ground lamella (*red arrow*); the vertical ground lamella has been opened with the anterior end of the superior turbinate (*white arrow*) visible.

bone of the floor of the sphenoid is seen. This marks the transition from the posterior to ethmoids to the sphenoid. Any coronal CT in which the horizontal bone is seen means that that scan is taken through the sphenoid sinus (**Fig. 8.5b,c**). In

Fig. 8.6a,b the crosshairs are placed in the two major posterior ethmoid air cells; in **Fig. 8.6c** the building blocks have been placed over these cells and one additional medial cell (green) so that the anatomical configuration of the posterior ethmoid cells can be understood. Finally, if a building block is placed over the sphenoid (**Fig. 8.7**, yellow block) and the drainage pathway of the sphenoid can be drawn onto the scans, a complete understanding of the posterior ethmoid and sphenoid complex is built (**Fig. 8.7**). Each configuration of the posterior ethmoids is different and each side of every patient needs to be independently assessed and the 3D picture built.

◆ Surgical Plan for the Posterior Ethmoids

Once a 3D reconstruction of the posterior ethmoids has been performed, a surgical plan is formulated as to how the dissection will be performed in the posterior ethmoids. The first step is to enter the superior meatus through the ground lamella in a region that can be easily identified on the CT scans. To achieve this, the transition from the posterior horizontal ground lamella to the vertical ground lamella needs to be identified. To positively identify the horizontal ground lamella, slide the endoscope under the middle turbinate toward the back end of the middle turbinate. As the posterior end of the middle turbinate is approached, the horizontal portion of the ground lamella is directly above the endoscope. The endoscope is brought anteriorly following the horizontal ground lamella until it turns vertically. At the point where it turns vertically, in the area directly adjacent to the middle

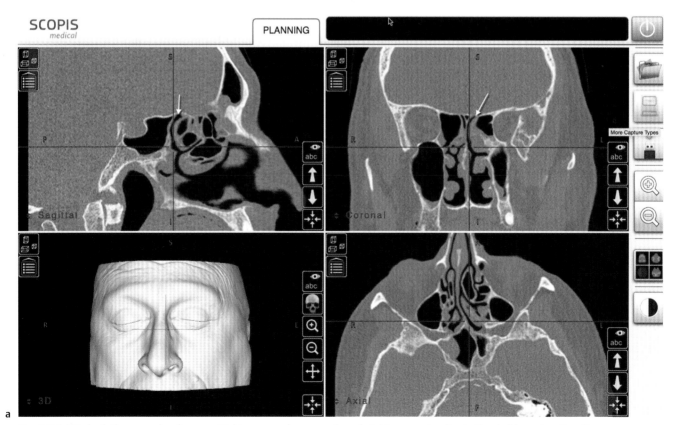

Fig. 8.5 (**a**) On both the coronal and parasagittal images, a clear space (*crosshairs*) is seen extending to the skull base. (*continued*)

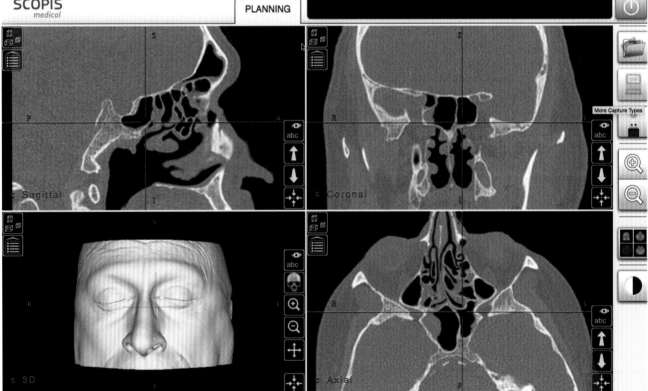

Fig. 8.5 (*continued*) (**b**) The crosshairs are placed on the bone of the anterior wall of the sphenoid. This marks the transition from the posterior to ethmoids to the sphenoid. In (**c**) the crosshairs are placed in the sphenoid.

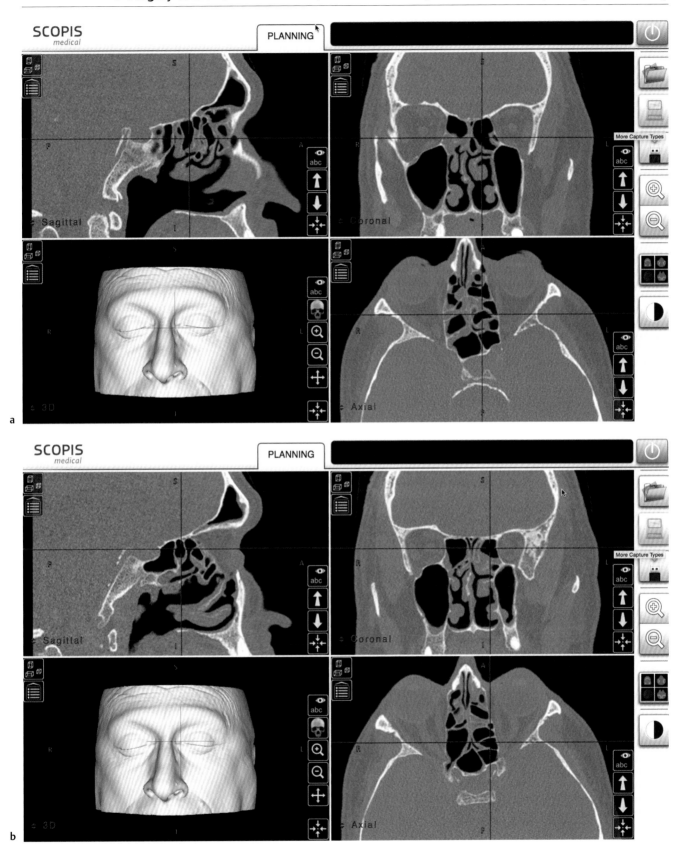

Fig. 8.6 (**a,b**) The *crosshairs* are placed in the two main posterior ethmoid air cells. (*continued*)

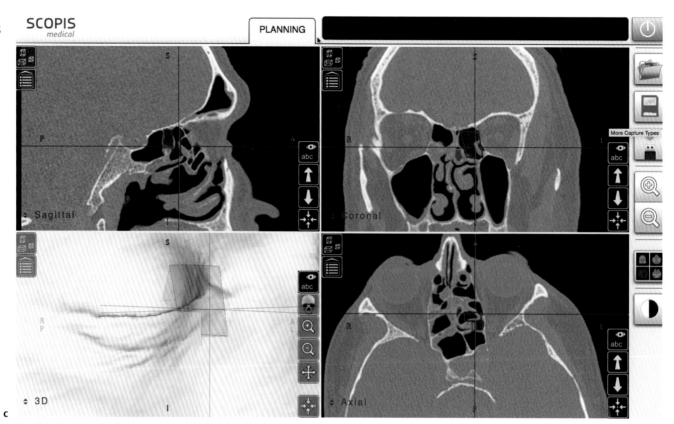

Fig. 8.6 (*continued*) (**c**) Illustrates how the building blocks can be used to understand the configuration of the cellular anatomy: blocks are placed over these cells and a 3D picture of the anatomy created.

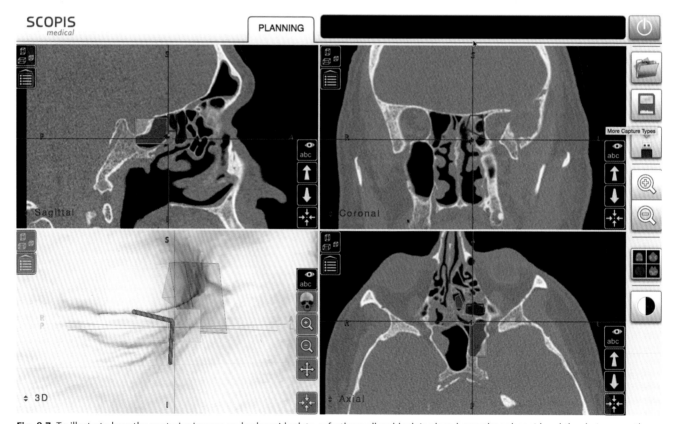

Fig. 8.7 To illustrate how the posterior images and sphenoid relate, a further yellow block is placed over the sphenoid and the drainage pathway of the sphenoid drawn in.

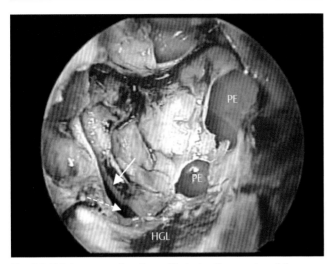

Fig. 8.8 This intraoperative picture illustrates the opening of the superior meatus on the left side (*broken white arrow*). The superior turbinate can be clearly seen (*solid white arrow*) and the partially opened posterior ethmoid (PE) cells are seen.

turbinate, the microdebrider or straight Blakesley is pushed through the ground lamella (**Fig. 8.8**, *broken white arrow*).

This access area is widened horizontally until the superior meatus and anterior edge of the superior turbinate are identified with certainty (**Fig. 8.8**, *solid white arrow*).

The surgeon can now place the point of dissection on the CT scans and knows how many and in what order the remaining cells are placed. These can then be sequentially entered and a complete dissection of the posterior ethmoids achieved. This low and medial entry into the posterior ethmoids minimizes the potential risk of damage to the skull base which may occur if entry is made higher on the vertical portion of the ground lamella.[1]

◆ The Middle Turbinate

In most patients, the middle turbinate is preserved. It is important that the middle turbinate is not destabilized during surgery. The most common cause for destabilization of the middle turbinate is fracturing its anterior vertical insertion from the skull base. The axillary flap is designed to preserve this insertion but does remove some support from the anterior insertion of the middle turbinate. The horizontal portion of the ground lamella should also be preserved to give posterior stability to the middle turbinate. However, excessive manipulation of the middle turbinate can fracture the turbinate's insertion on the skull base and result in it becoming floppy. The maneuver that should be avoided is placing the endoscope and instruments medial to the middle turbinate. The combination of a 4-mm endoscope and a 4-mm instrument will usually be enough to fracture the middle turbinate. Therefore, the techniques of posterior ethmoidectomy and sphenoidotomy are described through the middle meatus medial to the superior turbinate rather than medial to the middle turbinate. Despite all attempts to preserve the middle turbinate, there are some situations where partial or total resection of the middle turbinate is necessary.

Concha Bullosa

Patients with a concha bullosa need to have the lateral lamella of the middle turbinate removed to improve access to the middle meatus and, as this cell is often involved in the disease process, to clear the disease. In order to minimize damage to the lateral mucosa of the medial lamella, a scalpel is used to incise the anterior face of the concha bullosa vertically (**Fig. 8.9**).

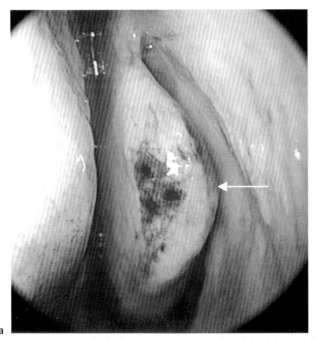

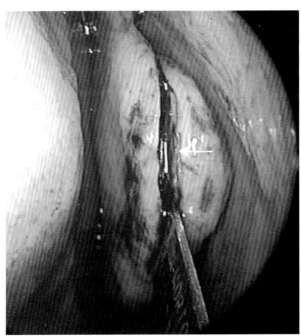

a   b

Fig. 8.9 (**a**) The concha bullosa is seen. Note the breadth of the middle turbinate (*white arrow*). (**b**) The scalpel has been used to vertically incise (*white arrow*) the concha separating the medial and lateral lamella.

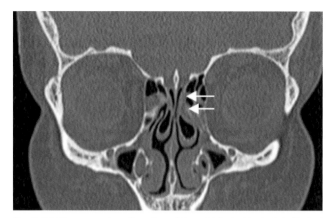

Fig. 8.10 The upward continuation of the middle turbinate is indicated with *solid white arrows*. Note the opacity medial to this upward continuation of the lateral lamella of the middle turbinate.

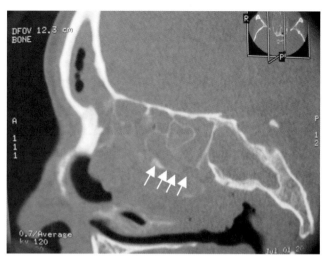

Fig. 8.11 The horizontal portion of the ground lamella is indicated by a series of *solid white arrows*. If this structure is maintained in patients with extensive nasal polyps it may result in underaeration of the posterior ethmoids and sphenoid.

A pair of 5-mm endoscopic scissors* (Integra) is used to continue the incision along the inferior margin of the middle turbinate to the lateral insertion of the turbinate on the lateral nasal wall. The scissors are used to continue the superior incision posterior as high as possible on the turbinate but progressively moving inferiorly as the posterior region of the turbinate is approached. Once the lateral lamella of the turbinate has been resected it is removed. The residual upward continuation of the lateral lamella of the middle turbinate needs to be removed as part of the frontal recess and bulla ethmoidalis dissection. Failure to remove this upward continuation can result in residual disease in the medial compartment of the anterior ethmoids (**Fig. 8.10**).

Revision Surgery with Extensive Nasal Polyposis

The most common indication for middle turbinate resection is revision surgery with extensive polyposis. In patients who have previously undergone posterior ethmoidectomy, contracture of the horizontal part of the ground lamella may drag the middle turbinate laterally, narrowing the ethmoidal space. This results in underventilation of the posterior ethmoid region and could precipitate secretion retention in the posterior ethmoids and sphenoid and polyp formation.[2,3] In patients with massive polyposis often from Samter's triad (aspirin sensitivity, asthma, and polyps) or fungal sinusitis, increased aeration of the posterior ethmoid cavity may be necessary to reduce polyp recurrence.[2,3] In these patients it may be necessary to partially resect the lower half of the middle turbinate and the horizontal portion of the ground lamella. This marsupializes the posterior ethmoids and sphenoid sinus (after a large sphenoidotomy) into the posterior nasal cavity with improved postoperative aeration of these sinuses (**Fig. 8.11**). This also facilitates the penetration of topical medications and nasal douches postoperatively.

Lateralized Atrophic Middle Turbinate

In some patients, especially those with long standing severe septal deflections into the nasal cavity, the turbinate may

be underdeveloped, very floppy, and lateralized (**Fig. 8.12**). In these patients, part of the turbinate may be resected at the time of surgery. When part of the middle turbinate is resected, then the horizontal portion of the middle turbinate should also be removed flush with the lateral nasal wall. This almost invariably exposes the middle turbinate branch of the sphenopalatine artery with resultant bleeding and requires bipolar cautery.

Lateral Displacement of the Middle Turbinate with Narrowing of the Frontal Recess

Particularly in patients who have had previous surgery or in patients with substantial olfactory fossa polyps, lateral displacement of the middle turbinates may occur (**Fig. 8.13**).

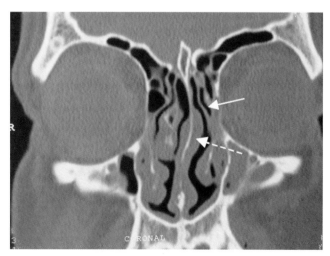

Fig. 8.12 CT scan illustrating a severe septal deflection (*broken white arrow*) and corresponding underdevelopment and lateralization of the middle turbinate on the left (*solid white arrow*).

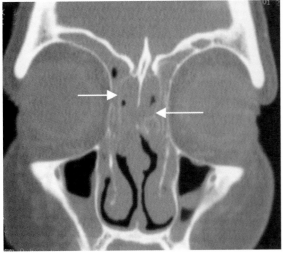
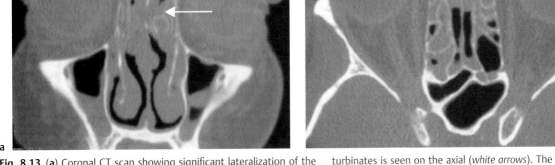

Fig. 8.13 (**a**) Coronal CT scan showing significant lateralization of the both middle turbinates (*white arrows*). Note opacified olfactory recesses in both (**a**) and (**b**). (**b**) The extent of the lateralization of the middle turbinates is seen on the axial (*white arrows*). The frontal recess is narrowed by at least 50% by this lateralization.

This narrows the outflow region of the frontal sinus substantially and creates two problems. The first is the very narrow lateral dimension of the frontal recess (**Fig. 8.13b**), which makes surgery in this region very difficult and increases the risk of damage to the lateral wall of the olfactory fossa. The degree of difficulty of the dissection increases if there is bleeding during the surgery. The lateralized portion of the middle turbinate is often thin and lacks rigidity and stability and this may result in this segment of the middle turbinate becoming unstable during surgery with resultant increased likelihood of postoperative lateralization and obstruction of the frontal ostium. The second problem is that as the sinuses heal after surgery, the narrow lateral dimension increases the likelihood of blood clot with subsequent fibrosis that leads to obstruction of the frontal ostium and consequently recurrent frontal sinusitis. If there are large polyps in the olfactory recess these may need to be resected to remove the lateral pressure that the polyps place on the middle turbinate. Care should be taken to limit the amount of raw tissue in the olfactory fossa to prevent scar formation in the olfactory fossa. This is best achieved by keeping the opening of the microdebrider blade facing only superiorly thereby preventing any lateral or medial mucosal damage.

Posterior Attachment of Middle Turbinate

The horizontal ground lamella attaches to the lateral nasal wall posterior to the maxillary sinus. Branches of the sphenopalatine artery traverse this region supplying blood to the middle turbinate. If this part of the ground lamella is removed, these vessels may bleed. This region is always meticulously inspected at the end of surgery and any bleeders cauterized with the suction bipolar forceps. Although the vessel may clot during surgery, coughing or straining in the postoperative period may dislodge the clot with consequent significant postoperative epistaxis.

Anatomical Configurations that Place the Patient at Risk During Surgery

Certain anatomical variations need to be sought on the CT scans prior to the dissection taking place. Identification of these may help avoid possible complications during the dissection of the posterior ethmoids.

Low Skull Base

A low skull base narrows the vertical height of the posterior ethmoids significantly. This is important for the surgeon to recognize before surgery in the posterior ethmoids is commenced. If the surgeon is unaware that the skull base is low, he or she may think that there may still be superior cells due to the low vertical height of the posterior ethmoids. Attempts to dissect further may injure the skull base associated dura and cause a CSF leak. The difference in vertical height with a normal skull base height and a patient with a low skull base is shown in **Fig. 8.14**.

It is critical in a patient with a low skull base that the approach into the posterior ethmoids is low and medial. A high entry through the vertical portion of the ground lamella in a patient with a low skull base would certainly put the skull base at risk[1] (**Fig. 8.15**).

A Curved Posterior Skull Base

Normally the posterior skull base is flat and the surgeon can dissect from the lamina papyracea medially along the skull base to the insertion of the superior turbinate with a minimum of risk. However, some patients may have a significant curve to the roof of the posterior ethmoids and the surgeon should assess the CT scans prior to surgery to establish the status of the posterior ethmoid fovea ethmoidalis before

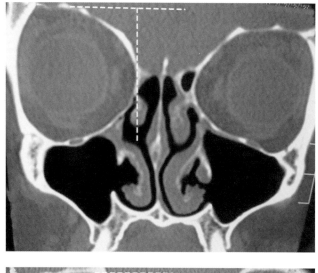

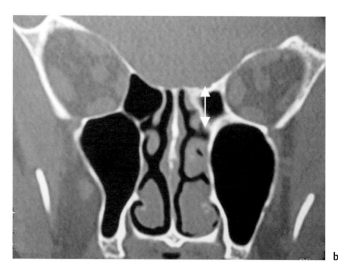

a

b

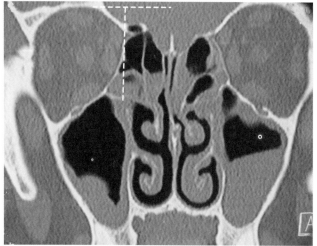

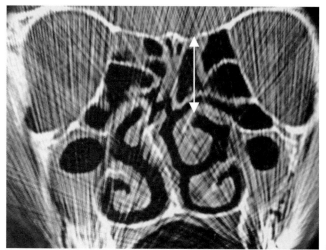

c

d

Fig. 8.14 (a,b) The skull base originates from a point almost halfway down the vertical height of the lamina papyracea of the orbit (*broken lines*), whereas (**c,d**) the more normal configuration is seen with the fovea ethmoidalis taking origin from the upper aspect of the lamina papyracea (*broken lines*). The vertical height of the ethmoid cavity (*solid double arrow*) is greater in scans (**c,d**) than in scans (**a,b**).

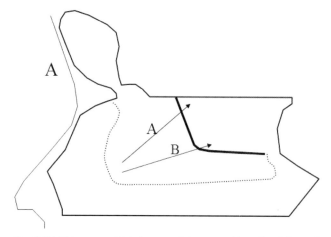

Fig. 8.15 This parasagittal diagram of the ground lamella of the middle turbinate illustrates the potential danger of entering the posterior ethmoids high on the vertical portion of the ground lamella (*A, arrow*) compared to the safety of entering the posterior ethmoids as low and medial possible (*B, arrow*).

surgery is performed in this area (**Fig. 8.16**). Failure to recognize this curvature may result in the surgeon thinking that there is another cell situated medially on the skull base and, if removal is attempted, injury to the skull base can occur.

Sphenoethmoidal Cell (Onodi Cell)

Previous descriptions of the sphenoethmoidal (Onodi) cell state that it is a pneumatization of the posterior ethmoid cell laterally[1,4] and that the incidence can be as high as 42%.[5] However, in most cases, this is not true as the sphenoethmoidal (Onodi) cell is rather a posterior pneumatization of the ethmoid cell over the sphenoid pushing the sphenoid inferiorly. To accurately identify a sphenoethmoidal (Onodi) cell, one must be able to recognize the transition from the posterior ethmoids to the sphenoid. This follows the theme of being able to recognize the transition from frontal sinus to anterior ethmoids (frontal recess), to recognize the transition from anterior to posterior ethmoids, and finally to be able to recognize

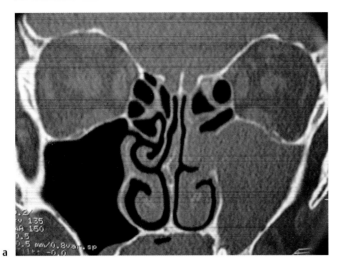

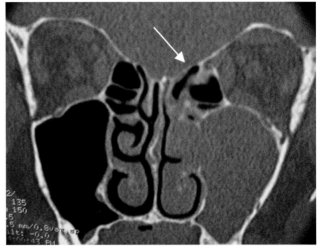

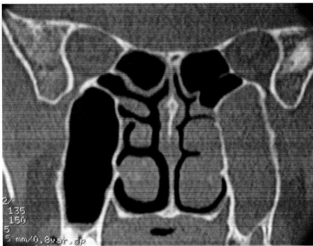

Fig. 8.16 (a) The fovea is horizontal, attaching to the vertical lateral wall of the olfactory fossa. (b) The *white arrow* indicates the curved fovea ethmoidalis at the level of the anterior ethmoidal artery. (c) Illustrates how the fovea flattens as the sphenoid is approached.

the transition from posterior ethmoids to sphenoid sinus. If sequential coronal CT scans of the posterior ethmoids are evaluated, the transition from posterior ethmoids to sphenoid starts on the first CT scan that the posterior bony choanae can be seen (see **Fig. 8.5**). Once the solid bony rim of the posterior choanae is identified, the cell sitting directly above this solid bone should be the sphenoid sinus. If there is any horizontal bony septation above this cell in this or subsequent more posterior coronal CT scans, this would be suspicious that there may be a sphenoethmoidal (Onodi) cell present (**Fig. 8.17**).

The posterior ethmoid cells should be followed in each sequential CT scan and one should establish whether a posterior ethmoid cell pneumatizes over the sphenoid. The parasagittal scan should always be checked as this can be very useful in recognizing a sphenoethmoidal (Onodi) cell. In **Fig. 8.18**, one can clearly see how the posterior ethmoid cell pneumatizes over the top of the sphenoid (SPH) which in turn creates the most useful characteristic of a sphenoethmoidal (Onodi) cell—the horizontal septum (*pink arrow*) seen on a scan that is taken through the sphenoid. In this patient, the optic nerve protrudes into the posterior sphenoethmoidal cell and would be vulnerable during surgery. Thus, the transition from the posterior ethmoids to the sphenoid is critical to establish

before the horizontal septation is sought. This septation is created by the anterior face of the sphenoid being pushed into a more horizontal plane by the sphenoethmoidal (Onodi) cell pneumatizing over the top of the sphenoid. Axial scans are of little value in diagnosing a sphenoethmoidal (Onodi) cell.

It is important to identify an Onodi cell as this cell has the optic nerve in its posterosuperior region (**Fig. 8.18**). If the cell is not recognized, the surgeon may not realize that the sphenoid sinus has been pushed inferiorly below the Onodi cell. If the access into the sphenoid is attempted through the Onodi cell, damage to the optic nerve, skull base, or carotid artery may result as these structures are adjacent to this cell whereas the sphenoid is below and more medial. The relationship between the Onodi cell and optic nerve can be clearly seen in **Fig. 8.18a**.

◆ Sphenoidotomy

After dissection of the posterior ethmoids, the sphenoid can be entered. The sphenoid ostium is located medial to the superior turbinate in 83% of patients.[6] If the sphenoid is normal (without disease visible on the CT scan), the sphenoethmoidal

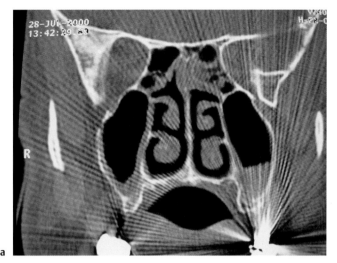

a

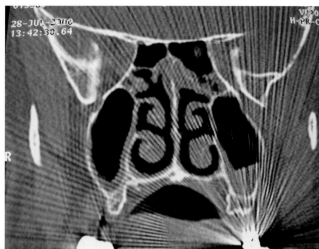

b

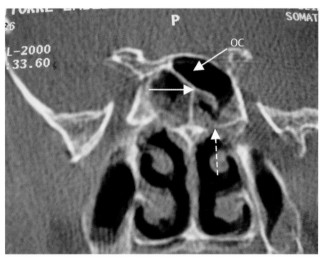

c

Fig. 8.17 The transition from the posterior ethmoids to the sphenoid occurs between CT scans (**b**) and (**c**). (**c**) The bony posterior choanae (*broken white arrow*) are seen. At the point where a complete bony posterior choana is identified, the sinus directly above this bony choanae should be the sphenoid sinus. The horizontal septation (*white arrow*) separates the sphenoid from the Onodi cell (OC) above it.

recess can be inspected through the middle meatus by gently moving the superior turbinate laterally and visualizing the recess. If there is no disease in the sphenoethmoidal recess, the sphenoid ostium should be visible in most patients. If the sphenoethmoidal recess is diseased (inflamed hypertrophic mucosa or the presence of polyps), then consideration can be given to clearance of the recess usually with sphenoidotomy. If significant mucosal trauma is created in the recess by clearance of disease, then it is likely that the sphenoid ostium may be closed by scar tissue formation during healing and a sphenoidotomy should be performed to prevent this occurrence. If the sphenoid is diseased on the CT scan, it should be opened. It is preferable to open the sphenoid through the posterior ethmoids rather than by passing the instruments and endoscope medial to the middle turbinate as previously emphasized.[7] The medial to the middle turbinate route to the sphenoid ostium is only used when no middle meatal surgery is necessary such as a patient with isolated sphenoid disease or for pituitary surgery. In the transethmoidal route, the already identified superior turbinate is used as the critical landmark for sphenoidotomy.[7,8] The lower third to half of the superior turbinate is removed either with a microdebrider or straight through-biting forceps (**Fig. 8.19**). Once the turbinate is removed flush with the anterior face of the sphenoid, the microdebrider is

used to palpate the face for the natural ostium of the sphenoid. It is usually found at the junction of the lower third and upper two-thirds but may be as high as the halfway point of the superior turbinate and is usually medial to the turbinate on the anterior face of the sphenoid[6] (**Fig. 8.19**).

In the majority of patients, the natural ostium will be located using the landmarks described above. However, in patients with a sphenoethmoidal (Onodi) cell, the natural ostium may be lower and more medial as the sphenoid is compressed by the sphenoethmoidal cell pneumatizing over the top of it. If the tip of the microdebrider does not fall into the natural ostium, a smaller straight suction is used to palpate this region. If the natural ostium can still not be located, then the CT scan is reviewed to confirm the position and size of the sphenoid sinus before proceeding further. If a sphenoid is present then the following measurement technique should be followed to open the sphenoid. The bony rim of the posterior choana is located by passing the 4-mm microdebrider blade through the posterior ethmoids and into the nasopharynx (**Fig. 8.20**). The tip of the microdebrider blade is pushed against the mucosa just above the bony choanae on the anterior face of the sphenoid. This creates a 4-mm indentation. Two further indentations are made above this one thereby measuring 12 mm from the bony rim of the posterior choana (**Fig. 8.20**).

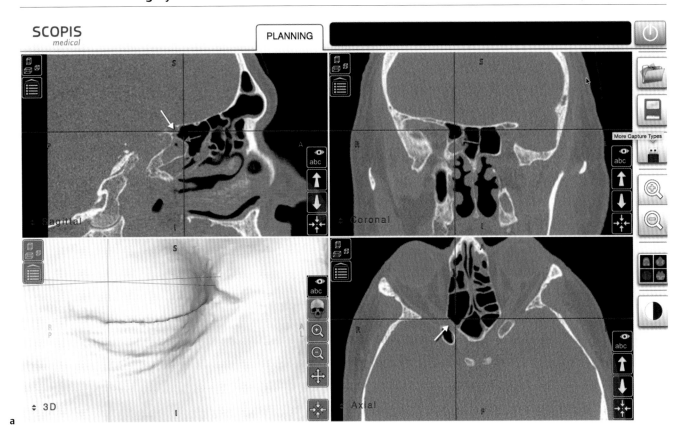

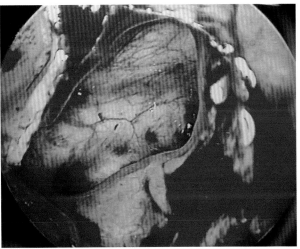

Fig. 8.18 (**a**) In the coronal CT, the horizontal septation is marked with a *red arrow*. The optic nerve can be clearly seen in the parasagittal and axial CT scans (*white arrow*). Note that the optic nerve is lying free in the posterior ethmoid cell with the cell having pneumatized around the nerve. (**b**) A clinical example of the optic nerve seen in an Onodi cell.

A Freer elevator is then used to push through the anterior face of the sphenoid directly above the third indentation. The tip of the instrument is pushed through the bone and once it has penetrated the sphenoid cavity, it is twisted to enlarge the opening. A microdebrider or Kerrison's punch is then used to further open the sinus. The natural ostium is opened with the punch or microdebrider initially inferiorly toward the floor of the sinus and then toward the lamina papyracea and into the posterior ethmoids (**Fig. 8.21**).

There should be at least 8 to 10 mm of anterior face of the sphenoid still above this lateral opening and this newly created opening should therefore be well below the optic nerve. The opening can be further enlarged directly superiorly from the natural ostium, medially and inferiorly as well (**Fig. 8.21**). Opening

of the natural ostium of the sphenoid invariably creates a circumferential raw surface around the natural ostium and therefore this opening needs to be enlarged into the posterior ethmoids to prevent postoperative stenosis. The anterior face of the sphenoid is removed up to the skull base and laterally to the lamina papyracea and then finally lowered to the floor of the sphenoid. The postnasal artery or vertical branch of the postnasal artery is often cut during widening of the sphenoid and requires bipolar cautery (**Fig. 8.22**). In patients with significant new bone formation, an inferiorly based mucosal flap can be elevated and the underlying bone drilled away before the flap is replaced.[9] This interrupts the circumferential raw area and prevents stenosis.

If the superior turbinate has been completely or partially removed by previous surgery, the measurement technique

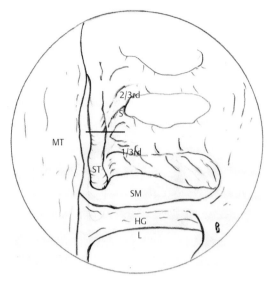

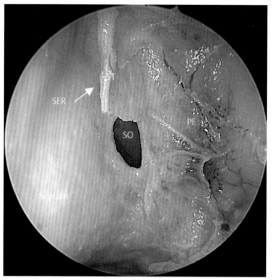

a

b

Fig. 8.19 (**a**) On the left side, the middle turbinate (MT), superior turbinate (ST), superior meatus (SM), and horizontal part of the ground lamella (HGL) are clearly identified before sphenoidotomy. In this figure, the posterior ethmoids have not as yet been opened. Once the posterior ethmoids have been sequentially opened, the superior turbinate is divided into the thirds. The lower third is removed with either a straight through-biting Blakesley or powered microdebrider up to the anterior face of sphenoid

and the sphenoid ostium identified before it is opened. (**b**) Cadaveric image taken with endoscope within the superior meatus on the left side. The lower third of the superior turbinate has been removed revealing the natural sphenoid ostium. Note how the anterior face of the sphenoid sinus is contributed by the sphenoethmoidal recess (*SER*) and the posterior wall of a posterior ethmoid cell (*PE*). *MT*, middle turbinate; *ST*, superior turbinate; *SM*, superior meatus; *HGL*, horizontal ground lamella.

described above is used to locate the position of the natural ostium of the sphenoid sinus. Resection of part of the superior turbinate may possibly remove some olfactory neurons so as much of this turbinate as possible is preserved. Studies done on olfaction after removal of the lower third of the superior turbinate have not been shown to adversely affect the sense of smell of the patient after surgery.[10] Sphenoidotomy for pituitary surgery is discussed in Chapter 13.

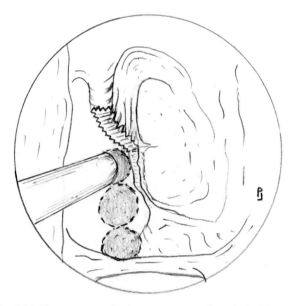

Fig. 8.20 Three sequential indentations are made with the blunt end of the 4-mm microdebrider blade starting at the medial upper limit of the posterior bony choana and moving directly superiorly medial to the cut edge of the superior turbinate.

Complications of Sphenoidotomy

Epistaxis

Bleeding is very common from the posterior nasal artery as it traverses the anterior face of the sphenoid on its way to the posterior septum. The posterior nasal artery is a branch of the sphenopalatine artery and travels horizontally just above the posterior choana (**Fig. 8.22**). It gives off a vertical branch that supplies the anterior face of the sphenoid. If this vertical branch is transected (and it often is as the sphenoid ostium is enlarged), a minor bleeder will be seen on the lower opening of the sphenoid. If the sphenoid ostium is further enlarged inferiorly toward the floor of the sphenoid sinus, the main trunk of the posterior nasal artery can be transected and result in a significant bleeder which usually spurts in a horizontal and medial direction. This is best managed with the suction-bipolar forceps* (Integra) as the blood can be suctioned and cautery rapidly applied before the active bleeding results in blood vessels being covered in blood and no longer visible for precise cautery. If a standard suction and standard bipolar forceps are used, the bleeder is usually so active that by the time the suction is removed and the bipolar forceps positioned the vessel can no longer be seen. Because the suction bipolar has integrated suction, this problem can be rapidly overcome.

Damage to the Optic Nerve and CSF Leak

The most common cause of injury to the optic nerve during ESS is when a sphenoidotomy is attempted too high and too lateral and damage is caused to the orbital apex and optic nerve. In **Fig. 8.22** a diagrammatic view of the posterior ethmoids and superior turbinate is presented. Attempted entry into the

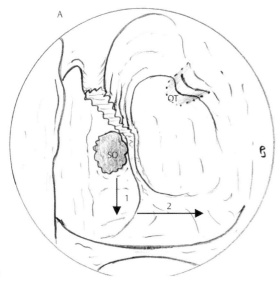

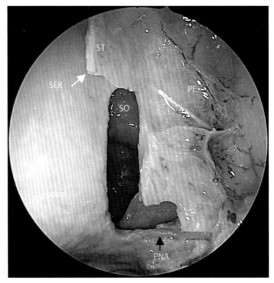

a

b

Fig. 8.21 (**a**) The sphenoid ostium (SO) is first opened inferiorly (*black arrow 1*) then laterally (*black arrow 2*). This should afford a clear view into the sphenoid sinus and the remaining anterior face of the sphenoid can be removed up toward the optic tubercle (OT) but usually stopping short of the tubercle to lessen the potential risk to the optic nerve. (**b**) A cadaveric image demonstrating technique for sphenoidotomy.

Note how the sphenoid is opened down to the posterior nasal artery as it transverses the anterior face of the sphenoid on its way to the posterior septum. *SO*, sphenoid ostium; *OT*, optic tubercle; *SER*, sphenoethmoidal recess; *PE*, posterior ethmoid cell; *ST*, superior turbinate; *PNA*, posterior nasal artery.

sphenoid in the superior lateral region will take the surgeon onto the orbital apex and optic nerve and even into the anterior skull base. This can result in a devastating complication of a damaged optic nerve with visual loss and a CSF leak with potential intracranial damage. In general, this situation begins when entry into the posterior ethmoids through the vertical portion of the ground lamella is made too high. The whole direction of surgery is then toward the skull base and if the surgeon is

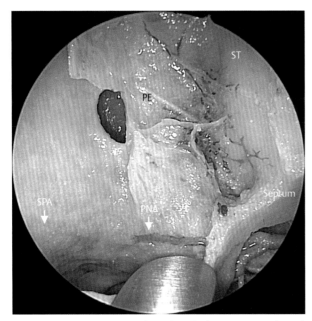

Fig. 8.22 Cadaveric image on the right side demonstrating the sphenopalatine artery (SPA) giving off the posterior nasal artery (PNA). This branch runs along the anterior face of the sphenoid, and can be inadvertently transected during sphenoidotomy. *PE*, posterior ethmoid cell; *ST*, superior turbinate; *SO*, sphenoid ostium.

inexperienced and does not recognize this, he or she may assume that the structure in front of them is a sloping anterior wall of the sphenoid sinus rather than the sloping wall of the skull base. If the skull base is thinner than usual, then entry into the anterior cranial fossa and/or damage to the optic nerve can occur. The key to preventing this devastating complication is to identify the superior meatus as the first step in the dissection of the posterior ethmoids immediately after the ground lamella is penetrated. This forces the surgeon to keep removing the ground lamella inferiorly until the superior meatus is clearly identified. If this dissection is continued and the anterior end of the superior turbinate is correctly identified, the surgeon is in the correct plane and place and so the risk of mistaking the skull base for the anterior face of the sphenoid should be minimized.

The other area that the optic nerve can be damaged is in the superolateral wall of the sphenoid sinus. The optic nerve is dehiscent in about 12%[5] of patients and inadvertent injury during surgery within the sphenoid sinus may lead to visual loss or blindness. It is tempting to use the microdebrider to remove polyps in the sphenoid but great care needs to be taken using the microdebrider in this sinus. In general, the microdebrider should only be used along the floor and medial wall of the sphenoid and not in the superior or lateral region. Surgeons are also concerned when the sphenoidotomy is widened in a lateral direction. There are a few rules to follow during sphenoidotomy that can minimize the risk to the optic nerve. The natural ostium of the sphenoid is generally around the lower third of the superior turbinate's insertion into the anterior face of the sphenoid. The forward biting Hajek Koeffler punch is used to enlarge this natural ostium first inferiorly toward the floor and then laterally toward the orbit. As the orbit is approached, the instrument should be well below the orbital apex and optic nerve (**Fig. 8.21**).

The second rule is that if the distal jaw of the biting mechanism of the Hajek Koeffler punch can be placed behind a bony septation it is generally safe to remove. Even a septation arising from the optic nerve can be safely removed onto the nerve by allowing the punch to rest on the nerve while the septation is engaged between the jaws of the punch and cleanly removed from the surface of the nerve. However, the superolateral region of the anterior face of the sphenoid is very carefully removed to lessen any possible risk to the optic nerve.

Damage to the Carotid Artery

The other major structure at risk during sphenoidotomy is the carotid artery. The bony wall covering the carotid is in most patients thin and dehiscent in 5–8%[5,11] of patients (**Fig. 8.23**).

This again emphasizes the risk of using a microdebrider with the cutting gate toward the lateral wall of the sphenoid. It only takes milliseconds for a dehiscent carotid artery wall to be damaged by the very effective cutting mechanisms in microdebriders with potentially catastrophic results. There are two other ways that the carotid artery may be damaged. In some patients, the natural ostium of the sphenoid sinus is very small and the surgeon is unable to identify it and thus allow a safe entry into the sphenoid sinus. If a small or narrow instrument is pushed hard onto the face of the sphenoid in an attempt to penetrate into the sphenoid, the bone may suddenly give way with the instrument being driven into the sinus with considerable force. This instrument can then inadvertently penetrate the thin or dehiscent bone or dehiscent carotid with subsequent massive hemorrhage. In the operative technique previously described, a blunt Freer elevator is used to push through the anterior face of the sphenoid sinus. The entry into the sphenoid can be well controlled with this instrument and the surgeon can easily feel as the bone is penetrated without risk of the instrument slipping inadvertently into the sinus. Also, the instrument has a large blunt surface and the penetration point is medial and inferior and is thus less likely to injure the carotid.

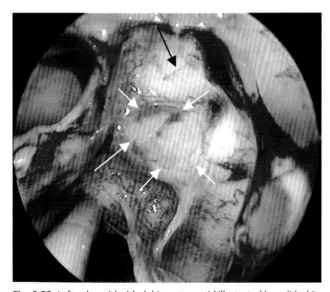

Fig. 8.23 Left sphenoid with dehiscent carotid illustrated by *solid white arrows* and optic nerve illustrated with *solid black arrow*.

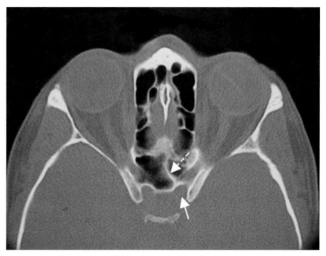

Fig. 8.24 This axial CT scan shows the sphenoid sinus septum (*broken arrow*) inserting into the anterior face of the left carotid artery (*solid arrow*). Rotation of this septum during removal may result in a tear of the wall of the carotid artery.

The second situation where a carotid injury may occur is if the intersinus septum of the sphenoid is attached to the anterior face of the carotid artery (**Fig. 8.24**).

If this septum needs to be taken down, as is often the case during pituitary surgery, and this attachment is grasped and rotated, it may fracture and bony spicules may damage the carotid wall. This can be avoided by using a through-biting instrument to sharply remove the septation. If the septation is too thick, a diamond bur can be used.

Management of a carotid artery hemorrhage is discussed in Chapter 22.

References

1. Edelstein DR, Liberatore L, Bushkin S, Han J.C. Applied anatomy of the posterior sinuses in relation to the optic nerve, trigeminal nerve and carotid artery. Am J Rhinol 1995;9:321–333
2. Klossek JM, Peloquin L, Friedman W, Ferrier J, Fontanel J. Diffuse nasal polyposis: postoperative long-term results after endoscopic sinus surgery and frontal irrigation. Otolaryngol Head Neck Surg 1997;117:355–361
3. DufourX, Bedier A, Ferrie J, Gohler C, Klossek JM. Diffuse nasal polyposis and endoscopic sinus surgery: long term results, a 65-case study. Laryngoscope 2004;114:1982–1987
4. Elwany S, Elsaeid I, Thabet H. Endoscopic anatomy of the sphenoid sinus. J Laryngol Otol 1999;113:122–126
5. Kainz J, Stammberger H. Danger areas of the posterior rhinobasis. An endoscopic and anatomical-surgical study. Acta Otolaryngol 1992;112:852–861
6. Kim H-U., Kim S-S, Kang S.S, Chung IH, Lee J-G, Yoon J-H. Surgical anatomy of the natural ostium of the sphenoid sinus. Laryngoscope 2001;111:1599–1602
7. Har-El G, Swanson R. The superior turbinectomy approach to isolated sphenoid sinus disease and to the sella turcica. Am J Rhinol 2001;15:149–156
8. Bolger W.E, Keyes A.S, Lanza D.C. Use of the superior meatus and superior turbinate in the endoscopic approach to the sphenoid sinus. Otolaryngol Head Neck Surg 1999;120:308–313
9. Donald P. Sphenoid marsupilization for chronic sphenoidal sinusitis. Laryngoscope 2000;110:1349–1352
10. Orlandi R, Lanza D, Bolger W, Clerico D, Kennedy D. The forgotten turbinate: the role of the superior turbinate in endoscopic sinus surgery. Am J Rhinol 1999;13:251–259
11. Unal B, Bademci G, Batay F, Avci E. Risky anatomic variations of sphenoid sinus for surgery. Surg Radiol Anat 2006;28:195–201

9 Extended Approaches to the Frontal Sinus: The Frontal Drillout or Modified Endoscopic Lothrop (Draf 3) Procedure

◆ Introduction

Chronic frontal sinusitis has challenged surgeons for many years. In the past, frontal sinus obliteration through an osteoplastic flap (OPF) approach was the gold standard for the management of recalcitrant frontal sinusitis.[1-3] Other external procedures such as frontoethmoidectomy have fallen into disfavor due to a failure rate of around 30%.[3,4] OPF and obliteration has a reported failure rate of around 10% but has a significant complication rate of around 65%.[3,5,6] The complications include cerebrospinal fluid (CSF) leak, frontal bossing, supraorbital neuralgia, chronic sepsis, mucocele formation, and chronic frontal bone osteitis with loss of the frontal sinus bone flap.[1-3,6] In recent years, the frontal drillout or modified endoscopic Lothrop (MEL) procedure/Draf 3 has been proposed as an alternative to the OPF with obliteration.[7-20] The frontal drillout procedure is based on the technique originally described by Lothrop in 1914.[21] This technique involves removal of the upper portion of the septum, the floor of the frontal sinus, and the inter-sinus septum. Removal of the floor was accomplished with the aid of a small external incision (similar to a Lynch incision) which created a window through which the drill can be observed. Although this procedure was successful in 29 out of 30 patients, the technique was considered too technically difficult for most surgeons to master and it was not until Draf in 1991[7] and Gross in 1995[8,9] published series of patients using a modified version of the technique that interest was renewed. The major modification to the frontal drillout technique is the absence of an external incision with the entire procedure performed endoscopically. The frontal drillout can be used as an alternative to OPF with obliteration with recent publications[12] showing excellent short-term success rates with minimal complications. The indications for the frontal drillout procedure should be the same as the indications for an OPF with obliteration and these are detailed here.[12]

◆ Indications for Frontal Drillout Procedure

Failed Endoscopic Sinus Surgery

The frontal drillout procedure is indicated in patients who have failed standard ESS techniques.[12] These include clearance of the frontal recess and removal of cells obstructing the frontal ostium.[20] In those very rare cases in which patients have a very large cell obstructing the frontal ostium (i.e., a very large supra agger frontal cell that extends into the frontal sinus significantly), management may include a primary frontal drillout procedure if the surgeon is certain that the cell is causing significant obstruction and that it is not possible to remove the cell with standard ESS techniques from below.[20] All patients should have had a standard ESS approach with an attempt to remove obstructing cells from the frontal ostium and improve the drainage of the frontal sinus. It is only if such techniques fail that the frontal drillout procedure should be considered for removal of a large supra agger frontal cell.[20] In **Fig. 9.1** the patient had undergone five previous standard ESS procedures and was still left with significant frontal sinus symptoms and a large supra agger frontal cell obstructing the frontal sinus ostium. This patient underwent a successful frontal drillout procedure.

Neo-Osteogenesis in the Frontal Recess and Frontal Ostium

Significant new bone formation in the regions of the frontal recess after ESS indicates probable osteitis. This can be difficult to manage with standard ESS techniques. The neo-osteogenesis results in a narrowed frontal sinus openings and increased vascularity in the region. Surgery to widen such narrowed ostia will often result in significant bleeding and

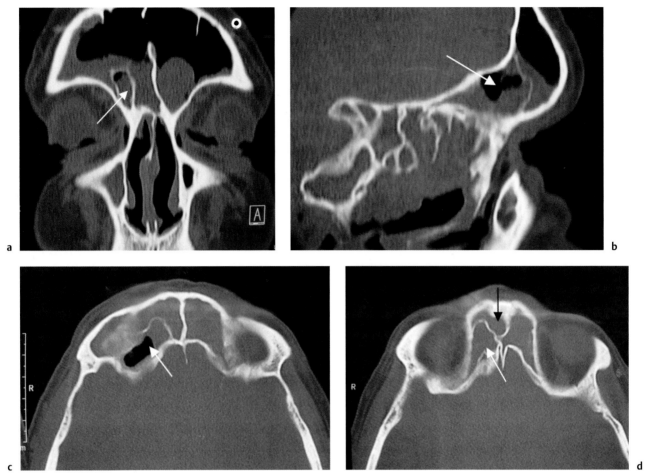

Fig. 9.1 (a–d) CT scans of a patient with a large supra agger frontal cell (*white arrow*) who had undergone multiple previous ESS procedures. (**d**) Note on the axial scan the significantly narrowed frontal sinus drainage pathway (*black arrow*) caused by the supra agger frontal cell (*white arrow*).

loss of mucosa. The healing process may produce significant re-stenosis as ongoing low-grade osteitis and sinusitis continues to stimulate new bone formation and fibrosis. The frontal drillout procedure overcomes this problem by drilling away a significant amount of the osteitic bone and creating the largest possible opening in the frontal sinuses. Even if some degree of re-stenosis occurs in the frontal drillout procedure, this should not affect the function of the frontal sinuses.[22] Recent work done on the frontal drillout procedure in our animal laboratory on the presence of neo-osteogenesis in a newly created frontal ostium suggests that most frontal ostia will re-stenose by an average of a third.[23] This figure was not affected by the presence of neo-osteogenesis that was found in 56% of animals. In addition, this re-stenosis did not affect the mucociliary drainage of the frontal sinuses as measured by the clearance of radioisotope from the frontal sinuses.[22] This average stenosis of the neo-frontal ostium was confirmed in subsequent human studies.[24] **Fig. 9.2** shows a patient with significant neo-osteogenesis in the left frontal ostium. This patient had undergone six previous standard ESS procedures in an attempt to maintain a patent left frontal ostium. In all cases the re-stenosis was rapid and associated with a return of frontal sinus symptoms.

Frontal Recess Adhesions

In patients who have previously undergone multiple ESS procedures, one will often find that the middle turbinates have been resected subtotally.[12] In this scenario, the middle turbinate remnant may lateralize and become adhesive to the lateral nasal wall in the frontal recess. This results in significant narrowing of the frontal drainage pathway and in some instances complete obstruction of the frontal ostium (**Fig. 9.3**). Standard ESS techniques will usually fail to re-create a mucosalized opening of sufficient diameter into the frontal sinuses and a frontal drillout procedure or OPF with obliteration should be considered.

Disease Processes with Resultant Loss of the Posterior Wall or Floor of the Frontal Sinus[18]

If the disease process results in bony erosion of either the posterior wall or floor of the frontal sinus, the mucosa of the sinus becomes adherent onto the dura or orbital periostium.[18] OPF with obliteration becomes extremely difficult in these patients as the mucosa cannot be safely or completely

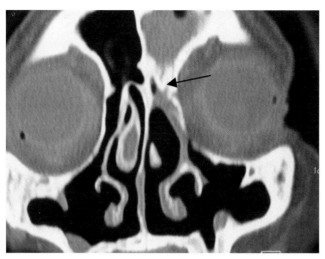
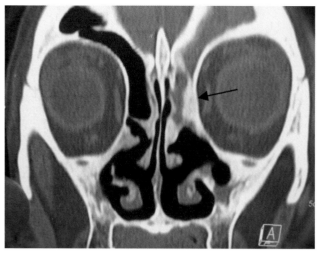

Fig. 9.2 (**a,b**) Coronal CT scans of a patient with multiple previous ESS procedures with neo-osteogenesis in the left frontal recess (*black arrow*) with associated chronic frontal sinusitis.

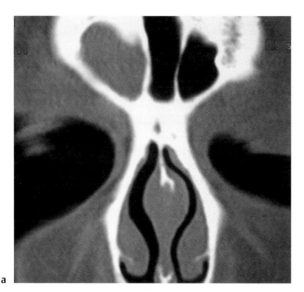
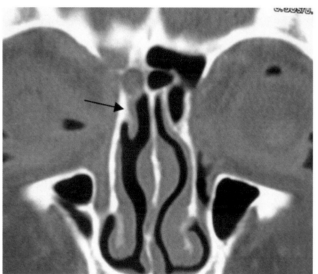

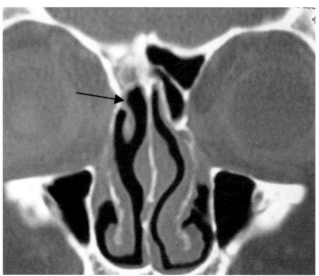

Fig. 9.3 (**a–c**) This patient has undergone previous middle turbinate resection and the stump (*black arrow*) has lateralized blocking the frontal ostium. (**c**) In addition, new bone formation can be seen above the middle turbinate.

removed from the dura or orbital periosteum and a recurrence of a mucocele is likely if the sinus is obliterated. These patients often have long-term severe chronic sinusitis and may have disease with a high incidence of recurrence such as fungal sinus disease. It is important to keep the frontal ostia open as obstruction of the frontal ostium may lead to either orbital or intracranial complications[18] (**Fig. 9.4**).

Failed Previous OPF with Obliteration with Mucocele Formation[13]

Frontal sinus obliteration has been the gold standard for the management of recalcitrant frontal sinusitis for many years. However, severe mucosal disease such as that seen in patients with Samter's triad (aspirin sensitivity, asthma, and nasal polyposis), allergic fungal sinusitis, and aggressive recurrent nasal polyposis is best managed endoscopically rather than with an OPF and obliteration.[14–18] There is now widespread agreement in the literature that the frontal drillout procedure should be the operation of first choice in this difficult group of patients.[14–18] One of the major problems with OPF and obliteration is the tendency for the adipose tissue placed in the frontal sinuses to resorb. Weber et al,[14] in a large study of 82 patients who underwent OPF and obliteration, showed that the majority of patients had less than 20% of the sinus obliterated after a median of 15.4 months.[14] In this patient group who aggressively form polyps, such space can be rapidly filled by even the smallest amount of residual mucosa inadvertently left in the frontal sinuses. In the postoperative period, this group tends to develop thick inspissated mucus amongst the regrowing polyps. Without a wide opening or marsupialization of the affected sinus, this mucus cannot be removed in the office. The inability to pass a large suction through the sinus ostium into the sinus cavity prevents this very tenacious mucus from being removed. A course of systemic prednisolone may loosen the mucus and lessen its tenacity, facilitating its removal. Clearance of this toxic material allows shrinkage of the polyps and reestablishment of the nasal airway with control of polyp growth. In most patients, it is a relatively simple procedure to create a wide maxillary antrostomy, completely remove

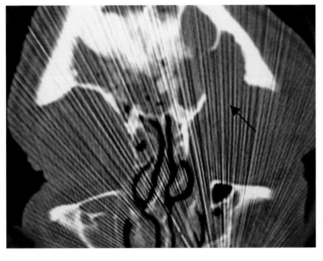
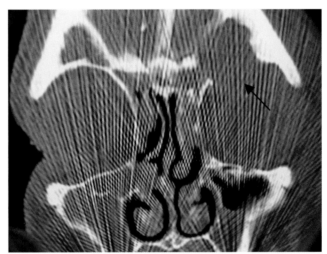
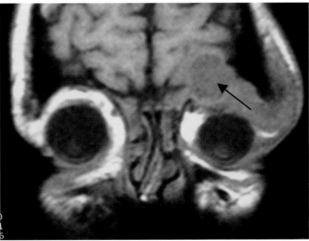
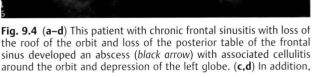
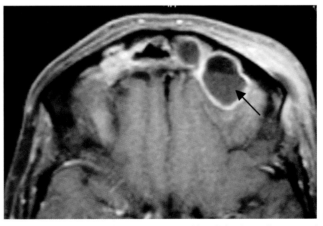

Fig. 9.4 (a–d) This patient with chronic frontal sinusitis with loss of the roof of the orbit and loss of the posterior table of the frontal sinus developed an abscess (*black arrow*) with associated cellulitis around the orbit and depression of the left globe. **(c,d)** In addition, this abscess had eroded the posterior table of the frontal sinus and compressed the anterior cerebral hemisphere. This was managed by a frontal drillout procedure with the creation of a large communal frontal ostium.

all ethmoid cells, and open widely the anterior face of the sphenoid sinus. However, the frontal sinuses are extremely difficult to access without the wide opening that the frontal drillout procedure creates. Naturally sized frontal ostia tend to be quickly obstructed by thickened mucosa and this results in a buildup of thick mucus in the frontal sinuses that may be resistant to aggressive prednisolone therapy and attempted suction clearance. One of the difficulties with OPF and obliteration in this group of patients is when there is loss

of bone over the orbit or dura. Due to the aggressive nature of the polyposis and in some cases aggravated by repeated surgeries, there may be loss of the anterior or posterior bony frontal sinus wall. This brings the mucocele lining in direct contact with the orbital periosteum and/or dura and makes it impossible to remove all the mucosa from these structures without resection.[15] Even microscopic mucosal remnants left on the periosteum or dura will lead to the development of a mucocele in the obliterated cavity (**Fig. 9.5**).

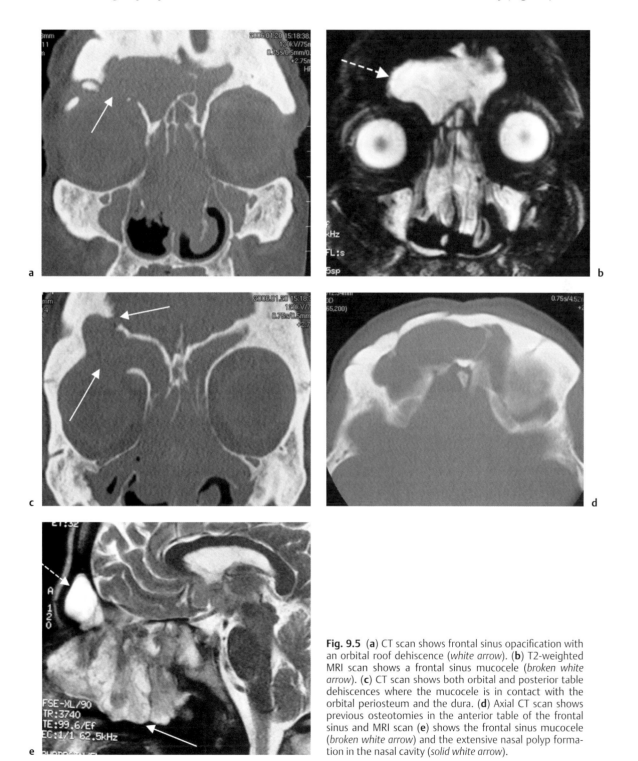

Fig. 9.5 (**a**) CT scan shows frontal sinus opacification with an orbital roof dehiscence (*white arrow*). (**b**) T2-weighted MRI scan shows a frontal sinus mucocele (*broken white arrow*). (**c**) CT scan shows both orbital and posterior table dehiscences where the mucocele is in contact with the orbital periosteum and the dura. (**d**) Axial CT scan shows previous osteotomies in the anterior table of the frontal sinus and MRI scan (**e**) shows the frontal sinus mucocele (*broken white arrow*) and the extensive nasal polyp formation in the nasal cavity (*solid white arrow*).

Another contraindication to OPF and obliteration is when the patient has very large pneumatized frontal sinuses.[15,18] In these patients it is extremely difficult to eradicate all the mucosa from the lateral and posterior recesses of the frontal sinus and this residual mucosa will form mucoceles that, if left untreated, will erode the bony walls of the sinus and may well give rise to either intracranial or orbital complications (**Fig. 9.6**). Mucoceles that form in a previously obliterated frontal sinus can be treated by a frontal drillout procedure.[13,14,18] The mucocele should be sufficiently large that it can be accessed through the frontal recess and marsupialized into the frontal recess[13,18] (**Fig. 9.6**). Mucoceles confined to the far lateral aspect of previously well-pneumatized sinuses maybe difficult to reach and, if the intervening space is filled with scar tissue, may be difficult to keep open postoperatively

Patients who have previously undergone an OPF with obliteration often present with frontal pain and it can be quite difficult to ascertain whether their pain is from a frontal sinus mucocele or from other causes. All these patients undergo MRI to ensure that there is indeed a mucocele present. If there is no mucocele present, surgery is usually not offered and the patient given treatment for neuralgic pain or myofascial pain syndrome. In order to assess if the pain is neuralgic or myofascial in origin, a trial of low-dose amitriptyline (10 mg per night) is prescribed for 6 weeks. If neuralgia or myofascial pain syndrome is contributing to the patient's pain, there should be an improvement in symptoms on this treatment.[19] Most patients will also undergo radioisotope screening to exclude osteomyelitis of the previous bone flap. If the radioisotope scan is positive, consideration may have to be given to removal of this bone flap.

Tumor Removal from the Frontal Sinus

The frontal drillout procedure is useful for the removal of benign tumors from the frontal sinuses. These tumors include

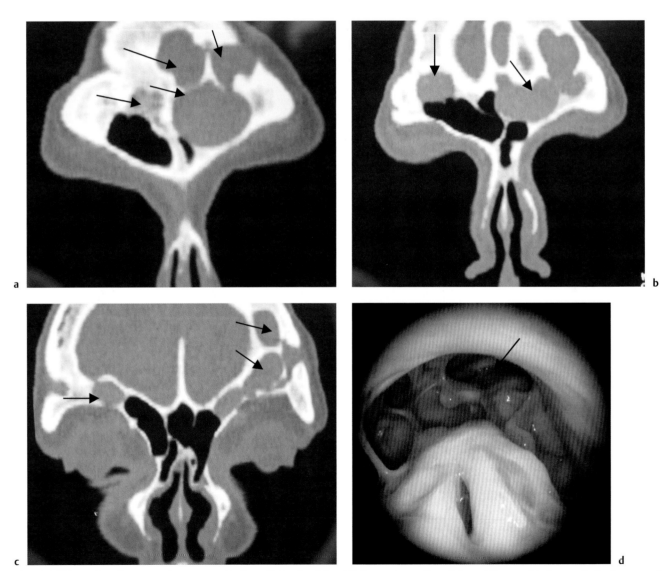

Fig. 9.6 This patient has extensive pneumatization of the frontal sinuses. (**a–c**) OPF with obliteration failed with resultant superior and lateral mucocele formation. This was addressed with a frontal drillout.

(**d**) The postoperative picture at 3 years; *black arrow* indicating one of the opened mucoceles.

osteomas and inverting papillomas. Fairly large osteomas can be removed through the frontal drillout opening.[12,15,18] **Fig. 9.7** illustrates a patient with a large frontal osteoma that has blocked the pathway of the right frontal sinus and resulted in the formation of a large lateral mucocele. This mucocele had eroded the bone over the roof of the orbit with the lining of the mucocele in contact with a large proportion of the orbital periosteum.

The patient underwent a frontal drillout procedure with removal of 90% of the osteoma and drainage of the mucocele. A free mucosal graft was placed on the circumferential raw area created after removal of the osteoma. The patient is now 3 years post surgery and has a nicely healed and patent right

frontal sinus with free drainage of the lateral mucocele into the nose (**Fig. 9.8**).

The frontal drillout procedure is also suitable for removing inverting papilloma from the frontal sinus.[12,15,20] **Fig. 9.9** shows a recurrent inverting papilloma entering the frontal sinus on the left. This had previously been removed via a lateral rhinotomy procedure. The tumor is seen in the left frontal recess and sinus.

The entire tumor was removed after a frontal drillout procedure until direct visualization. As a large area of frontal sinus mucosa was removed in association with the tumor, a free mucosal graft was placed. **Fig. 9.10** shows the patient 4 years after the procedure. Excellent visualization of the

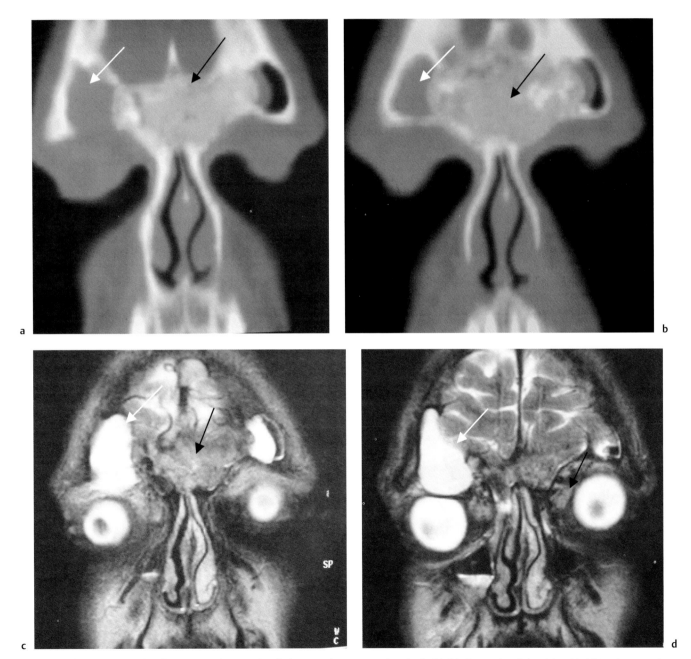

Fig. 9.7 (**a,b**) CT scans and (**c,d**) MRI scans (T2-weighted) showing the osteoma (marked with *black arrow*) and the right-sided lateral mucocele (marked with *white arrow*) with associated proptosis and inferolateral displacement of the eye. (*continued*)

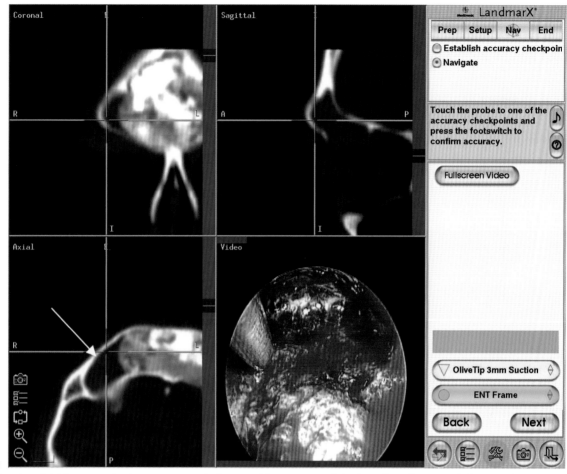

e

Fig. 9.7 (*continued*) (**e**) Intraoperative images seen on the image-guidance system of the large frontal osteoma (*white arrow*) occupying the vast majority of the frontal sinuses. The laterally based mucocele is under the crosshairs that are formed from the tip of the suction.

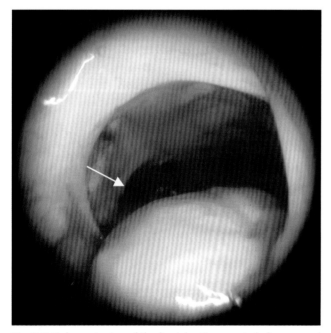

Fig. 9.8 Endoscopic view of the frontal ostium created after removal of the large frontal osteoma shown in **Fig. 9.7a,b**. The *white arrow* indicates the lateral pathway created into the laterally based mucocele indicated in **Fig. 9.7** on the CT scans.

site of the tumor is provided by the large frontal ostium and recurrences can be detected early.

◆ Relative Contraindications for the Frontal Drillout Procedure

Poorly Pneumatized Frontal Sinuses

In patients who have poorly developed (pneumatized) frontal sinuses, the bone of the frontal beak and the inter-sinus septum is very thick[12,18,20] (**Fig. 9.11**). This can make creation of a large frontal sinus ostium difficult as more bone needs to be taken away. In most cases this results in a larger raw bony surface as there is less residual mucosa in the region of the frontal sinus. In the postoperative period there is a tendency for the frontal ostium to cicatrize. We routinely now harvest a free mucosal graft from the region where the septal window is created and create anterior base pedicled mucosal flaps which we place in the neo-ostium at the end of surgery. No glue is used to hold the grafts in place; it sticks well within a few hours. The pedicled and free grafts prevent the circumferential laying down of fibroblasts and results in less postoperative

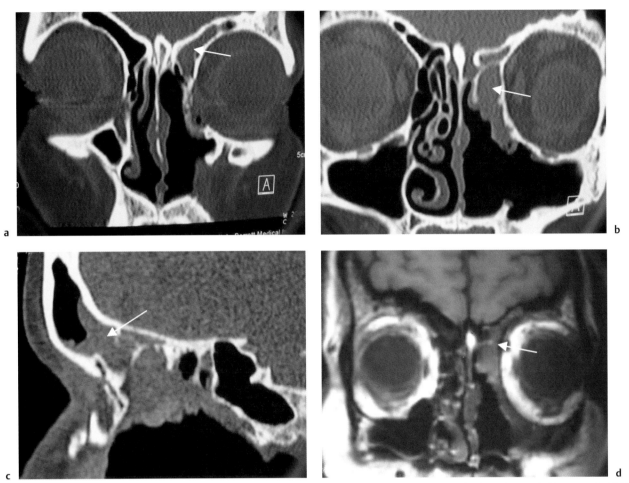

Fig. 9.9 (**a–c**) The CT scans show recurrent inverting papilloma on the lamina papyracea entering the frontal sinus (*white arrows*). (**d**) This is confirmed with a MRI scan that shows that the opacity within the frontal sinus is not just retained secretions.

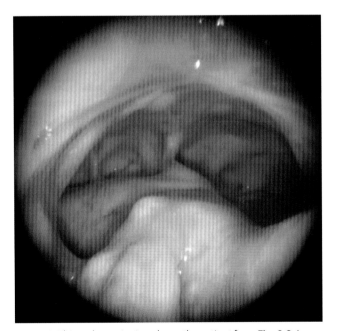

Fig. 9.10 This endoscopic view shows the patient from **Fig. 9.9** 4 years postoperatively with a nicely healed common opening into both frontal sinuses. The entire area of previous tumor involvement can be easily surveyed endoscopically for any recurrences.

stenosis and less granuloma formation than if the bone was left bare. In **Fig. 9.11** the patient has very underdeveloped frontal sinuses with a thick frontal beak and intersinus septum.

If the postoperative frontal ostium is viewed after 24 months (**Fig. 9.12**) the smaller than usual frontal ostium can be seen. This case illustrates the importance of creating the largest possible bony ostium at the time of surgery and that although underdeveloped frontal sinuses may be a relative contraindication, the patient can still have a successful frontal drillout procedure if these principles are adhered to.

Narrow Anteroposterior Diameter of the Frontal Sinus[12,18,20]

In some patients, the skull base comes farther forward than normal and narrows the anteroposterior width of the frontal ostium and sinus. This in turn limits the anteroposterior width that can be created during surgery and increases the likelihood of postoperative scarring and closure of the frontal ostium. In **Fig. 9.13** the patient has a very narrow anteroposterior diameter of the frontal sinus. This limits the opening that can be surgically created.

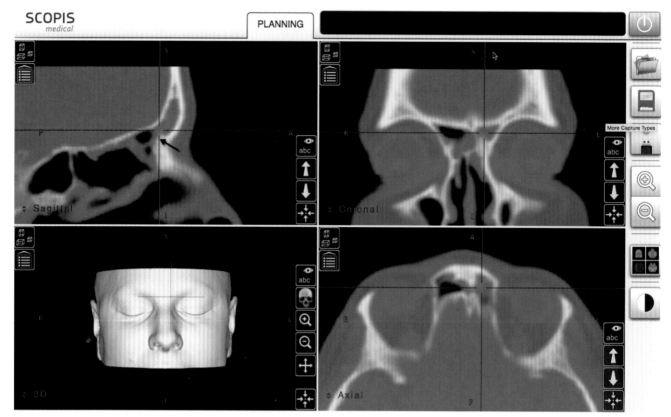

Fig. 9.11 A CT scan illustrating the thick frontal beak resulting from underpneumatized frontal sinuses. Note the thick posteriorly projecting frontal beak (*black arrow*).

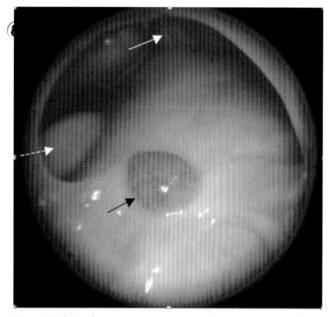

Fig. 9.12 This is the postoperative picture taken of the patient shown in **Fig. 9.11** 3 years after surgery. The *black arrow* reveals a small granulation on the anterior skull base which was subsequently removed. The *white solid arrow* indicates the frontal intersinus septum and the *broken white arrow* indicates a small amount of mucus present in the right frontal sinus. The patient is currently asymptomatic.

◆ Surgical Technique[12,13,17,18,25–30]

It is currently our routine to use image-guidance equipment for all our frontal drillout procedures.[12,13,18,20,24–30] Image guidance helps to identify the olfactory fossa projections and aids in the creation of the largest possible frontal sinus ostium. This ability to create the largest possible opening is critical for the success of this procedure. Image guidance is set up before surgery. Once the accuracy of the system is verified, surgery begins. The first step is to surgically revise, as necessary, the maxillary, ethmoid, and sphenoid sinuses. It is important that this is done before the frontal sinus surgery as the frontal sinus component can be relatively time-consuming and the surgical field tends to worsen progressively as the operation proceeds. Visualization of the anatomy of the maxillary, ethmoid, and sphenoids can be difficult due to excessive bleeding if this is left to the end of the surgical procedure.

Infiltration with lidocaine and adrenaline is performed in the region above the axilla of the middle turbinate and the vault of the nose. The adjacent septum anterior to the middle turbinate is also infiltrated. A 0-degree scope is used for the majority of the dissection and a 30-degree used to maximize the removal of bone of the anterior wall of the frontal sinus. The first step is to harvest the mucosa of the septum on both sides in the region where the septal window will be created (**Fig. 9.14a**). In **Fig. 9.14a** the *dotted lines* outline the incisions

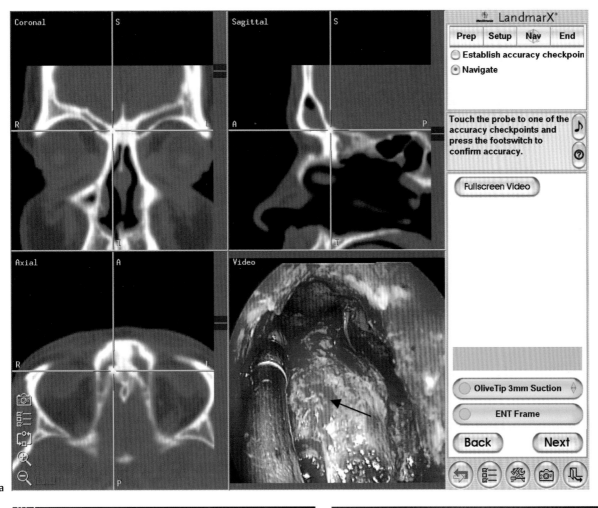

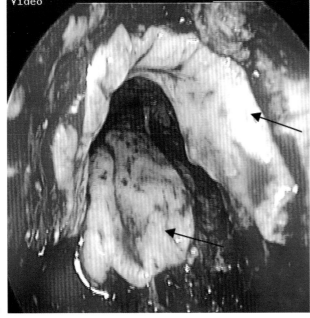

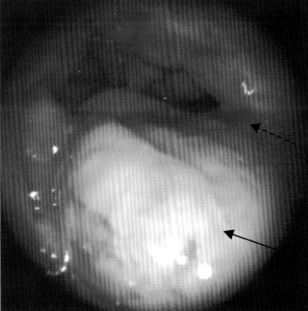

Fig. 9.13 (**a**) This image taken from the computer-assisted surgical navigation (CAS) system shows the very narrow anteroposterior dimension of the frontal sinuses. The *black arrow* on the operative view indicates the relatively large area of bone removed from the forward extending anterior skull base. The only residual mucosa in this newly created frontal ostium is in the posterolateral regions. (**b**) Shows the anterior and posterior free mucosal grafts (*black arrows*) that were put in place at the end of the surgery. (**c**) Shows the frontal ostium after 3 months. The adhesion between the upper and lower grafts is indicated by the *black broken arrow*. (*continued*)

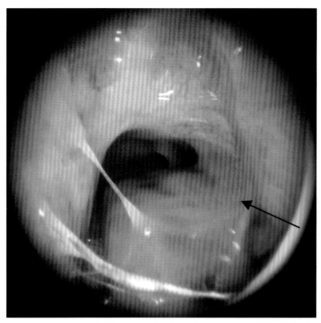

d

Fig. 9.13 (*continued*) (**d**) shows the frontal ostium at 5 years with the adhesion indicated by the *black arrow*. This adhesion can be seen in the early postoperative period in (**c**) marked by the *broken black arrow*. The patient is currently asymptomatic.

window and under the axilla of the opposite side. When making the mucosal incisions for the septal flap graft, look at the level of the axilla on the ipsilateral side to estimate where the inferior incision should be placed. The anterior edge of the window is estimated and if necessary once the window is created it can be brought forward until about a centimeter of the frontal process of the maxilla anterior to the middle turbinate is seen from the opposite side of the nose with a zero scope. The superior margin of the window is the roof of the nose[12] (**Fig. 9.14b**). This mucosa is harvested as a free mucosal graft using a scalpel as illustrated in **Fig. 9.14a**. We attempt to take the graft as a partial thickness mucosal graft rather than to incise onto the perichondrium and harvest in the subperichondrial plane. We find that the take rate of the graft is better if the perichondrium is not harvested as part of the graft. Next the mucosa above the middle turbinate that overlies the agger nasi cell is raised as an anteriorly based pedicled mucosal graft (**Fig. 9.15a**). A vertical incision is made just posterior to the middle turbinates behind the axilla and the superior horizontal incision runs along the roof of the nose with the inferior horizontal incision running just above the axilla of the middle turbinate. This is illustrated in **Fig. 9.15b** by the *dotted lines* overlying the mucosal incisions (**Fig. 9.15a**). A malleable suction curette is used to raise these flaps starting posteriorly and using the sharp edge of the curette to make sure the incisions are onto bone and that the flap is raised in the subperiosteal plane (**Fig. 9.15b**). This mobilization of the flaps continues until the flaps are mobilized past the septal window and the ends of the flaps are brought out of the nose. This prevents the mobilized flaps from obstructing the view of the dissection during the drill-out. At the end of surgery, the flaps are placed into the neo-ostium with the free flaps lining the raw bone. This lessens

to be made for the harvesting of the free mucosal septal graft. The landmarks for the septal window are important—the posterior edge of the window is at the level of the middle turbinates, and the inferior edge of the window is made just below the axilla of the middle turbinate so that an instrument can be passed from the one side of the nose across the

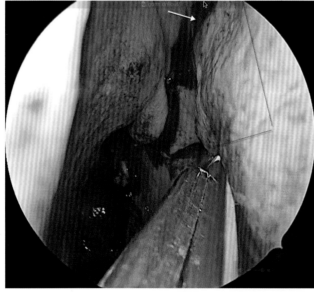

a

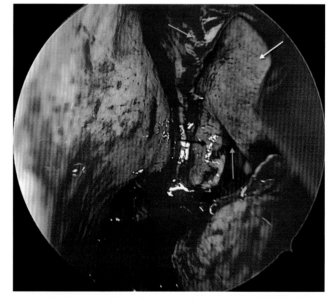

b

Fig. 9.14 (**a**) The patient's right side of the nose illustrating the incisions for the septal window (*dotted lines*). The upper incision (*white arrow*) is high on the septum with the lower horizontal incision just below the axilla of the middle turbinate. The anterior vertical incision is far enough anteriorly so that when the opposite nasal wall is viewed the frontal process of the maxilla is visible. (**b**) The septal window has been

removed and the middle turbinate on the opposite side is seen (*black arrow*), the frontal process of the maxilla is seen (*white arrow*), and the axilla and pathway under the axilla across the septum is illustrated with an *orange arrow*. The *green arrow* illustrates the superior edge of the septal window.

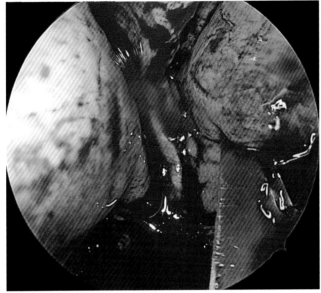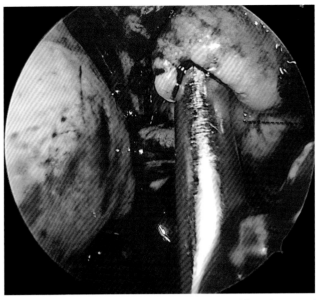

a   b

Fig. 9.15 (**a**) The *dotted lines* and scalpel illustrate the incision for the anterolateral-based pedicled flaps performed from the patient's right nostril across the septal window on the left side. (**b**) A malleable suction curette is used to mobilize the flap from above the middle turbinate with the pedicle based anteriorly.

the granulation formation postoperatively and improves the healing. After harvesting of the free mucosal grafts, the cartilage and bone in the septal window is removed. An instrument should be able to be passed from the one side of the nose through the septal window and under the axilla of the middle turbinate on the other side[12] (**Fig. 9.16**).

If this is not possible, the septal window should be lowered until this can be easily done. If there is a pathway between the frontal sinus and the frontal recess (i.e., there is no mucocele present with complete separation of the frontal sinus and frontal recess), a frontal sinus mini-trephine can be placed in each frontal sinus (**Fig. 9.17**). Flushing the frontal sinus mini-trephine will result in fluorescein-stained saline being seen under the axilla of the middle turbinate. This step is done early as it increases the safety of the dissection but is not absolutely necessary as the ostium can be palpated with a right-angled probe or the image guidance can be used to check the position of the ostium. Regular flushing with fluorescein through the frontal ostium allows the surgeon to have a constant posterior reference point and thus keep the

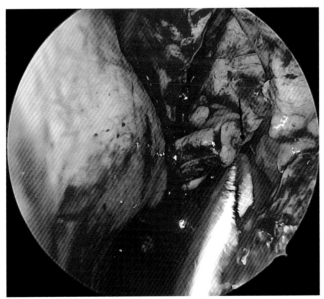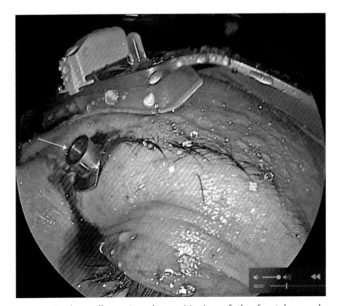

Fig. 9.16 Picture illustrating the anterolateral mucosal flap has been raised off of the frontal process of the maxilla above the axilla of the middle turbinate (*black arrow*) with a suction curette being passed from the right nostril across the septum and under the axilla of the left side.

Fig. 9.17 Photo illustrating the positioning of the frontal cannula (*white arrow*) through the medial end of the eyebrow into the lumen of the frontal sinus (FS).

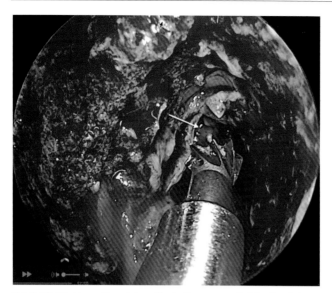

Fig. 9.18 Intraoperative picture illustrating removal of the frontal process directly above the axilla of the middle turbinate with the frontal ostium with fluorescein in the ostium visible (*white arrow*).

dissection away from the skull base. The fluorescein-stained saline (**Fig. 9.18,** *white arrow*) delineates the frontal ostium and we can therefore dissect the bone anterior to the ostium (but not medial) knowing that the dissection is anterior to the skull base.

The CT scans of both frontal recesses are viewed in three planes and the anatomy of the frontal recess is reconstructed using the building block software as previously described.[31,32] The 4-mm angled cutting bur or rough diamond bur is used to remove the frontal process of the maxilla directly above the axilla (**Fig. 9.19**). In **Fig. 9.19,** the *white arrow* indicates the position of the frontal ostium with drilling only occurring in a lateral and superior direction but not medially. Medtronic ENT has 30,000 rpm burs that cut extremely fast and if the surgeon is inexperienced in the frontal drillout procedure, a rough diamond bur is much safer as the 30,000 rpm cutting bur can get you into trouble very quickly. A zero-degree endoscope is used for most of the dissection. Both the scope and the bur are placed from the one nostril across the septal window and dissection begins on the opposite frontal process. This working from one nostril across the septum and onto the opposite side improves the angle of dissection, affording a much better view of the frontal process and improving the angle at which the bur contacts the frontal process, making the dissection safer. In the initial stages of this dissection the bur is swept from the frontal ostium anterior across the frontal process of the maxilla removing both anterior and lateral bone. This opens the access to the frontal ostium in a funnel shape. This process is analogous to performing a front to back mastoidectomy by removing the outer cortical bone and creating a funnel-shaped access to the antrum. As this lateral and superior bone removal continues anterior and superior to the axilla of the middle turbinate a small amount of skin is exposed to define the lateral extent of the dissection.

Dissection is continued superiorly using regular flushes of the fluorescein to identify the anterior lip of the frontal ostium (**Fig. 9.19**) and to allow the bone anterior to the frontal ostium

(the bone which forms the frontal "beak") to be removed. Care is taken to ensure that drilling is done in only a superior and lateral direction without drilling medially as this may endanger the skull base. It is important to accurately define the lateral extent of the dissection by exposing a small area of skin. As long as the exposure of the skin is done directly above the axilla of the middle turbinate, the drill will be anterior to the orbit. This dissection is in the same coronal plane as the lacrimal sac and the lacrimal sac maybe exposed if bone is removed laterally within 8 mm of the axilla of the middle turbinate. The skin exposure is done bilaterally to define the lateral limits of dissection and to ensure achievement of maximal ostial width. Drilling continues superiorly until the floor of the frontal sinus is entered and the frontal sinus can be seen. Once the floor of the frontal sinus is opened on one side, the endoscope and drill are transferred into the opposite nostril and the process repeated until the floor of the second frontal sinus is exposed (**Fig. 9.20**). Note that up until this point no medial dissection has taken place. If the dissection is brought medially before the frontal sinus is entered, the surgeon is likely to damage the forward projections of the olfactory fossae and cause a CSF leak. The olfactory neurons (**Fig. 9.21,** *black arrows*) can be exposed in the region medial to the middle turbinate and they mark the anterior projection of the olfactory fossae (skull base) and drilling can only proceed medially once the ostium is brought anterior to these neurons.

The dissection is now brought medially from both sides until the frontal intersinus septum is seen (**Fig. 9.20**). Note that this medial dissection takes place at the upper limit of the opening of the frontal sinuses and that drilling in a medial direction lower down can still potentially injure the skull base. This dissection is alternated from side to side thereby connecting the two frontal sinuses by taking down the intersinus septum (**Fig. 9.22**). Once this is done the frontal sinus opening is in the shape of a crescent.

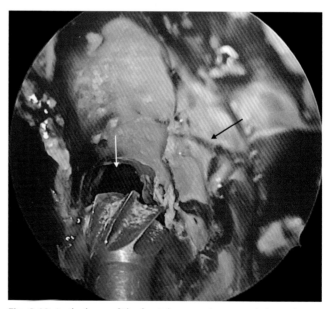

Fig. 9.19 As the bone of the frontal process is removed above the axilla, the dissection is also taken laterally until the skin's undersurface is exposed with a blood vessel seen on this surface (*black arrow*). The frontal ostium is always kept in view (*white arrow*).

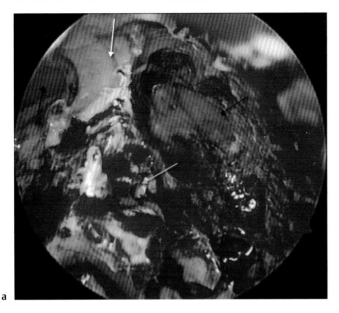

Fig. 9.20 (**a**) The floor of both frontal sinuses has been removed (*black arrows*); note the frontal septal cell (*green arrow*) has also been opened. The intersinus septum (*white arrow*) is seen separating the two frontal sinuses. (**b**) The CT image of this patient the frontal septal cell is illustrated with the *crosshairs*.

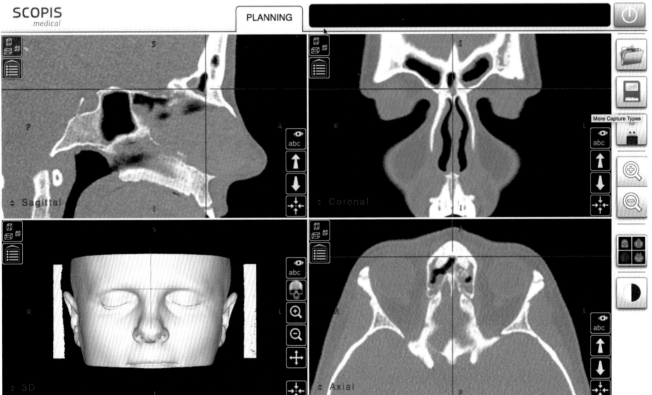

The aim of the surgery is now to transform this crescent opening into an oval opening thereby creating the largest possible anteroposterior and lateral diameters for the frontal ostium. The most dangerous step of the operation is to remove the bone over the forward projection of the skull base. This forward projection forms the frontal "T" (**Fig. 9.23**, *black arrow*). The "T" is made up by the two middle turbinates attaching to the septum (**Fig. 9.23**). The frontal sinus intersinus septum, nasal septum, and associated middle turbinates are drilled posteriorly toward the skull base. At the "T," the olfactory fossae project forward from the skull base and great care needs to be taken so that the "T" is lowered as far as possible without exposing the dura of these olfactory projections. These projections can most clearly be seen on the axial scan (**Fig. 9.24**). The position of these forward projections or horns can be identified in two ways. First, the image guidance suction can be used to determine the exact position of these forward projections of the skull

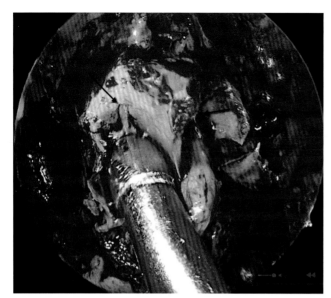

Fig. 9.21 This picture demonstrates the first olfactory neuron (*black arrow*) as the mucosa is peeled away from the skull base identifying the most anterior projection of the skull base. The frontal T can be lowered onto this first olfactory neuron but not beyond it.

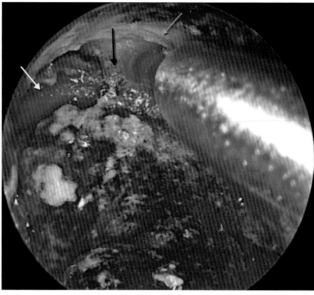

Fig. 9.22 This picture shows how the anterior wall of the frontal sinus (*green arrow*) is drilled away until the anterior wall of the frontal sinus runs smoothly into the nasal cavity without any ridges (*white arrow*); this ensures that the frontal ostium obtains its maximum anteroposterior dimension. The intersinus septum (*black arrow*) is removed up to the roof of the sinus. This prevents loculations forming as the sinus heals.

base. However, these should always be clinically correlated by sliding a suction Freer elevator between the bone and mucosa in the roof of the nose medial to the middle turbinates and gently pushing the mucosa downward. The anterior ethmoidal nerve and first olfactory fibers are easily visible and indicate the most anterior position of the olfactory bulb (**Fig. 9.21**). It is important to clinically correlate findings of the image guidance as the headframe can shift with resultant inaccuracies.

Once the position of the forward projections of the anterior skull base are located, the bone over the anterior skull base is lowered to within 1 mm of the olfactory fibers. This is done either with a diamond bur or if the surgeon is very experienced with a cutting bur. If a cutting bur is used, the bone should be lightly brushed with the bur spinning at maximum revolutions. The technique is similar to that used when removing the final bone from the facial nerve during facial nerve decompression. Lowering this forward projection of the olfactory fossa is crucial for the largest possible opening to be created into the frontal sinuses. Failure to remove this projection gives a narrow anteroposterior dimension and a crescent-shaped opening which has a greater tendency to stenose. Lowering the bone over the olfactory fossa gives the widest possible anteroposterior dimension to the new common frontal sinus ostium (**Fig. 9.25**).

The scope is now changed to a 30-degree scope and intersinus septum is removed up to the roof of the frontal sinus. Once this is done, the anterior frontal bone is removed until there is no longer an anterior ridge or lip of bone separating the frontal sinus from the nasal cavity (**Fig. 9.26**, *white arrow*). When the anterior table of the frontal sinus is viewed with a 30-degree scope, the transition from the frontal sinus to nasal cavity should be smooth. Any bony ridges should be removed (**Fig. 9.26**).

In most patients, an oval-shaped frontal sinus ostium is created. The average dimensions should be about 18 mm in the anteroposterior plane and 20 to 24 mm from side to side. The size of the opening is determined by the patient's anatomy but should be made as large as possible.

To ensure healing of the neo-ostium with minimal granulations, the anteriorly based pedicled grafts are rolled back

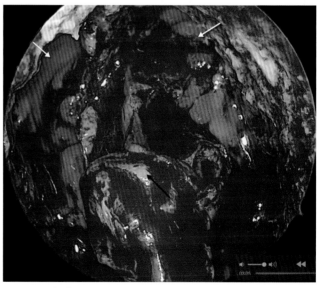

Fig. 9.23 The forward projection of the olfactory fossa forms a frontal T (*black arrow*). The T is formed by the middle turbinates attaching to the septum. The left and right frontal sinuses are marked with *white arrows*.

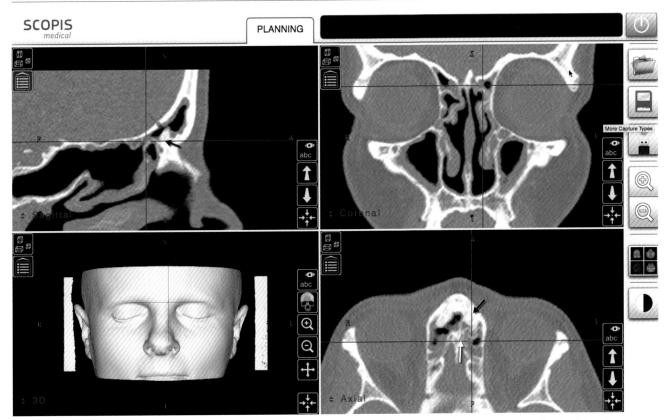

Fig. 9.24 CT scan of patient from **Fig. 9.14** to **Fig. 9.23** with the *crosshairs* on the axial CT indicating if the drill was moved medially then the skull base (*white arrow*) would be entered with a subsequent CSF leak.

Note on the parasagittal scan how narrow the frontal ostium (*orange arrow*) with the frontal beak (*black arrow*) protruding posteriorly.

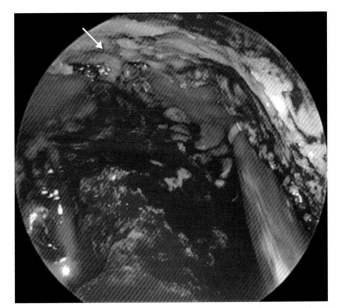

Fig. 9.25 The scope is changed to a 30-degree scope and anterior wall taken down until the anterior wall runs smoothly out into the nose. Note the intersinus septum has been removed to the roof of the sinus (*white arrow*).

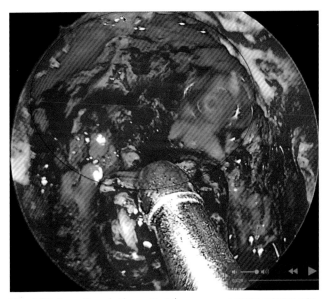

Fig. 9.26 Even though the patient has a very narrow anteroposterior (AP) as seen in **Fig. 9.24**, a large oval frontal ostium is able to be created with the maximum AP and lateral dimensions.

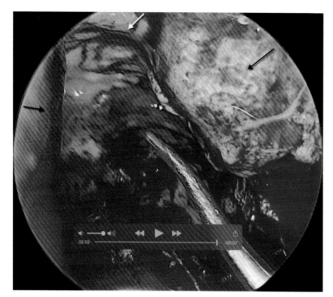

Fig. 9.27 The pedicled anteriorly based anterolateral flaps (*black arrows*) are laid back into the frontal sinus neo-ostium. The septal free mucosal graft is placed on the raw bone between these flaps (*white arrow*).

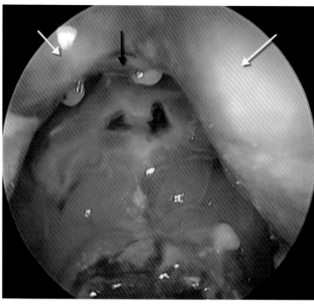

Fig. 9.28 At 2 weeks postsurgery, the two anterolateral pedicled flaps (*white arrows*) line the neo-ostium. The septal free mucosal graft (*black arrow*) is slightly edematous but still healthy.

into the neo-ostium and cover the anterolateral aspects of the ostium (**Fig. 9.27**). One of the free mucosal grafts that was harvested from the septum is positioned between these pedicled grafts and the other laterally, usually on exposed skin as they seem to take better on the exposed skin (**Fig. 9.27**). These grafts and flaps are not secured as they stick onto the bone very well and do not shift despite the nasal and sinus douches that are started the following day.

At the end of the procedure, the suction bipolar forceps are used to achieve hemostasis. Particular attention is paid to the posterior edge of the septal window and region of the first olfactory neuron where the anterior nasal artery (a branch of the anterior ethmoidal artery) is seen. In most cases, the lower half of the middle turbinates are trimmed to improve ventilation of the posterior ethmoids and sphenoids. If the remnant middle turbinates are unstable, they are sutured with a dissolving suture through the septum. This allows their lateral surfaces to heal before the suture dissolves and they lateralize. This prevents adhesions from forming.

◆ **Postoperative Care**[12,13,18,24–28]

The frontal sinus cannulae are removed at the end of surgery. Saline nasal washes are started the next day and are performed with a 240-mL squeeze bottle wash four to six times a day. Half the bottle is administered through each nostril with the top half of the body parallel to the floor with the head tilted up, as this position maximizes frontal sinus penetration. In the last saline wash of the day, one 2-mL ampule of budesonide 1 microgram/mL (Pulmicort Respules) is added to the saline before douching. The Pulmicort wash is continued once daily for a few months post-

operatively until the sinuses have healed. The patient from **Fig. 9.27** is seen at 2 weeks after surgery (**Fig. 9.28**). Note the anterior-based pedicled septal flaps (*white arrows*) line the neo-ostium while the free mucosal graft (*black arrow*) is more edematous and paler (**Fig. 9.28**). Depending on the patient's diagnosis this may need to be continued long term (allergic fungal sinusitis or Samter's triad). The patients are reviewed again at 2 weeks when all crusts and blood clots are meticulously removed from the frontal sinus ostium. This process is crucial because if these adherent clots are left, they form the framework into which collagen is laid, encouraging fibrosis of the frontal sinus ostium. **Fig. 9.29**

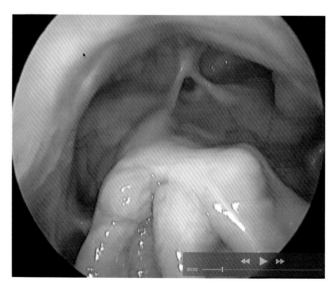

Fig. 9.29 The same patient as **Fig. 9.14** to **Fig 9.28** with a healthy healed frontal sinus neo-ostium 6 months postoperatively.

shows a well-healed frontal neo-ostium with both left and right frontal sinuses visible. In our animal model, postoperative douching of the frontal sinus after a frontal drillout procedure tended to improve the mucociliary drainage of the frontal sinuses at 2 and 4 months after surgery.[22] This trend was not statistically significant.

◆ Stenosis of the Frontal Neo-Ostium[23–28]

In both studies done on the sheep animal model and on long-term review of 80 frontal drillout patients, the frontal ostium narrowed to about a third of its original size.[23,24] It was also apparent that this narrowing occurred within the first 12 months after surgery and that thereafter the frontal ostium was stable.[24,25] The time course of how the frontal ostium narrow is presented in **Fig. 9.30**.

The factors in the patients who eventually developed frontal ostial stenosis were the size of the original ostium at the time of the initial surgery, more than five previous surgeries, and aspirin exacerbated respiratory disease (AERD).[24–28] Other factors such as fungal sinusitis and presence of *Staphylococcus aureus* infection at the time of surgery were found to be significant.[28] This emphasizes the importance of creating the largest possible opening at the time of the original surgery (exposure of skin on each side and removal of the frontal beak, lowering of the frontal T). These results also emphasize the success that the frontal drillout has in the management of patients with these very difficult conditions. One would expect that aspirin triad and fungal sinusitis that aggressively form polyps would develop postoperative stenosis as the high likelihood of polyp regrowth in these conditions would narrow the frontal ostium significantly necessitating re-operation. Analysis of the AERD patients showed that only 58% of these patients developed a recurrence of polyps with only 22% requiring revision surgery.[26] It appears that the frontal drillout is one operation that can break the ongoing cycle of repeated polyp regrowth and revision surgery.

This may be due to the surgeon's ability to remove the fungal and/or eosinophilic mucus from the frontal sinuses and then to be able to clear the frontal sinus in the office. If the patient is then given a course of prednisolone, the mucosa of the frontal sinus and ethmoids may return to normal. Repeated suction clearance and prednisolone may be required and, as long as the patient is having four or fewer courses of prednisolone every 12 months, this regimen is continued and gives good control of the patient's symptoms. Once the patient requires more than four courses of prednisolone a year, revision surgery is offered.

◆ Results[12,13,18,24–28]

Our department has published the largest series of frontal drillout procedures to date.[12,13,18,24–28] The most recent study included 213 primary frontal drillouts (all had undergone previous ESS which had failed) and 19 revision drillouts (prior frontal drillout). Of the primary drillouts, 8.9% failed and required revision surgery whereas in the revision drillout group 21% failed and required further surgery. Further surgery was mostly for polyp recurrence (73%) with 27% of patients having frontal ostial stenosis.[27] **Fig. 9.31** shows a patient with frontal ostial stenosis.

In most of the studies the patency rate for a primary frontal drillout varied between 87.5% and 95% and at 30 months' follow-up.[12,24–28] Thus, the overall incidence of frontal ostium stenosis (5–12.5%) is low if attention is paid to creating the largest possible frontal sinus opening at the time of surgery. **Fig. 9.32** shows three examples of healthy frontal sinus ostia at more than 12 months after a frontal drillout.

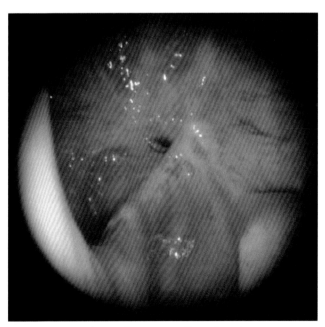

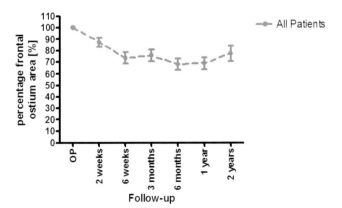

Fig. 9.30 Time course for 80 patients in whom the frontal ostium was measured at the time of surgery and at regular time points in the postoperative period.[24] All patients start with the biggest possible frontal ostium (100%) and each subsequent reading is a percentage of this original measurement.

Fig. 9.31 Patient has undergone significant frontal ostium stenosis until the residual ostium is only 2 × 4 mm. This will cause retention of secretions within the frontal sinuses and symptoms and needs to be revised.

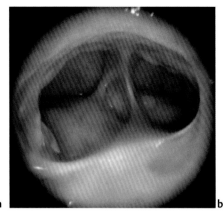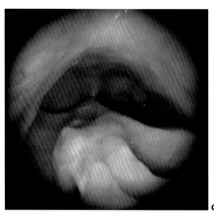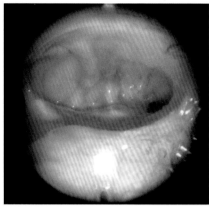

a   b   c

Fig. 9.32 (**a–c**) Three patients post frontal drillout procedure with oval-shaped frontal ostia and healthy frontal sinuses.

◆ Revision Surgery

Revision frontal drillout is conducted along similar lines to the primary surgery. Frontal trephine cannulae are usually not placed as the bony work on the ostium had been previously done. The frontal ostium is widened by removal of all scar tissue. If the repeat CT scan shows any areas of bone which are still significantly thick, then these are lowered until the maximum-sized frontal sinus ostium is created. Postoperative care is similar to what has been described above other than all patients receive postoperative prednisolone, antibiotics, and saline douches. If a circumferential raw area is created, free mucosal grafts are placed in the ostium but pedicled flap are usually not possible due to the prior surgery. We have also found the use of CHITODEX gel* (Wellington, New Zealand) to be very helpful in maintaining patency in both primary and revision frontal drillout patients.[33,34] This gel is made up of chitosan and dextran, and it is important to remove all crusts and blood clots at the 2-week postoperative visit. CHITODEX gel has been shown both in vitro and in vivo in human trials to be very successful in preventing scar tissue formation. Failure to properly debride and clean the frontal ostium at this point can lead to the formation of adhesions which may in turn contribute to long-term closure of the frontal ostium.

References

1. Casiano RR, Livingston JA. Endoscopic Lothrop procedure: the University of Miami experience. Am J Rhinol 1998;12(5):335–339
2. Becker DG, Moore D, Lindsey WH, Gross WE, Gross CW. Modified transnasal endoscopic Lothrop procedure: further considerations. Laryngoscope 1995;105(11):1161–1166
3. Wormald PJ. The axillary flap approach to the frontal recess. Laryngoscope 2002;112(3):494–499
4. Close LG, Lee NK, Leach JL, Manning SC. Endoscopic resection of the intranasal frontal sinus floor. Ann Otol Rhinol Laryngol 1994;103(12):952–958
5. Alsarraf R, Kriet Jd, Weymuller EA Jr. Quality-of-life outcomes after osteoplastic frontal sinus obliteration. Otolaryngol Head Neck Surg 1999;121(4):435–440
6. Catalano PJ, Lawson W, Som P, Biller HF. Radiographic evaluation and diagnosis of the failed frontal osteoplastic flap with fat obliteration. Otolaryngol Head Neck Surg 1991;104(2):225–234

7. Draf W. Endonasal micro-endoscopic frontal sinus surgery, the Fulda concept. Oper Tech Otolaryngol—Head Neck Surg 1991;2(4):234–240
8. Gross WE, Gross CW, Becker D, Moore D, Phillips D. Modified transnasal endoscopic Lothrop procedure as an alternative to frontal sinus obliteration. Otolaryngol Head Neck Surg 1995;113(4):427–434
9. Gross CW, Gross WE, Becker D. Modified transnasal endoscopic Lothrop procedure: frontal drillout. Oper Tech Otolaryngol—Head Neck Surg 1995;6(3):193–200
10. Schlosser RJ, Zachmann G, Harrison S, Gross CW. The endoscopic modified Lothrop: long-term follow-up on 44 patients. Am J Rhinol 2002;16(2):103–108
11. Ulualp SO, Carlson TK, Toohill RJ. Osteoplastic flap versus modified endoscopic Lothrop procedure in patients with frontal sinus disease. Am J Rhinol 2000;14(1):21–26
12. Wormald PJ. Salvage frontal sinus surgery: the endoscopic modified Lothrop procedure. Laryngoscope 2003;113(2):276–283
13. Wormald PJ, Ananda A, Nair S. Modified endoscopic lothrop as a salvage for the failed osteoplastic flap with obliteration. Laryngoscope 2003;113(11):1988–1992
14. Weber R, Draf W, Keerl R, et al. Osteoplastic frontal sinus surgery with fat obliteration: technique and long-term results using magnetic resonance imaging in 82 operations. Laryngoscope 2000;110(6):1037–1044
15. Javer AR, Sillers MJ, Kuhn FA. The frontal sinus unobliteration procedure. Otolaryngol Clin North Am 2001;34(1):193–210
16. Hosemann W, Kühnel T, Held P, Wagner W, Felderhoff A. Endonasal frontal sinusotomy in surgical management of chronic sinusitis: a critical evaluation. Am J Rhinol 1997;11(1):1–9
17. Weber R, Draf W, Kratzsch B, Hosemann W, Schaefer SD. Modern concepts of frontal sinus surgery. Laryngoscope 2001;111(1):137–146
18. Wormald PJ, Ananda A, Nair S. The modified endoscopic Lothrop procedure in the treatment of complicated chronic frontal sinusitis. Clin Otolaryngol Allied Sci 2003;28(3):215–220
19. West B, Jones NS. Endoscopy-negative, computed tomography-negative facial pain in a nasal clinic. Laryngoscope 2001;111(4 Pt 1):581–586
20. Wormald PJ, Chan SZX. Surgical techniques for the removal of frontal recess cells obstructing the frontal ostium. Am J Rhinol 2003;17(4):221–226
21. Lothrop HA. XIV. Frontal Sinus Suppuration: The Establishment of Permanent Nasal Drainage; the Closure of External Fistulae; Epidermization of Sinus. Ann Surg 1914;59(6):937–957
22. Rajapaksa SP, Ananda A, Cain T, Oates L, Wormald PJ. The effect of the modified endoscopic Lothrop procedure on the mucociliary clearance of the frontal sinus in an animal model. Am J Rhinol 2004;18(3):183–187
23. Rajapaksa SP, Ananda A, Cain TM, Oates L, Wormald PJ. Frontal ostium neo-osteogenesis and restenosis after modified endoscopic Lothrop procedure in an animal model. Clin Otolaryngol Allied Sci 2004;29(4):386–388
24. Tran KN, Beule AG, Singal D, Wormald PJ. Frontal ostium restenosis after the endoscopic modified Lothrop procedure. Laryngoscope 2007;117(8):1457–1462
25. Naidoo Y, Bassiouni A, Keen M, Wormald PJ. Risk factors and outcomes for primary, revision, and modified Lothrop (Draf III) frontal sinus surgery. Int Forum Allergy Rhinol 2013;3(5):412–417

26. Morrissey DK, Bassiouni A, Psaltis AJ, Naidoo Y, Wormald PJ. Outcomes of modified endoscopic Lothrop in aspirin-exacerbated respiratory disease with nasal polyposis. Int Forum Allergy Rhinol 2016;6(8):820–825

27. Morrissey DK, Bassiouni A, Psaltis AJ, Naidoo Y, Wormald PJ. Outcomes of revision endoscopic modified Lothrop procedure. Int Forum Allergy Rhinol 2016;6(5):518–522

28. Naidoo Y, Bassiouni A, Keen M, Wormald PJ. Long-term outcomes for the endoscopic modified Lothrop/Draf III procedure: a 10-year review. Laryngoscope 2014;124(1):43–49

29. Gross CW. Surgical treatments for symptomatic chronic frontal sinusitis. Arch Otolaryngol Head Neck Surg 2000;126(1):101–102

30. Loehrl TA, Toohill RJ, Smith TL. Use of computer-aided surgery for frontal sinus ventilation. Laryngoscope 2000;110(11):1962–1967

31. Wormald PJ. The agger nasi cell: the key to understanding the anatomy of the frontal recess. Otolaryngol Head Neck Surg 2003;129(5):497–507

32. Wormald PJ. Surgery of the frontal recess and frontal sinus. Rhinology 2005;43(2):82–85

33. Athanasiadis T, Beule AG, Robinson BH, Robinson SR, Shi Z, Wormald PJ. Effects of a novel chitosan gel on mucosal wound healing following endoscopic sinus surgery in a sheep model of chronic rhinosinusitis. Laryngoscope 2008;118(6):1088–1094

34. Valentine R, Athanasiadis T, Moratti S, Robinson S, Wormald PJ. The efficacy of a novel chitosan gel on hemostasis after endoscopic sinus surgery in a sheep model of chronic rhinosinusitis. Am J Rhinol Allergy 2009;23(1):71–75

10 Sphenopalatine Artery Ligation and Vidian Neurectomy

◆ Introduction

Epistaxis may be classified clinically into anterior and posterior bleeds.[1] If the vascular supply of the nose is reviewed, it is apparent that anterior epistaxis would originate from the vascular anastomosis of vessels around Little's (or Kiesselbach's) area or from the anterior ethmoidal artery. Little's plexus is formed by branches from the sphenopalatine artery (via the posterior nasal artery branch) anastomosing with branches from the greater palatine, nasolabial (a branch of the facial artery), and anterior ethmoidal arteries. Bleeding from Little's area is usually easily visible and managed by either local cautery or an anterior nasal pack. Bleeding from the anterior ethmoidal artery is rarely spontaneous and usually seen after trauma with associated skull base fractures or intraoperative injury. Posterior bleeding is often seen from under the inferior turbinate where branches of the sphenopalatine artery anastomose with branches from the pharyngeal artery. This area is termed Woodruff's area. Bleeders in this region can be difficult to visualize due to their location under the posterior end of the inferior turbinate. Other posterior bleeders may arise from the lateral nasal wall, posterior choana, or posterior septum.

◆ Postoperative Epistaxis

Significant postoperative epistaxis (as opposed to the blood-stained ooze usually seen in the first 24 hours after nasal surgery) typically occurs when a vessel of significant diameter bleeds. Logically, this would be either in the region of the sphenopalatine or anterior ethmoidal artery. Intraoperative damage to the anterior ethmoidal artery is almost always visible during surgery and would in most patients need to be dealt with immediately as the resultant bleeding usually obscures the surgical field, making further surgery difficult if not impossible. However, vessels divided in the region of the sphenopalatine artery may bleed for a short period of time and then undergo spasm and thrombose. As these vessels are located posteriorly, the blood will drain into the nasopharynx and not come to the notice of the surgeon who may then not seek out the bleeding vessel and cauterize it. By the time the surgery is completed, the vessel may either be in spasm or thrombosed. If the patient strains or becomes hypertensive in the immediate postoperative period, significant epistaxis can result, which may necessitate the placement of a nasal pack or return to theatre to cauterize the bleeding vessel. On occasion, epistaxis may occur days or even weeks postoperatively. In this situation, the patient has likely developed a postoperative infection with increased vascularity and if the blood clot detaches from the vessel or is dislodged by coughing or straining, epistaxis may result.

In order to prevent postoperative epistaxis, close inspection of the region of the sphenopalatine artery is performed at the end of surgery. Particular attention is paid to the region of the horizontal insertion of the ground lamella into the lateral nasal wall, especially if the ground lamella has been resected and to the lateral nasal wall in the superior meatus (**Fig. 10.1**). In addition, close inspection is made of the anteroinferior region of the sphenoid at the lower edge of the sphenoidotomy. If the sphenoid has been widely opened, then the posterior nasal artery or its vertical branch may have been divided (**Fig. 10.1**). Bipolar cautery is applied with the suction bipolar forceps* (Integra) until the field is dry. If the patient is still hypotensive at this stage, the anesthesiologist is asked to raise the blood pressure into the normal range before the patient is awakened. During this time, this region is inspected regularly on both sides and any vessels that bleed as the pressure is raised are cauterized.

Comorbidities for Spontaneous Epistaxis

The majority of patients (69%) presenting with severe epistaxis have associated comorbidities.[1] These usually

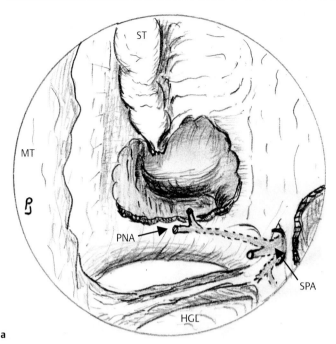

Fig. 10.1 (**a**) The vessels branching from the sphenopalatine artery (*SPA*) commonly bleed after ESS. Branches supplying the horizontal portion of the ground lamella (*HGL*) and the anterior wall of the sphenoid (posterior nasal artery [*PNA*]) need to be cauterized using a suction bipolar at the end of surgery to ensure that no bleeding occurs in the postoperative period. (**b**) Cadaveric image demonstrating the SPA, within the pterygopalatine fossa, giving off the PNA. This branch runs along the anterior face of the sphenoid, and can be inadvertently transected during sphenoidotomy. *PE*, posterior ethmoid cell; *ST*, superior turbinate; *SO*, sphenoid ostium; *MT*, middle turbinate.

include hypertension, cardiovascular disease, and clotting abnormalities. Over 60% of patients managed in our series were either on aspirin or on warfarin as part of their ongoing medical treatment.[1] As the effects of aspirin and aspirin-like drugs are not immediately reversible, no specific treatment is given for these clotting abnormalities. However, in patients who are on warfarin, this is stopped and, if necessary, a transfusion of fresh frozen plasma is given to rapidly lower the INR (below 2) before proceeding to surgery.

◆ Indications for Sphenopalatine Artery Ligation

Before sphenopalatine artery (SPA) ligation is considered, it needs to be established that the bleeding is coming from the posterior region of the nose. Patients who are assessed for possible SPA ligation are asked to forcefully blow their nose to expel all blood clots from the nose. The nose is then sprayed with a combination of lidocaine and epinephrine. The patient keeps their head forward after the nose blowing, allowing blood to drip into a kidney dish held below the nose. A rigid nasal endoscope and suction are then passed into the nose to assess where the bleeding is coming from. If the vessel is clearly visible, cautery is attempted.[2] If the vessel is not visible but bleeding is confirmed to be posterior, then an inflatable or expanding nasal posterior nasal pack is placed and the patient prepared for surgery.

Surgical Technique

This procedure can be performed under either local anaesthetic or general anaesthetic. The first step is to put the bleeding vessel into spasm. A pterygopalatine block is placed transorally. The greater palatine canal is located by palpation of the hard palate. A finger is passed along the hard palate until the junction of the hard and soft palate is felt. The finger is slowly slid anteriorly along the midpoint between the midline and teeth. The depression created by the greater palatine foramen is felt. This is usually opposite the second molar tooth[1,3] (**Fig. 10.2**).

With the finger still on the mucosal depression, an endoscope is slid into the mouth and the location of the depression endoscopically confirmed. The finger is then removed while the endoscope position is maintained. A 2-mL syringe with 1:80,000 lidocaine and adrenaline is attached to a 25-gauge needle that has been bent 25 mm from the tip at a 45-degree angle. The detailed anatomy of the greater palatine canal is presented in Chapter 2. The greater palatine canal is on average 18 mm long and the overlying soft tissue has an average depth of 7 mm. Therefore, bending the needle at 25 mm ensures that the needle does not enter the pterygopalatine fossa for any significant distance.[3] This lessens the risk of damage to the maxillary nerve or artery by the needle. The foramen and canal are located with the tip of the needle and the needle slid up into the canal to the bend. After aspiration has been performed 2 mL of lidocaine and adrenaline are injected. Spasm of the sphenopalatine artery with cessation of active bleeding was achieved in all the patients in our published series who were actively bleeding at the time of surgery.

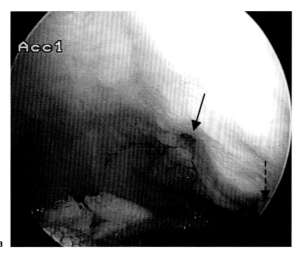
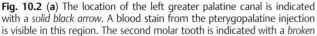
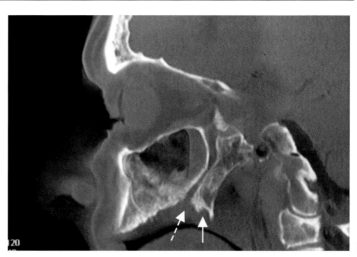

a

b

Fig. 10.2 (**a**) The location of the left greater palatine canal is indicated with a *solid black arrow*. A blood stain from the pterygopalatine injection is visible in this region. The second molar tooth is indicated with a *broken* *black arrow*. (**b**) The posterior edge of the hard palate is indicated with a *solid white arrow*. This is the first landmark. The finger is slide anteriorly until the depression of the greater palatine canal is felt (*broken white arrow*).

The nasal cavity is decongested using the combination of cocaine and adrenaline–soaked neuropatties. The lateral wall of the nose anterior to the posterior end of the middle turbinate is infiltrated with lidocaine and adrenaline. A right-angled suction is used to palpate the membranous posterior fontanelle of the maxillary sinus and the junction of the vertical portion to the palatine bone (see **Fig. 10.4**). Once the palatine bone is identified, a U-shaped incision is made onto bone (see **Fig. 10.4**). The incision is started under the horizontal portion of the ground lamella, down the palatine bone, and continued along the insertion of the inferior turbinate posteriorly[1] (**Figs. 10.3** and **10.4**).

The suction Freer elevator is used to elevate the mucosal flap. It is important to establish the subperiosteal plane at the point of incision as this allows a relatively bloodless dissection and also allows the periosteum to be stripped off the underlying bone in a manner similar to that used in raising a subperichondrial flap during a septoplasty. The initial elevation is done in the inferior region of the flap just above the insertion of the inferior turbinate on the lateral nasal wall[1] (**Fig. 10.4**).

Keeping the dissection low initially keeps the surgeon under the SPA. This dissection should be carried posteriorly until the anterior face of the sphenoid is reached. This is an important landmark as it allows the surgeon to be sure that the dissection has been carried far enough posterior before the dissection is taken superiorly. As the flap is lifted superiorly, the SPA is visualized exiting the sphenopalatine foramen. It is tented by the flap[1] (**Fig. 10.5**).

An additional landmark that can be sought is the ethmoidal bony process/crest of the palatine bone.[4,5] This bony projection is seen directly anterior to the sphenopalatine foramen (**Figs. 10.4** and **10.5**). It can be curetted away to improve visualization of the foramen. The artery is contained within the tissues exiting the foramen. Dissection with the suction Freer elevator is performed above the pedicle and the artery identified within the pedicle (**Fig. 10.5**). Once it is clearly delineated, two ligar clips are placed on the artery. Care should be taken to ensure that the clip is placed all the way across the artery. The artery may divide before exiting the foramen

and it is not uncommon for there to be a posterior branch exiting the foramen behind the anterior branch.[5] This posterior branch may exit through its own foramen in up to 16% of patients.[5] This branch (called the posterior nasal artery) travels across the posterior choana to the posterior aspect of the septum to supply the majority of the blood to the septum (**Fig. 10.1**). Endoscopic Ligar clip applicators should be used as they are easier to manipulate in the posterior region of the nasal cavity. The Ligar clip should be placed across the pedicle as the front of the clip applicator is pushed until it touches the anterior face of the sphenoid. As the clip is closed, the tips are moved slightly anterior to the sphenoid face so that they do not rub against the bone during closure. If, despite this maneuver, the clip does not sit properly across the pedicle, then further dissection may be needed before further clips are applied. When the pedicle is first exposed, there is too great a volume of tissue to be clipped and the vessels should be dissected out and clipped individually. A malleable suction Freer elevator or standard suction Freer elevator can be of value for this as the pedicle tends to ooze during this dissection before the clip is applied. Continuous suction through the instrument allows dissection to continue despite any oozing of blood. Clipping is recommended in spontaneous epistaxis as the caliber of the SPA is large in these patients and bipolar cautery alone may not be as effective. However, the vessel is usually cauterized after clipping to make sure no bleeding results if the clip is dislodged during the dissection for the posterior nasal artery (PNA). The PNA is sought in all patients as it may significantly contribute to a spontaneous posterior bleed and if not sought may contribute to failure of the procedure. Such dissection may dislodge the clip from the SPA and if the artery had not been cauterized in addition to being clipped, may result in a significant bleed that can be difficult to manage. Once the PNA is identified, it is cauterized with the suction bipolar. It is difficult to clip as it sits on the anterior face on the sphenoid and so the clip will often not sit over the vessel properly. The mucosal flap is replaced and held in place by a 2 cm by 2 cm piece of fibrillar Surgicel (Ethicon; Somerville, NJ). This is used as a considerable

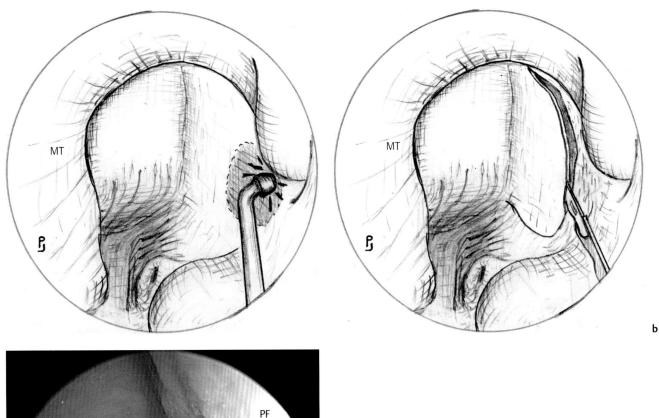

Fig. 10.3 (**a**) The right-angled curved suction palpating the posterior fontanelle of the maxillary sinus. (**b**) The U-shaped incision extending from the inferior surface of the horizontal part of the middle turbinate to just above the insertion of the inferior turbinate. (**c**) A cadaver image of palpation of the posterior fontanelle.

proportion of patients are either on aspirin or warfarin and it helps control oozing from the incision. No other packing is placed in the nose. The patient is discharged soon after recovery if no further bleeding is noted.

Results

In a recently published series of 13 consecutive patients,[1] four patients underwent SPA ligation under local anesthetic and nine under general anesthetic. The four who had local anesthetic were considered to be at risk if given general anesthetic.

The average age was 55.9 years (range 23–79) with an approximate equal sex distribution (males 7: females 6). All patients presented with intractable posterior epistaxis and underwent SPA ligation. One patient developed further epistaxis during the 12-month follow-up period, resulting in a 92% primary success rate in the treatment of the epistaxis.[1] The patient who re-bled was on aspirin and had a platelet abnormality with widespread ecchymosis on his arms and legs.

To date, a further 56 patients have undergone SPA ligation in our department. Similar incidences of comorbidities and anticoagulation were seen. The success at 12-month follow-up remains in the region of 90%.

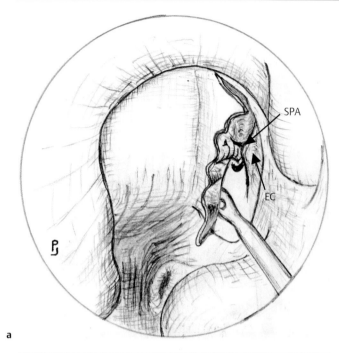

a

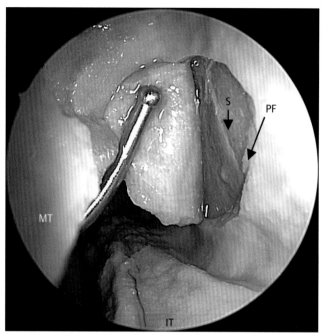

b

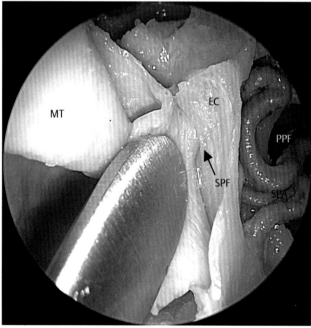

c

Fig. 10.4 (**a**) A suction Freer elevator is used to elevate the mucosal flap in the subperiosteal plane, keeping the initial dissection low just above the insertion of the inferior turbinate until the anterior face of the sphenoid is reached. As the dissection is taken superiorly the ethmoidal crest (*EC*) and sphenopalatine artery (*SPA*) are seen. (**b**) A cadaveric image of a U-shaped incision from the middle turbinate to just above inferior turbinate. This image clearly identifies the suture between the maxilla and the palatine bone (*S*). (**c**) Further dissection with the posterior maxillary sinus wall removed revealing the sphenopalatine artery (*SPA*) within the pterygopalatine fossa (*PPF*). The ethmoid crest (*EC*) is seen directly anterior to the sphenopalatine foramen (*SPF*). *MT*, middle turbinate; *IT*, inferior turbinate; *PT*, posterior fontanelle.

Bleeding From a Large Vessel in the Nose or Sinuses

A spurting artery in the region of the frontal recess will usually indicate damage to the anterior ethmoidal artery. The region should be packed with neuropatties soaked in adrenaline and cocaine. After waiting several minutes, the area can be checked. If the bleeding is from the skull base or from the region of the orbital periosteum associated with the skull base, suction bipolar cautery can be used to control the bleeding. Unipolar diathermy should not be used as it can arc to exposed dura and cause a cerebrospinal fluid (CSF) leak. If the bleeding is from the medial region of the frontal

recess, Surgicel and Gelfoam (Pfizer; Kalamazoo, MI) soaked in thrombin should be placed over the artery and the area firmly packed. Our preference is to use ribbon gauze soaked with bismuth iodoform paraffin paste (BIPP). This allows pressure to be placed over the Gelfoam and Surgicel. The BIPP gauze can be removed after a day or two. Cautery (bipolar or unipolar) should be avoided as there is a significant risk that any cautery (higher risk with unipolar) may burn a hole through the dura and cause a CSF leak.

Arterial spurting from the region of the SPA should be controlled with suction bipolar forceps* (Integra). If this is not available, a pterygopalatine fossa block will usually put the

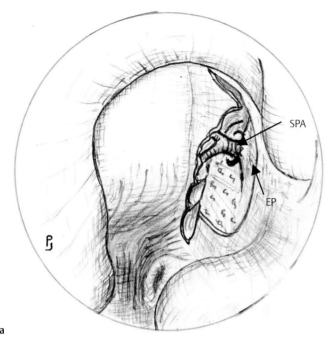

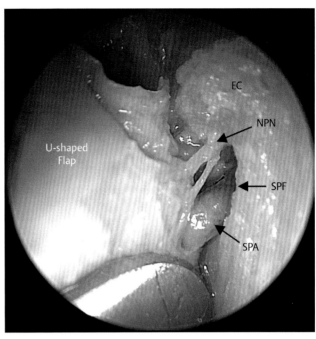

a

b

Fig. 10.5 (**a**) The flap is elevated superiorly and the sphenopalatine artery (*SPA*) is tented as it exits the sphenopalatine foramen. The ethmoidal crest (*EC*) of the palatine bone has been curetted to further expose the sphenopalatine foramen (*SPF*) and SPA. (**b**) The U-shaped mucosal flap has been elevated in a mucoperiosteal plane, and the contents of the sphenopalatine foramen (*SPF*) have been dissected demonstrating the nasopalatine nerves (*NPN*) and the SPA.

vessel in spasm and allow bipolar diathermy (without suction) to be used to control the bleeder (Chapter 2). Arterial bleeding is usually from the posterior nasal artery or the sphenopalatine artery (**Fig. 10.1**).

Key Points

The management of intractable epistaxis can either be with a nasal pack and postnasal balloon or ligation of the artery. If packing is used, the balloon will usually occlude the nasopharyngeal airway.[6] In elderly patients this may produce hypoxic episodes which may in turn precipitate fatal arrythmias.[7-10] The alternative to endoscopic SPA ligation is ligation of the maxillary artery through a Caldwell Luc approach.[11-13] Although this has a good success rate (87–90%), there are significant associated morbidities, with cheek and teeth pain and paresthesia being the most common (28%).[11-13] The nonsurgical option of management is to embolize the bleeding vessel.[13] Again, this is usually a successful procedure but has significant associated morbidities including hemiplegia, facial pain and facial paraesthesia, ophthalmoplegia, and blindness.[11-13] The overall complication rate of this procedure is 29%. The advantages of endoscopic SPA ligation are that it can be done under either local or general anesthetic, is relatively quick and straightforward with minimal associated morbidity, and has a good success rate. Our policy is that the nose should not be packed after the procedure and, if possible, the patient should be discharged from the hospital within 12 hours of the procedure. This dispenses with the need to keep patients in the ward with a packed nose, resulting in a better utilization of hospital resources.

◆ Vidian Neurectomy

Vidian neurectomy was established by Golding-Wood in the 1960s for the management of intractable vasomotor rhinitis, allergic rhinitis, and nasal polyposis.[14] The Vidian nerve supplies the nasal cavity with parasympathetic secretomotor fibers and sectioning of this nerve was found to improve symptoms of rhinorrhea, sneezing, postnasal space discharge, and nasal obstruction.[14-16] The initial enthusiasm for this technique was tempered by recurrence of symptoms after a 2-year follow-up and by complications. The surgical technique for severing the nerve has varied[14-16] and in some cases the nerve was never accurately identified before it was either cut or cauterized.[16] It is interesting that even though there have been a number of reports regarding the success of this technique over many years[13-18] in the management of chronic rhinorrhea and in some cases of nasal polyposis, this technique has not been widely adopted. One of the reasons for this may be the lack of a reliable and safe surgical technique for identifying and sectioning the nerve.

The Anatomy of the Vidian Canal

The Vidian canal connects the foramen lacerum with the pterygopalatine fossa, and is formed just anterior to the foramen lacerum where the carotid artery turns vertically toward its vertical segment in the sphenoid sinus. The greater superficial petrosal nerve and fibers from the sympathetic plexus around the carotid artery join to form the Vidian nerve which then enters the Vidian canal just anterior to the foramen lacerum. To aid understanding of the course of the

Vidian canal, a series of coronal CT scans are presented starting in the foramen lacerum and progressing forward, allowing the Vidian canal to be identified and followed anteriorly and slightly medially to where the canal opens in a funnel fashion into the pterygopalatine fossa (**Fig. 10.6**). If the parasagittal CT scan of this region is viewed, the Vidian canal can be clearly seen traversing the floor of the sphenoid sinus into the pterygopalatine fossa (**Fig. 10.6**).

Understanding the anatomy of the Vidian canal is very important in the endoscopic management of tumors infiltrating the pterygopalatine fossa and particularly in the management of juvenile nasopharyngeal angiofibromas (JNA). JNA tend to track down the Vidian canal and widen the canal toward the carotid artery. If this is not looked for, both on the imaging and during surgical removal of JNA, residual tumor can be left in the canal and may form the nidus for tumor regrowth. **Fig. 10.7** demonstrates the anatomical relationship between the Vidian canal, the pterygopalatine fossa,

and the carotid artery. This dry bone dissection illustrates the relationship between the Vidian canal, floor of the sphenoid sinus, and carotid artery (**Fig. 10.7**). In this specimen, the carotid artery has been exposed. The Vidian canal can be seen as it travels along the floor of the sphenoid from the Vidian canal foramen to the paraclival carotid artery.

Fig. 10.8 illustrates the palatovaginal canal and how this can be confused with the Vidian canal; their close relationship is not recognized.

Surgical Technique for Vidian Neurectomy

The nasal preparation and injection of the pterygopalatine fossa through the mouth is performed as previously described (Chapter 2). The mucosal incisions for Vidian neurectomy are the same as for SPA ligation. The artery is localized and cauterized with the suction bipolar diathermy forceps. Cautery is

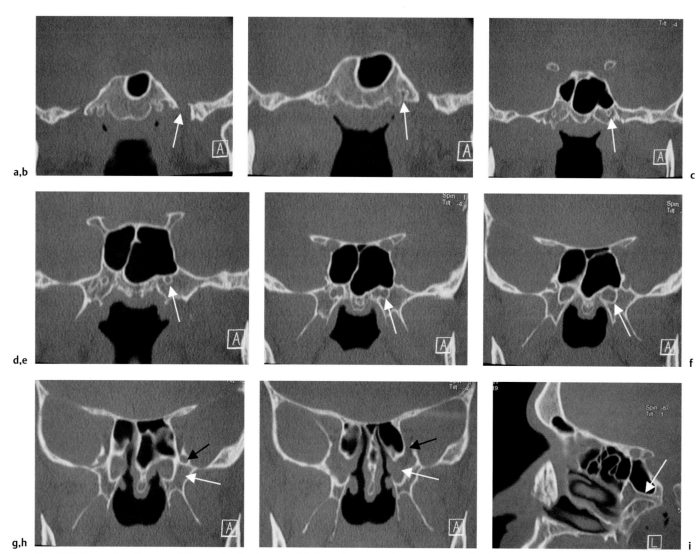

a,b

c

d,e

f

g,h

i

Fig. 10.6 The series of coronal CT scans begin with scan (**a**) through the foramen lacerum (*white arrow*) and as the scans move anteriorly (**b–h**), the Vidian canal can be followed along the floor of the sphenoid (*white arrows*) into the pterygopalatine fossa (**g,h**). Note the foramen rotundum in scan (**g**) (*black arrow*) and the supra orbital fissure (*black arrow*) in scan (**h**). (**i**) A parasagittal scan and shows the Vidian canal from the foramen lacerum to the pterygopalatine fossa (*white arrow*). Note how the canal funnels outward as it enters the fossa.

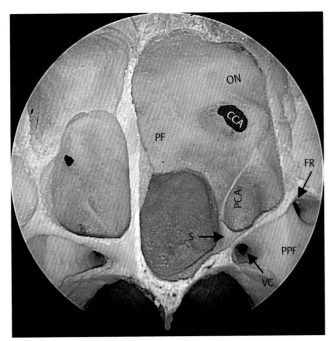 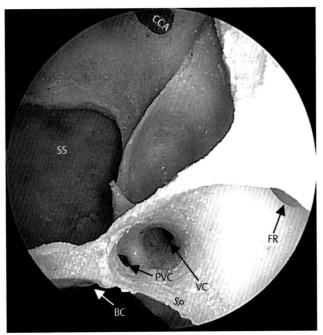

Fig. 10.7 This dry bone image of the sphenoid sinus within the body of the sphenoid. It clearly demonstrates how the Vidian canal (*VC*) communicates with the pterygopalatine fossa (*PPF*) anteriorly, and the foramen lacerum posteriorly. The Vidian canal runs in the floor of the sphenoid sinus, and frequently has a sphenoid sinus septation (*S*) attaching to the roof of the canal. The foramen lacerum is the location of the supralacerum genu of the carotid artery, where the horizontal petrous carotid artery turns upward to become the paraclival carotid artery (*PCA*). The Vidian canal and nerve is a vital landmark in surgical dissection in this area. *PF*, pituitary fossa; *FR*, foramen rotundum; *CCA*, anterior genu of the cavernous carotid artery.

Fig. 10.8 This dry bone specimen has had the sphenoidale process (*SP*) of the palatine bone drilled (the posterior bony contribution to the sphenopalatine foramen). This allows visualization of the palatovaginal canal (*PVC*) and Vidian canal (*VC*), both running along the floor of the sphenoid sinus (*SS*) and emanating at the anterior face of the sphenoid sinus. Note the more medial position of the PVC, and the smaller diameter when compared to the Vidian canal (*VC*). Also note the gutter formed from the SP and indicated underlying the letter VC as this forms the floor of the Vidian canal, which widens as it enters the pterygopalatine fossa. *FR*, foramen rotundum; *BC*, boney choana; *CCA*, anterior genu of the carotid artery.

preferred as the clips tend to slip off or are knocked off as the surgery progresses to the area behind the sphenopalatine foramen. The SPA is significantly larger in patients with active epistaxis than in patients undergoing elective surgery (Vidian neurectomy) and therefore bipolar cautery is effective for obtaining hemostasis in the latter cases.

Once the SPA foramen is identified, the mucosal flap is raised behind the foramen until the face of the sphenoid sinus is identified (**Fig. 10.9**). One of the first structures seen as this flap is elevated is the posterior pharyngeal nerve emanating from the pterygopalatine ganglion and running superficial to the Vidian canal laterally into the palatovaginal canal. This nerve can easily be mistaken for the Vidian nerve (**Fig. 10.9**). The posterior pharyngeal nerve travels through the palatovaginal canal (**Fig. 10.9**) and then onto the pharynx to provide sympathetic and parasympathetic fibers to this region (**Fig. 10.9**).

If a successful Vidian neurectomy is to be performed, it is vitally important to understand the relationship between the palatovaginal canal (PVC) and the Vidian canal. These two canals both transmit sizable nerves and both travel along the floor of the sphenoid sinus, emanating from the anterior aspect of a widening Vidian canal as it approaches the pterygopalatine fossa, and separated by only a few millimeters. Important differences allowing accurate identification of each of these structures are the more medial position of the PVC, the relatively smaller nerve passing through the

PVC, and the significantly smaller diameter of the PVC compared to the Vidian canal (**Figs. 10.9** and **10.10**).

The posterior pharyngeal nerve is divided and the anterior face of the sphenoid is identified and perforated with a Freer elevator (**Fig. 10.11a**). This opening is enlarged until a clear view into the sphenoid sinus is obtained and the floor of the sphenoid sinus identified. This gives certainty regarding the horizontal location of the Vidian canal as it always runs along the floor of the anterior aspect of the sphenoid sinus (**Fig. 10.8**). The key landmark is the palatine bone. If a line is drawn vertically up the posterior aspect of the palatine bone and the intersection of this line with a line drawn through the floor of the sphenoid sinus, the intersection of these two lines marks the Vidian canal (**Fig. 10.10**). Check the coronal CT scans in **Fig. 10.6** and the cadaver dissection in **Fig. 10.9** to confirm this.

In order to expose the Vidian canal, the posteroinferior margin (sphenoidale process of the palatine bone) of the sphenopalatine foramen needs to be removed (**Fig. 10.12**). This is best done with either a straight through-biting Blakesley forceps or a forward-biting 2-mm Kerrison's punch. This will remove the medial wall of the pterygopalatine fossa and allow the Vidian canal to be clearly identified. In some patients, this bone can be thick and difficult to remove and can be removed with a DCR diamond bur. Note that the periosteum overlying the pterygopalatine fossa is still intact and if this is torn the yellow fat within the fossa

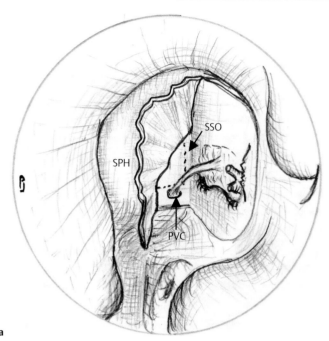

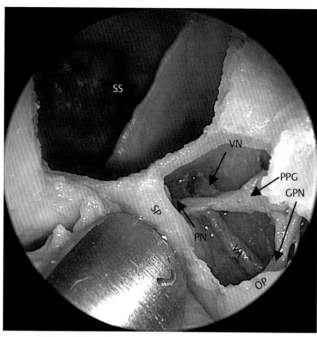

a

b

Fig. 10.9 (**a**) The anterior face of the sphenoid sinus (*SPH*) is exposed and the outline of the sinus marked (*SSO*) with *dotted lines*. The palatovaginal canal (*PVC*) is seen with the posterior pharyngeal branch of the pterygopalatine ganglion entering the canal. (**b**) Cadaver picture of the sphenoid sinus (*SS*) opening maximized down to the floor of the sphenoid. The sphenopalatine foramen is made up of the sphenoidale process (*SP*) and the orbital process (*OP*) of the palatine bone, and drilling these allows wide exposure of the medial contents of the pterygopalatine fossa. The pharyngeal nerve (*PN*) is the first nerve visualized and is the most medial nerve, running to the pterygopalatine ganglion (*PPG*). Just lateral to this the vidian nerve (*VN*) can also be seen joining the PPG. *GPN*, greater palatine nerve; *VA*, Vidian artery.

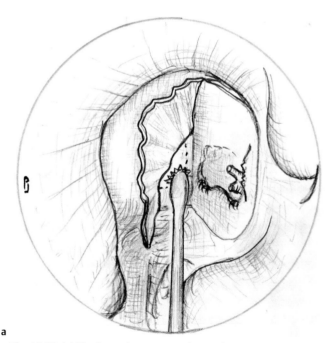

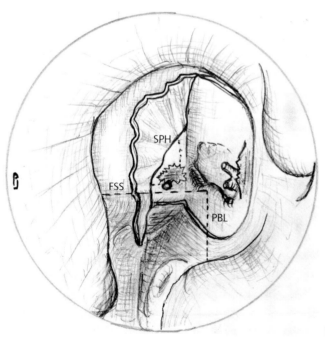

a

b

Fig. 10.10 (**a**) The Freer elevator is used to perforate the anterior face of the sphenoid sinus just above the floor of the sinus. This opening is enlarged and a clear view into the sphenoid sinus obtained so that the floor of the sphenoid sinus (*FSS*) can be clearly seen, (**b**) A line is drawn in continuation with the posterior margin of the palatine bone (*PBL*).

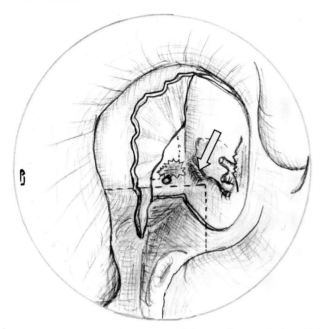

Fig. 10.11 The poster inferior region of the SPA foramen (sphenoidal process) needs to be removed to identify the Vidian canal (*block arrow*).

should be visible. This should be expected and should not be confused with orbital fat. Removal of the posteroinferior wall of the sphenopalatine foramen will allow identification of the floor of the funnel-shaped opening of the Vidian canal. This floor forms a "gutter" in which the Vidian nerve

runs (see **Fig. 10.9**). A sickle knife is used in the subperiosteal plane to slide from the removed edge of the foramen along the "gutter" to the lateral wall of the funnel-shaped opening of the Vidian canal. Once this maneuver has been performed, the Vidian nerve lies directly above the sickle knife.

A sickle knife is again used to stay on the bone of the anterior face of the sphenoid above the Vidian canal and to continue this subperiosteal dissection over the Vidian nerve until the lateral aspect of the canal is identified. The fat of the pterygopalatine fossa is exposed and the sickle knife is used to probe the fat and expose the Vidian nerve. Note that the nerve is large (3–4 mm in diameter). Also note that the Vidian canal travels directly posteriorly toward the vertical part of the carotid artery. If there are additional septations within the sphenoid sinus, these septations will in most cases attach to the roof of the Vidian canal in the floor of the sphenoid sinus (providing an additional landmark; **Fig. 10.7**). The nerve is usually immediately visible after it exits the Vidian canal at the level of the floor of the sphenoid sinus. It is dissected free until it is seen to move laterally toward the pterygopalatine ganglion in the pterygopalatine fossa (**Figs. 10.9** and **10.12**).

Extensive lateral dissection can allow the maxillary nerve to be visualized but this not recommended for the standard Vidian nerve section (**Fig. 10.12**). Once the nerve is identified, confirmation that it is the Vidian nerve is made by following the nerve into the Vidian canal. This canal runs in an anteroposterior direction and the nerve can be visualized exiting the canal. The normal procedure to cut the nerve is to

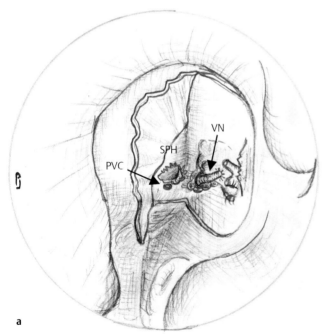

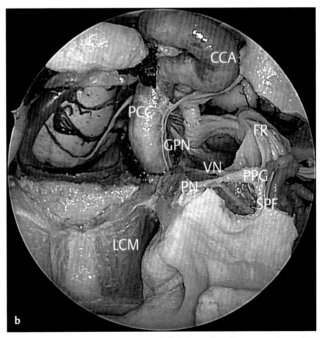

Fig. 10.12 (**a**) The Vidian nerve is seen exiting the Vidian canal running toward the sphenopalatine foramen before moving laterally toward the maxillary nerve in the pterygopalatine fossa. Cadaver dissection (**b**) shows more extensive dissection. The superior third of the clivus and the planum sphenoidale have been drilled and dura removed, along with exposure of the junction between the lateral sphenoid wall and the pterygopalatine fossa. The floor of the sphenoid sinus has been drilled up to the Vidian nerve (*VN*).

The VN can be visualized running in a slightly laterally, after it exits the Vidian canal, to join the pterygopalatine ganglion (*PPG*), as opposed to the pharyngeal nerve (*PN*) that runs in a lateral direction to join the PPG. The PPG can be seen to hang medially off the maxillary nerve just after it exits the skeletonized foramen rotundum (*FR*). *IT*, inferior turbinate; *LCM*, longus capitis muscle; *PCA*, paraclival carotid artery; *CCA*, anterior genu of the cavernous carotid artery; *SPA*, sphenopalatine foramen; *GPN*, greater petrosal nerve.

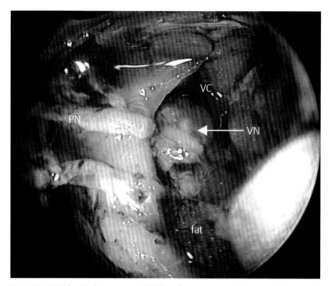

Fig. 10.13 The Vidian nerve (*VN*) has been cut and the entire bone of the Vidian canal (*VC*) around the nerve can be seen. The stump of the nerve should then be cauterized with a bipolar forceps. The pharyngeal nerve (*PN*) and fat of the pterygopalatine fossa can be seen.

either use the sickle knife with the tip tracking subperiosteally along the gutter until the nerve sits in the natural curve of the sickle knife and then to cut upward or to use a curved skull base scissors (Integra) angled from medial to lateral to cut the nerve. A 2- to 3-mm section of the nerve is removed and the remaining nerve exiting the Vidian canal is cauterized with bipolar diathermy. Unipolar diathermy is not recommended as the infraorbital canal and maxillary nerve are in relative close proximity and damage can occur with injudicious usage of unipolar diathermy in this region. Optic nerve injury has also been described after blind attempts were made to cauterize the Vidian nerve. Therefore, we advocate clear visualization and positive identification followed by section of the nerve and bipolar diathermy of the nerve root (**Fig. 10.13**). To ensure that the nerve has been cut, 360 degrees of bone must be visible around the Vidian canal with the cut nerve end clearly visible in the canal. Once this is achieved, the mucosal flap is replaced. If it tends to fall away from the lateral nasal wall, a small piece of Gelfoam is placed under the middle turbinate over the flap to hold it in place. No other packing is placed in the nose.

Results with This Technique[19]

Over the past 5 years, nine patients have undergone 14 operations. The mean follow-up was 25 months. Most of the patients suffered intractable rhinorrhea (80%) with nasal obstruction (72%), postnasal drip (64%), and sneezing (57%) also prominent. Postoperatively, there was a significant improvement in rhinorrhea and nasal obstruction at the last follow-up (mean greater than 2 years). In three patients, there was a worsening of sneezing postoperatively. In addition, 35% of patients suffered a variable amount of dry eye and 28% had nasal crusting. Half of the Vidian neurectomies were deemed to be highly successful by the patients at a mean follow-up time of 2 years.[19]

Key Points

Vidian neurectomy has been shown to result in significant histological changes in the nasal mucosa including mast cell depletion.[20] The exact mechanism by which Vidian neurectomy results in improvement in symptoms postoperatively is unknown. As most previous studies have not histologically confirmed the sectioning of the nerve, there may be patients who have not actually had their Vidian nerve sectioned but have been included among patients who have undergone Vidian neurectomy. A significant amount of research on the outcomes after Vidian neurectomy needs to be performed before the role of Vidian nerve neurectomy in endoscopic sinus surgery is properly defined.

References

1. Wormald PJ, Wee DTH, van Hasselt CA. Endoscopic ligation of the sphenopalatine artery for refractory posterior epistaxis. Am J Rhinol 2000;14(4):261–264

2. Sharp HR, Rowe-Jones JM, Biring GS, Mackay IS. Endoscopic ligation or diathermy of the sphenopalatine artery in persistent epistaxis. J Laryngol Otol 1997;111(11):1047–1050

3. Mercuri LG. Intraoral second division nerve block. Oral Surg Oral Med Oral Pathol 1979;47(2):109–113

4. Snyderman CH, Goldman SA, Carrau RL, Ferguson BJ, Grandis JR. Endoscopic sphenopalatine artery ligation is an effective method of treatment for posterior epistaxis. Am J Rhinol 1999;13(2): 137–140

5. Wareing MJ, Padgham ND. Osteologic classification of the sphenopalatine foramen. Laryngoscope 1998;108(1 Pt 1):125–127

6. McGarry GW, Aitken D. Intranasal balloon catheters: how do they work? Clin Otolaryngol Allied Sci 1991;16(4):388–392

7. Jacobs JR, Dickson CB. Effects of nasal and laryngeal stimulation upon peripheral lung function. Otolaryngol Head Neck Surg 1986;95(3 Pt 1): 298–302

8. Shaheen OH. Epistaxis in the middle aged and elderly. Thesis for the master of Surgery. University of London; 1967

9. El-Guindy A. Endoscopic transseptal sphenopalatine artery ligation for intractable posterior epistaxis. Ann Otol Rhinol Laryngol 1998;107(12): 1033–1037

10. Papsidero MJ. The role of nasal obstruction in obstructive sleep apnea syndrome. Ear Nose Throat J 1993;72(1):82–84

11. Metson R, Lane R. Internal maxillary artery ligation for epistaxis: an analysis of failures. Laryngoscope 1988;98(7):760–764

12. Premachandra DJ, Sergeant RJ. Dominant maxillary artery as a cause of failure in maxillary artery ligation for posterior epistaxis. Clin Otolaryngol Allied Sci 1993;18(1):42–47

13. Strong EB, Bell DA, Johnson LP, Jacobs JM. Intractable epistaxis: transantral ligation vs. embolization: efficacy review and cost analysis. Otolaryngol Head Neck Surg 1995;113(6):674–678

14. Golding-Wood PH. Observations on petrosal and vidian neurectomy in chronic vasomotor rhinitis. J Laryngol Otol 1961;75:232–247

15. Kamel R, Zaher S. Endoscopic transnasal vidian neurectomy. Laryngoscope 1991;101(3):316–319

16. Fernandes CM. Bilateral transnasal Vidian neurectomy in the management of chronic rhinitis. J Laryngol Otol 1988;102:894–895

17. Greenstone MA, Stanley PJ, Mackay IS, Cole PJ. The effect of vidian neurectomy on nasal mucociliary clearance. J Laryngol Otol 1988;102(10): 894–895

18. Krajina Z. Critical review of vidian neurectomy. Rhinology 1989;27(4): 271–276

19. Robinson SR, Wormald PJ. Endoscopic vidian neurectomy. Am J Rhinol Am J Rhinol 2006;20(2):197–202

20. Konno A, Togawa K. Vidian neurectomy for allergic rhinitis. Evaluation of long-term results and some problems concerning operative therapy. Arch Otorhinolaryngol 1979;225:67–77

11 Powered Endoscopic Dacryocystorhinostomy

◆ Introduction and Anatomy

Endoscopic dacryocystorhinostomy (DCR) was initially described by Caldwell in the 19th century.[1] However, it fell into disrepute as surgeons experienced problems with visualization of the surgical site. In the early 20th century, Toti described the external DCR procedure and with a few modifications this procedure remains largely unchanged from those early descriptions.[2] As the technique has developed, so the success rate for the external procedure has improved until today, in the hands of properly trained oculoplastic surgeons, success rates of between 90% and 95% can be expected.[3] As endoscopic sinus surgery became popular in the late 1980s, there was renewed interest in endoscopic DCR with the initial descriptions having appeared in the late 1980s and early 1990s.[4–6] As could be expected of a new and developing technique, the initial success rates were lower than that of external DCR and varied between 65% and 90%.[4–6] Laser endoscopic DCR was promoted in the mid-1990s but success rates were disappointing and tended to be at the lower end of the spectrum (around 75%).[7–9] This was probably due to the technique creating only a small opening into the posterior inferior lacrimal sac through the thin lacrimal bone. It is well recognized within the literature on external DCR that a small ostium does not achieve the same success rates as a large openings of the lacrimal sac.[10]

The original endoscopic DCR technique was described as follows: a mucosal flap anterior to the middle turbinate was raised and the junction between the lacrimal bone and frontal process of maxilla established. A Hajek Koeffler punch was used to remove what bone one could over the lacrimal sac.[4] In the early 1990s, I reviewed my own results with this technique and found a disappointing long-term patency rate of only 83%.[11] On review of the literature on external DCR, the critical factor necessary for achieving the 90 to 95% success rate was a wide bone removal so that the entire lacrimal sac was exposed.[10,12–14] Following this, the mucosa of the lacrimal sac and nasal mucosa were anastomosed with sutures allowing primary intention healing without significant granulation. This raised the question: Could the external DCR technique be duplicated by a similar intranasal technique? If this were to be done, the first step was to define the intranasal anatomy of the lacrimal sac.[13] The early descriptions of the intranasal anatomy of the sac placed the sac anterior to the middle turbinate with minimal extension of the sac above the insertion of the middle turbinate on the lateral nasal wall (the so-called axilla of the middle turbinate as it resembles an armpit).[13,15,16] To investigate the precise location of the sac, a series of CT dacryocystograms (DCGs) in patients undergoing DCR were performed and the relationship of the lacrimal sac and the axilla of the middle turbinate evaluated.[13] This study showed that the anatomy of the sac on the lateral nasal wall was significantly different to what had been previously described in the literature (**Fig. 11.1**). The sac was not only anterior to the middle turbinate but a significant proportion was located above the axilla of the middle turbinate. On average, the sac extended 8 mm above the axilla of the middle turbinate.[13] Therefore, if the external DCR principles were to be applied to endoscopic DCR, a different technique was required. This led to the design of a new technique (powered endoscopic DCR), which is presented here.[14,17,18]

◆ Preoperative Assessment of the Patient Presenting with Epiphora

Examine the Eye and Look for Other Causes of Watery Eye

Excess Tear Production

◆ *Conjunctival disease.* Patients with conjunctivitis present with sticky secretions or pus in the eye that is often worse when they wake in the morning. Antibiotic eye drops are used to treat bacterial infections and prevent colonization in patients with viral conjunctivitis.

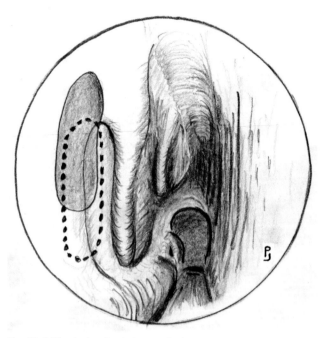

Fig. 11.1 The *broken line* indicates the location of the sac prior to our studies on the intranasal anatomy of the lacrimal sac. The shaded area is the actual intranasal position of the lacrimal sac on the lateral nasal wall. Note it extends between 8 to 10 mm above the axilla of the middle turbinate.

◆ *Dry eye.* Patients may have significant dryness that will irritate the eye and produce tearing. Application of artificial tears is usually all that is necessary.
◆ *Lid malposition.* Ectropion or entropion cause the puncta to not be properly positioned in the tear lake. A floppy lower eyelid (increased lid laxity) may also place the puncta in a position where tear collection is impaired. Surgical repositioning or tightening of the lid is required.
◆ *Blepharitis.* Blepharitis causes a mucoid discharge from the eye. In this condition, there is an alteration in the bacteriology of the mucous glands in the hair follicles of the eyelashes that results in a mucoid discharge from the eye.

The vision will be blurred and the eye often burns. Treatment is to rub the eyelid margin with gauze soaked in warm, soapy water twice a day. This will need to be done for about 3 months before the condition resolves.

Epiphora

◆ *Punctal stenosis.* Obliteration or narrowing of the superior or inferior punctum
◆ *Canalicular stenosis or obstruction.* Superior or inferior canalicular stenosis or obstruction may follow trauma or viral infection.
◆ *Nasolacrimal duct blockage.* Usually from unknown cause.

Nasolacrimal Duct Obstruction

In epiphora caused by nasolacrimal duct obstruction (NLDO), tears will frequently run down the cheek. This is more noticeable in conditions that stimulate tear formation such as walking in a cold wind. During examination, the position and size of the puncta should be assessed. The lid laxity and positioning of the puncta in the tear lake should be determined. In order to assess the patency of the inferior, superior, and common canaliculi, the upper lacrimal system should be probed (**Fig. 11.2**). The punctum is dilated with a punctum dilator. A Bowman's lacrimal probe is then used to probe the inferior canaliculus and common canaliculus.

Differentiating between a soft and a hard stop on probing helps assess the patency of the canalicular system. If a common canaliculus stricture is present, it should be diagnosed preoperatively so appropriate steps can be taken to correct it during surgery. Additionally, the patient can be informed that the likelihood of a successful procedure is significantly less than is the case with a DCR performed for nasolacrimal duct obstruction.

Syringing of the lacrimal system will also help assess the patency of the nasolacrimal system. In NLDO there will be significant reflux through the upper punctum with no saline penetration into the nose. In partial NLDO there will be reflux through the upper punctum with saline penetration into the

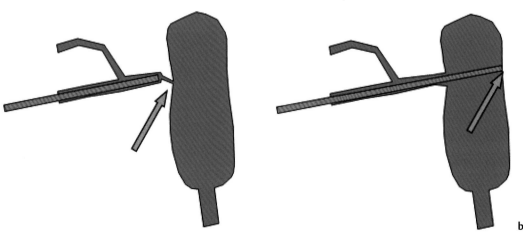

a   b

Fig. 11.2 (**a**) A soft stop is felt as the probe rests against a common canaliculus stricture or obstruction, whereas in (**b**) a hard stop is felt as the probe comes to rest against the bone encasing the lacrimal sac.

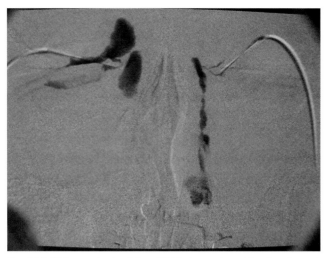

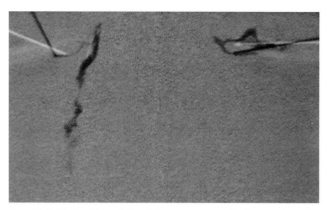

Fig. 11.4 Obstruction of the left common canaliculus–sac junction with reflux of dye into the conjunctival region.

Fig. 11.3 Right nasolacrimal duct (NLD) obstruction with reflux through the superior punctum into the conjunctiva with patent left NLD system.

nose but only with increased syringing pressure. Penetration into the nasal cavity without reflux through the upper punctum indicates a patent (but not necessarily functional) lacrimal system. It is sometimes confusing to determine exactly where the saline is refluxing as some may reflux from the punctum that has been injected, or from the other punctum or a combination.

Examine the Nasal Cavity

Rigid nasal endoscopy is performed on all patients presenting with epiphora. A significant proportion (15%) of patients require surgery for nasal pathology at the same time as the DCR. Mostly this is for associated chronic sinusitis. All patients need to be questioned regarding nasal symptoms and endoscopy performed to assess the nasal cavity. If there is evidence of nasal and sinus disease, appropriate investigations are performed and treatment instituted. If medical

therapy fails to resolve the problem, surgery is performed at the same time as the DCR.

Dacryocystogram and Lacrimal Scintillography

We routinely perform a DCG to assess the patency of the canalicular system and penetration of dye into the nasolacrimal sac.[17] If the patient has a hard stop on probing with a blocked system on syringing, this investigation can be omitted. Filling of the sac but failure of the dye to penetrate the nasal cavity confirms the diagnosis of NLDO (**Fig. 11.3**).

Patency of the NLD system without reflux through the canalicular system normally indicates an anatomically patent system (**Fig. 11.3**, left side). Failure of the dye to penetrate the lacrimal sac may indicate a common canalicular obstruction (**Fig. 11.4**).

To assess the function of the NLD system, lacrimal scintillography is performed. DCG assesses anatomy but not function. A radioisotope is placed in the conjunctival fornix and regular scanning performed for 30 minutes. If the isotope penetrates the lacrimal sac and not the nasal cavity, NLDO exists (**Fig. 11.5**).

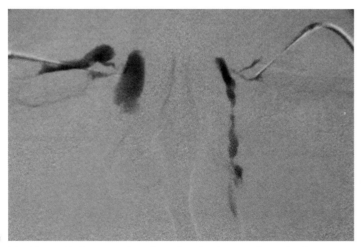

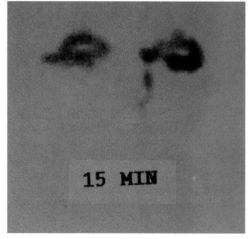

a

b

Fig. 11.5 DCG shows NLDO on the right side. The scintillography shows penetration of the radioisotope on the left into the nasal cavity but shows holdup on the right with no nasal cavity penetration. This confirms the diagnosis of NLDO.

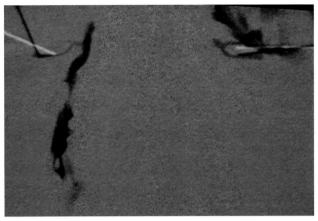
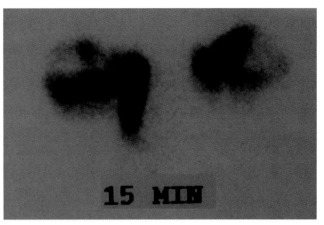

a   b

Fig. 11.6 Obstruction of left common canaliculus on DCG with radioisotope penetrating the lacrimal sac on scintillography indicating likely distention of sac kinking common canaliculus–sac junction.

In some patients, the DCG may show no filling of the lacrimal sac, whereas scintillography shows filling of the sac (**Fig. 11.6**). This may occur when the sac is full of mucus and the distended sac kinks the common canaliculus just before it enters the sac.

Scintillography also helps identify a functional obstruction when the DCG is normal (patent) in a symptomatic patient. If the scintillography confirms lack of nasal cavity penetration of the isotope, then a functional NLDO exists (**Fig. 11.7**). These patients can be managed by performing an endoscopic DCR but the outcome is not as successful as with anatomical obstruction of the NLD system (see results of functional NLDO).

◆ Surgical Technique[14,17–19] (see Video)

After nasal decongestion with neuropatties and infiltration with lidocaine and adrenaline, a no. 15 scalpel blade is used to make the initial mucosal incisions. It is important that these incisions are correctly placed as they form the borders for the subsequent bone removal and lacrimal sac exposure. The first incision is made horizontally 8 to 10 mm above the axilla of the middle turbinate, starting about 3 mm posterior to the axilla and coming forward about 10 mm onto the frontal process of the maxilla (bony prominence in the lateral nasal wall just anterior to the middle turbinate). The blade is then turned vertically and a vertical incision made to about two-thirds of the vertical height of the middle turbinate, stopping just above the insertion of the inferior turbinate into the lateral nasal wall (**Fig. 11.8**). The blade is turned horizontally and the inferior incision is started at the insertion of the uncinate process and brought forward to meet the vertical incision (**Fig. 11.9**).

Using a 30-degree endoscope, a suction Freer elevator is used to elevate the mucosal flap while ensuring that the tip of the instrument always maintains contact with the bone (**Fig. 11.10**). Be particularly careful to keep the tip of the suction Freer on bone as it rides over the prominence of the frontal process of the maxilla because the bone contour can

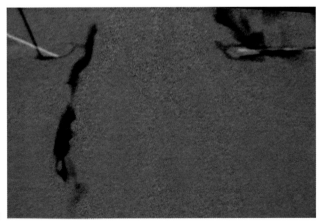
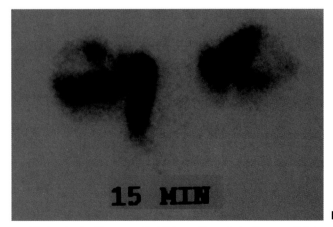

a   b

Fig. 11.7 This is the same DCG and scintillogram as seen in **Fig. 11.6**. If the right side is examined on the DCG, the system appears normal. However, on the scintillography, although the sac fills nicely with radioisotope, no penetration of the nasal cavity occurs. Later time points need to be checked to ensure that this continues to be the case. This is a functional obstruction of the nasolacrimal system on the right side and an anatomical obstruction on the left side.

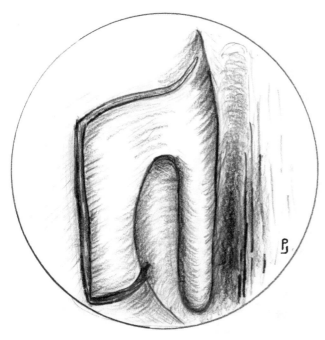

a

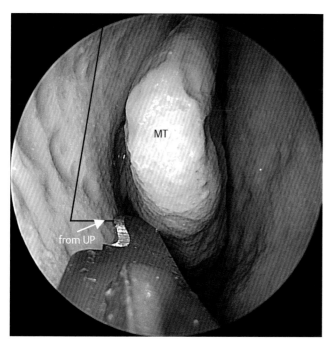

b

Fig. 11.8 (**a**) Mucosal incisions 8 to 10 mm above and anterior to the axilla of the middle turbinate. (Adapted with permission from Wormald PJ. Powered endoscopic DCR. Otolaryngol Clin North Am 2006;39:539–549.) (**b**) Cadaveric dissection demonstrating the horizontal and vertical incisions.

The horizontal superior incision is made 8 to 10 mm above the axilla of the middle turbinate (*MT*), started 3 mm behind the axilla of the MT, and continued 10 mm in front. The vertical incision is continued for two-thirds of the MT height.

fall away abruptly and contact with the bone and surgical plane can be lost. At this point the bone should be palpated so that the junction of the soft lacrimal bone and hard bone of the frontal process can be identified (**Fig. 11.10c**). This is a key landmark and must be sought in all primary surgeries. Note that the lacrimal bone is sought at the bottom

Fig. 11.9 Cadaveric image of left nasal cavity demonstrating the inferior horizontal incision. This incision begins from the insertion of the uncinate process (*UP*) forward to meet the vertical incision. *MT*, middle turbinate.

of the region from which the mucosal flap has been raised, just above the insertion of the inferior turbinate. The thin lacrimal bone is 2–5 mm wide before the insertion of the uncinate process is reached (**Fig. 11.11**). Dissection stops at the uncinate and the uncinate insertion should not be disturbed. A round knife (Storz, Germany; from the standard ear tray of instruments) is used to flake the soft lacrimal bone away from the posteroinferior region of the sac. If this is difficult, the frontal process can be removed first before the lacrimal bone is flaked away.

Once the lacrimal bone has been removed, a forward biting Hajek Koeffler punch (Storz, Germany) is used to remove the lower portion of the frontal process of the maxilla (**Fig. 11.12**). The tip of the punch is used to push the lacrimal sac away before the punch is engaged and the bone is removed. The lacrimal sac may be inadvertently grasped as the punch is closed. The punch should be opened after the initial bite to allow any sac wall that may have been pinched in the jaws of the punch to be released. After this maneuver, the punch is closed over the loose bone and this bone removed. This avoids tearing the sac with the punch. Bone removal continues both anteriorly and superiorly until the punch can no longer be seated on the bone. Removal of the frontal process of the maxilla uncovers the anteroinferior portion of the lacrimal sac (**Fig. 11.12**), and only stops when the bone becomes too thick for the punch to engage. At this point a 25-degree curved 2.5-mm rough diamond bur (Medtronic ENT; Minneapolis, MN) is attached to the microdebrider and used to remove the rest of the bone up to the superior mucosal incision (**Fig. 11.13**). In the vast majority of cases, an agger nasi cell is present and the mucosa of this cell will be exposed as the sac is followed superiorly above the

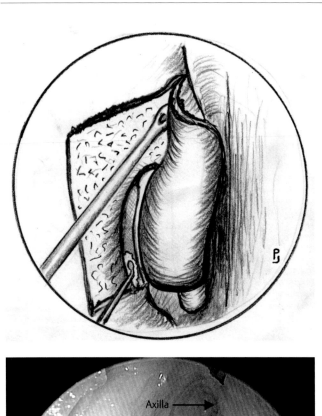

a

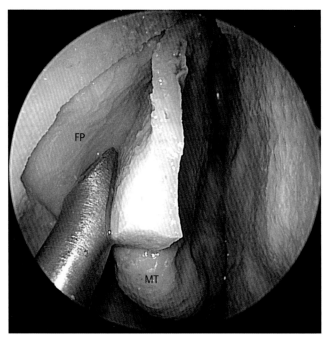

b

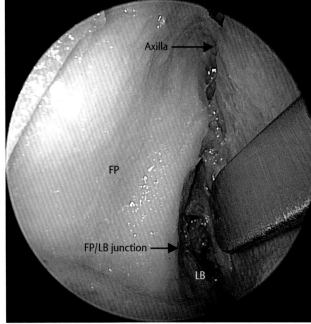

c

Fig. 11.10 (**a**) Illustrates elevation of the flap with a suction Freer elevator. Note the round knife removing the thin lacrimal bone in the inferior region of the dissection. The cadaveric photo (**b**) shows the suction freer hard against the frontal process (*FP*), elevating the mucoperiosteal flap. (**c**) Shows the junction where the hard frontal process can fall away to become the soft lacrimal bone (*LB*); care must be taken when elevating in this region. *MT*, middle turbinate. (**a**, Adapted with permission from Wormald PJ. Powered endoscopic DCR. Otolaryngol Clin North Am 2006;39:539–549.)

axilla of the middle turbinate (**Fig. 11.12b**). The diamond bur can be brought into light contact with the lacrimal sac lining without damaging the sac. Significant pressure by the diamond bur on the sac will cause damage. A cutting bur will remove the bone faster; however, it does cause significant damage to the sac wall and will often result in a hole in the sac wall. The bone is removed until the entire sac is exposed. The sac should stand proud of the lateral nasal wall so that when the sac is incised and the mucosal flaps are rolled out, they will lie flat on the lateral nasal wall (**Fig. 11.13**). Thus, the sac will be marsupialized into the wall rather than an ostium being created in the sac.

Next the inferior punctum is dilated with a punctum dilator and a Bowman's lacrimal probe is passed into the sac (**Fig. 11.14**). When the probe is moved up and down in the sac its tip should be able to seen moving behind the sac wall. This confirms that the probe is indeed within the sac (**Fig. 11.15**). Movement of the sac without visualization of the tip of the probe usually indicates that the probe is still at the common canaliculus–sac junction and the lateral wall has been pushed onto the medial wall with some movement of the medial wall. Cutting down on the probe, if it is not in the sac lumen, can result in damage to the common canaliculus opening. With the tip of the

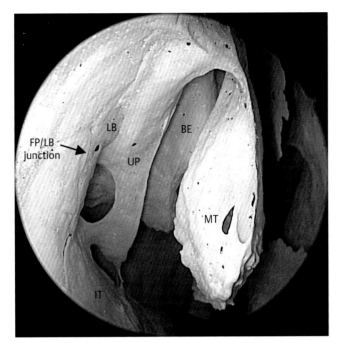

Fig. 11.11 Dry bone image demonstrating the junction between the hard frontal process (*FP*) and soft lacrimal bone (*LB*). The common boundary shared between the lacrimal bone and the uncinate process (*UP*) can be clearly visualized. *IT*, inferior turbinate; *MT*, middle turbinate; *BE*, bulla ethmoidalis.

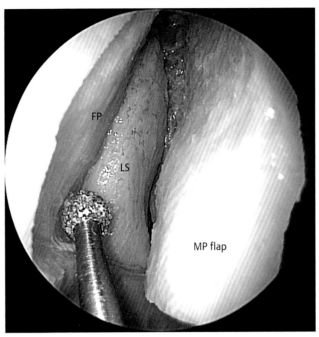

Fig. 11.13 Cadaveric photo of the right side demonstrating further exposure of the lacrimal sac (*LS*) by drilling the frontal process (*FP*) of the maxilla and superiorly. *MP flap*, mucoperiosteal flap.

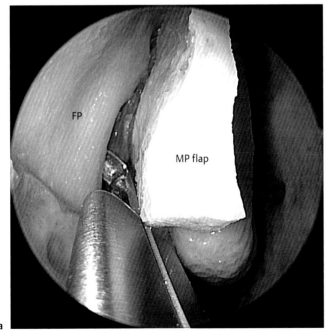

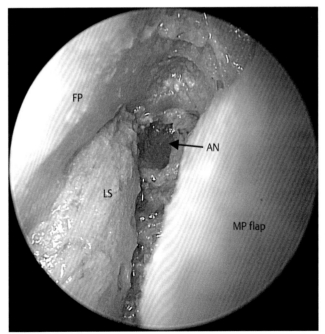

a

b

Fig. 11.12 (**a**) A cadaveric image of the right side showing removal of the bone of the frontal process (*FP*) of the maxilla by Hajek Koeffler punch (lower end) and DCR diamond bur (upper end). (**b**) The exposure of the lacrimal sac (*LS*) with exposure of the agger nasi cell (*AN*) mucosa. *MP flap*, mucoperiosteal flap.

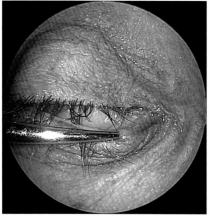
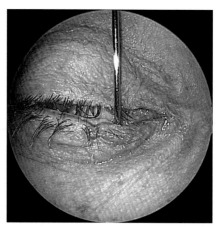
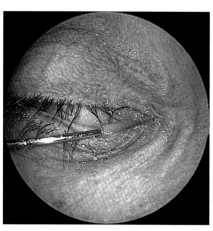

a,b   c

Fig. 11.14 Cadaveric images of the right lower eyelid. (**a**) The punctum dilator has been passed into the inferior punctum. (**b**) When passing the dilator, and then the lacrimal probe, it is important to firstly pass the probe 90 degrees to the lower eyelid. (**c**) Then the probe is rotated parallel with the lower lid and inserted until the probe tip is seen within the lacrimal sac.

probe visible through the sac wall, a DCR spear knife* (Integra) is used to make a vertical incision as far posteriorly as possible through the sac wall (**Fig. 11.15**). This results in the largest possible anterior flap. The tip of the spear knife is pushed into the tented sac wall just underneath the region of the probe and the sac wall is opened using a rotating motion (**Fig. 11.15**). Do not place the entire blade of the spear knife into the sac but rather cut with the anterior two-thirds of the blade. The sac is slit from top to bottom. The DCR mini-sickle knife* (Integra) is used to make upper and lower releasing incisions in the anterior flap so that the flap can be rolled out on the lateral nasal wall (**Fig. 11.16**).

Three-millimeter soft tissue scissors from the skull base set (Integra) are used to make upper and lower releasing incisions in the posterior flap and this flap is also rolled out (**Fig. 11.16**). The sac should now be completely marsupialized and lie flat on the lateral nasal wall (**Fig. 11.16**).

To determine the width of the mucosal flaps, the amount of raw bone above and below the sac is estimated. The original mucosal flap repositioned over the opened sac so that the areas of raw bone can be measured up against the original flap. Once the width of flap is determined, the flap is trimmed with a pediatric through-biting Blakesley forceps leaving the upper and lower limb of this flap the same thickness as the exposed bone above and below the marsupialized sac (**Fig. 11.17**). Most of the middle section of the original flap is removed to allow the posterior wall of the flap and mucosal edge of the mucosal flap to be approximated. The posterosuperior region of lacrimal and nasal mucosa is difficult to approximate because the middle turbinate holds the nasal mucosal flap away from the sidewall. In this region, the agger nasi cell is opened and the mucosa from this cell approximated to this region of the lacrimal mucosa. This results in a U-shaped flap and the surgeon should aim to achieve approximation of

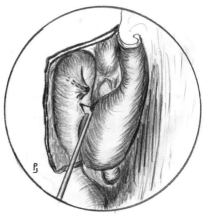
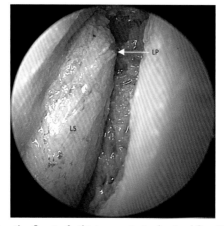
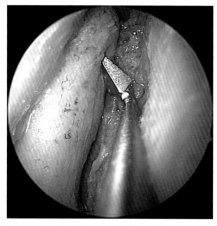

a,b   c

Fig. 11.15 (**a**) Bowman's lacrimal probe tenting the flap to facilitate incision with the DCR spear knife. Cadaveric dissection demonstrating the lacrimal probe (*LP*) tenting (**b**) the lacrimal sac (*LS*), and DCR spear knife incision (**c**) as far posteriorly as possible to allow for the largest anterior lacrimal flap. This incision should be made along the posterior third of the tented sac wall to ensure the largest possible anterior lacrimal flap. (**a**: Adapted with permission from Wormald PJ. Powered endoscopic DCR. Otolaryngol Clin N Am 2006;39:539–549.)

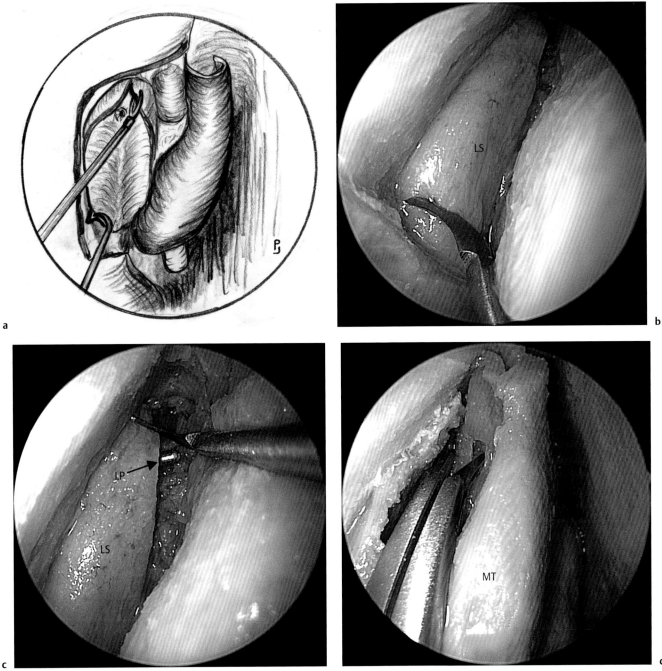

Fig. 11.16 (**a**) The mini-sickle knife is used the make the inferior and superior releasing incision on the anterior mucosal flap to allow the flap to be rolled out onto the frontal process of the maxilla. The superior and inferior releasing incisions are cut in the posterior flap with the scissors from the skull base set. (Adapted with permission from Wormald PJ. Powered endoscopic DCR. Otolaryngol Clin North Am 2006;39:539–549.) Cadaveric dissection images showing the mini-sickle knife being used to perform the inferior (**b**) and superior (**c**) releasing incision on the anterior lacrimal flap, with superior and inferior incision on the posterior flap performed with skull base scissors (**d**). *LS*, lacrimal sac; *MT*, middle turbinate; *LP*, lacrimal probe.

lacrimal and nasal mucosa superiorly, posteriorly, and inferiorly. This mucosal flap can be difficult to fashion with standard through-biting Blakesley forceps so the pediatric Blakesley forceps are kept for DCR surgery alone and only used on this flap. This keeps them sharp and allows the mucosa to be cut without tearing of the mucosa and losing the flap. Approximating the lacrimal and nasal mucosa should result in a first intention healing rather than a secondary intention healing and should reduce the formation of granulation tissue and scarring and therefore lessen the potential risk of closure of the sac and failure of the surgery (**Fig. 11.18**).

Next the tightness of the common canaliculus is evaluated by placing a Bowman's canalicula probe through the

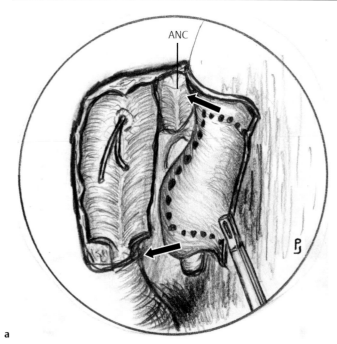

a

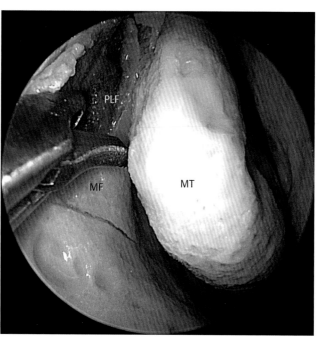

b

Fig. 11.17 (a) The mucosal flap is trimmed with the pediatric through-biting forceps. The superior and inferior mucosal flaps are matched to the raw bone above and below the opened lacrimal sac (*block arrows*). The agger nasi cell (*ANC*) mucosa is exposed and opened to allow apposition in this area. (Adapted with permission from Wormald PJ. Powered endoscopic DCR. Otolaryngol Clin N Am 2006;39:539–549.)

(b) Cadaveric dissection image demonstrating the trimming of the mucosal flap (*MF*) centrally to allow for raw bone coverage superiorly and inferiorly. This allows mucosal apposition between the posterior (*PLF*) and anterior lacrimal sac mucosa to the nasal mucosal and primary intention wound healing. *MT*, middle turbinate.

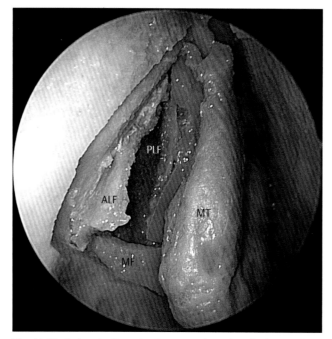

Fig. 11.18 Cadaveric dissection image on the right side showing both the anterior (*ALF*) and posterior (*PLF*) lacrimal flaps opened and lying along the lateral nasal wall. Apposition of the mucosal flap (*MF*) with the lacrimal sac mucosa, both anterior and posterior lacrimal flaps, can be seen. *MT*, middle turbinate.

common canaliculus and the probe is visualized entering the sac through the common canaliculus. If the common canaliculus holds the probe tightly then lacrimal tubes should be placed to dilate the common cannaliculus.[20] If the probe passes easily through the common canaliculus and is not firmly gripped then no tubes are placed. If the gripping of the probe is equivocal then tubes are placed in patients with functional NLDO but not placed in patients with anatomical NLDO. For placement of tubes the puncta are dilated and silastic lacrimal intubation tubes (O'Donoghue tubes) are placed through the upper and lower puncta and retrieved endosnasally (**Fig. 11.19a**). A square of Gelfoam (Pfizer; Kalamazoo, MI) is slid over the tubes into the nasal vestibule (**Fig. 11.19b**). A spacer of silastic tubing is slid over the tubes and used to push the Gelfoam onto the mucosal flaps (**Fig. 11.19c,d**). This spacer is about 10 mm long and 4 mm in diameter. This tubing acts as a spacer below which Ligar clips are placed to secure the tubes (**Figs. 11.19d** and **11.20**). Before placing the clips, ensure a loop of tubing is pulled in the medial canthus of the eye so that the tubes are not tight (**Fig. 11.21**). If the loop is tight, the tubes can cheese-wire through the puncta.

The silastic tubing is cut and the Gelfoam gently lifted off the flaps and the position of the flaps checked before it is replaced (**Fig. 11.22**). The postnasal space is cleared of blood.

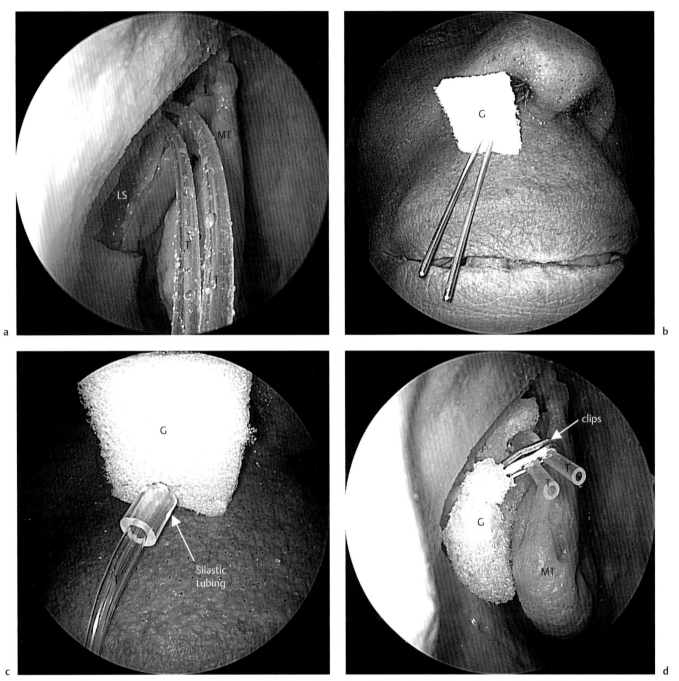

Fig. 11.19 Cadaveric dissection images taken on the right side. O'Donoghue lacrimal intubation tubes (*T*) have been passed through the superior and inferior canaliculus, then through the common canaliculus, the nasal cavity (**a**), and then the right nostril (**b**). The lacrimal tubes (*T*) are passed through a small square of Gelfoam (*G*) followed by a 10-mm piece of 4-mm silastic tubing (**c**). The silastic tubing and Gelfoam is then passed up into the middle meatus so that the Gelfoam square secures the lacrimal flaps and mucosal flap into position (**d**). Ligar clips are then placed below the silastic tubing to hold the Gelfoam in position (**d**).

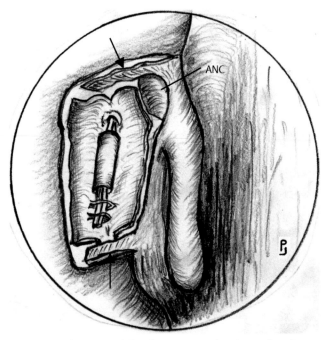

Fig. 11. 20 Placement of the silastic O'Donoghue lacrimal intubation tubes with a silastic sleeve space and Ligar clips to hold the tubes in place. The superior and inferior mucosal flaps are indicated with *black arrows*. (Adapted with permission from Wormald PJ. Powered endoscopic DCR. Otolaryngol Clin N Am 2006;39:539–549.)

◆ **Postoperative Care**

Saline nasal washes are started within 3 to 4 hours of surgery. This aids in clearing any residual blood clots and keeping the nasal cavity moist and clear of secretions.

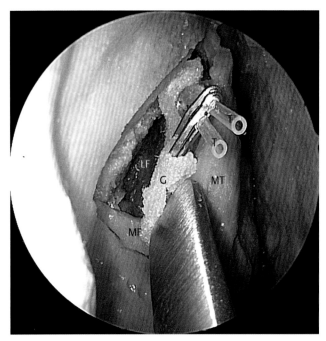

Fig. 11.22 Cadaveric dissection image of the right-sided demonstrating that the Gelfoam square (*G*) is lifted and the position of the lacrimal (*LF*) and mucosal flaps (*MF*) are checked after the O'Donoghue tubes (*T*) have been cut. *MT*, middle turbinate.

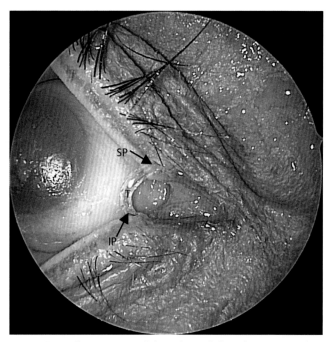

Fig. 11.21 Cadaveric image of the right medial canthus. O'Donoghue lacrimal intubation tubes (*T*) have been placed through the superior (*SP*) and inferior puncta (*IP*). Care is taken to ensure that tubes are not positioned too tight, making eye opening difficult.

Gentle blowing of the nose is allowed without closing the nasal vestibule. The patient is placed on broad-spectrum antibiotics for 5 days and antibiotic eye drops are used for 10 days. If O'Donoghue tubes were placed, they are removed in the clinic after 4 weeks and the patency of the nasolacrimal system checked by placing a drop of fluorescein in the conjunctiva and endoscopically monitoring the flow of fluorescein from the conjunctiva to the nose. It is rare to see any granulations but if they are present they should be removed. The patient is reviewed for a further 18 months.

◆ **Results**

The results of this technique have been published in peer-reviewed journals.[14,17–22] When discussing the success rate of DCR, it is important to clearly define "success." In many previous studies "success" was defined as either a symptomatic improvement, a complete absence of symptoms, or as an anatomically patent nasolacrimal system after surgery. For a DCR to be called successful, both criteria (symptoms and anatomical patency) need to be fulfilled: the patient should be completely asymptomatic and there should be an endoscopically confirmed patent nasolacrimal system. The lacrimal sac should be marsupialized and well healed, forming part of the lateral nasal wall (**Fig. 11.23a**). Once fluorescein has been placed in the conjunctiva, it should be visualized immediately in the marsupialized sac (**Fig. 11.23b**).

One of the recent published series included 162 consecutive DCRs with a minimum follow-up of 12 or more months.[18]

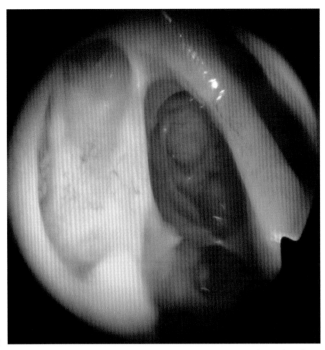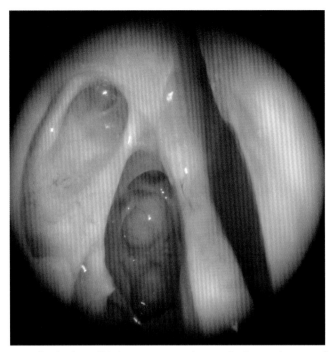

Fig. 11.23 (**a**) Lacrimal sac marsupialized into the lateral nasal wall in a patient that had ESS. (**b**) Fluorescein seen draining freely into the opened lacrimal sac.

Patients who had a nonfilling lacrimal sac on DCG—which may suggest a common canaliculus problem but had otherwise normal canaliculi—were included. Only patients who had a 3-4 mm long obliteration of the common canaliculus on both DCG and probing were excluded. There were four patients who were excluded for significant common canaliculus stenosis/obstruction. Patients who have a nonfilling lacrimal sac on DCG may have a large or distended lacrimal sac that may cause the common canaliculus to kink at its insertion to the sac. These patients can be successfully managed with an endoscopic DCR. To examine the results of this technique, the patients have been divided into those who underwent a primary DCR (no previous surgery), revision DCR, and those who filled the criteria for a pediatric DCR (less than 10 years old).

◆ **Results in Primary DCR**[14,17,18,20,21]

In one of the larger series[18] with 162 patients, 126 were primary DCRs, 19 revision DCRs, and 18 pediatric DCRs. In the primary DCR group, there were 115 patients who had a successful outcome (90%). Of the 11 patients considered failures, six had an anatomically patent nasolacrimal system with a free flow of fluorescein from the conjunctiva to the nose (such as demonstrated in **Fig. 11.23b**). This gives and anatomical patency rate of 96% (121/126). However, symptomatic patients are still classified as failures even if the surgery was technically successful. The primary DCR patient group can be further divided into anatomical or functional obstruction according to their preoperative investigations (DCG and scintillography). In the anatomically obstructed group, the success rate was 95%, whereas in the functional

group it was 81%. This functional group still had a 95% anatomical patency but a few patients with a patent system still had symptoms and were therefore classified as failures. If success is defined as complete absence of symptoms with anatomical patency, functional obstruction of the lacrimal system does not have as good a prognosis as anatomical obstruction and this should be kept in mind when consenting patients with functional obstruction. An important caveat to this is that all patients who had residual postoperative symptoms in the functional group stated that the symptoms were significantly improved after the DCR.

Results and Technique Modifications in Revision DCR[14,17,18]

There were 19 revision DCRs performed in this series. The success rate was 83% but increased to 89% with a second revision operation. The surgical technique for revision DCR is the same as for primary DCR with a few minor modifications. A variably sized bony ostium would have been created at the time of the primary DCR. The sac remnant may be significantly smaller and scarred than is the case with a primary DCR and this may make the creation of nasal mucosa and lacrimal sac mucosa apposition more difficult. The initial mucosal incisions are still placed as previously described with the reservation that the anterior vertical incision must be placed anterior to the previously created bony ostium. In other words, the anterior vertical incision must be placed onto bone. If you are unsure of the anterior limit of the previous bony ostium, palpate the frontal process of the maxilla. Start anteriorly on the frontal process and move posteriorly until the junction of the hard bone and soft ostium can be palpated. Once the initial mucosal incisions have been made, use the suction Freer elevator to elevate the mucosal flap from the bone anteriorly, above, and below the previous bony ostium. The plane of the already elevated mucosa should be continued posteriorly using a scalpel. Sharp dissection is necessary as the mucosa is attached to the underlying sac by fibrous tissue. Once the mucosal flap is raised, bony removal and the rest of the DCR technique is as previously described. If the sac was seen to be scarred with a small sac volume then once this sac had been opened, the preserved nasal mucosa that has been previously elevated from the sac can be trimmed so that the nasal mucosa still abuts the lacrimal mucosa even if the lacrimal mucosa was small on marsupialization. This leaves little exposed tissue and bone and should result in a successful revision DCR.

Results and Technique Modifications in Pediatric DCR[14,17–23]

In the most recent series there were 21 consecutive pediatric DCRs. The success rate was 92%. Patients included in this group were under the age of 14 years. In the pediatric age group, especially the patients in the 18 months to 6 year age group, there are important anatomical differences that the surgeon needs to be aware of. The nasal vestibule is much smaller and there can be some initial difficulty getting a 4-mm endoscope and an instrument in the nasal cavity simultaneously. The same sized scopes and instruments are used for the pediatric and adult endoscopic DCRs with the exception of the Hajek-Koeffler punch, which is replaced by a 2-mm Kerrison's forward-biting punch. However, as surgery continues, the nasal vestibule stretches and nasal vestibule narrowness was never more than an initial concern. The other anatomical variation is the underdevelopment of the turbinates with a relatively small vertical height of the nasal cavity. This puts the axilla of the middle turbinate in relative close proximity to the skull base and increases the risk to the skull base. The initial mucosal incisions remain similar to those described in adults and the superior incision is still placed about 8 mm above the axilla. This will be just below the skull base in a 2-year-old so the surgeon must be aware of this proximity while removing bone from over the sac. The remainder of the procedure is the same as was previously described. Pediatric DCR is a very successful operation with 100% anatomical success rate in our series[20] (patency of the lacrimal ostium on endoscopy). However, only 92% of these patients were completely symptom free.[20] The postoperative management for patients under 10 years of age is different to that previously outlined. We electively do a postoperative evaluation under general anesthesia after 4 weeks. The intranasal lacrimal ostium is evaluated and the O'Donoghue tubes are removed. There may be granulations around the ostium, especially on the anterior wall as this is the region where lacrimal and nasal mucosa are most difficult to approximate, and there is often a little exposed bone after draping of all the mucosal flaps (**Fig. 11.24**). These granulations should be removed and this region should subsequently heal well. In some patients there may be minor adhesions between the lateral nasal wall and septum, and these are also divided. This occurs because the nasal cavity is small and we do not perform a septoplasty unless there is significant septal deviation. In those patients with significant septal deviation, a Killian's incision is performed and the septum mobilized from the maxillary crest and from the bony septum. No cartilage or bone is excised. This mobilization is usually sufficient and allows surgery to proceed in the previously obstructed nasal cavity. Mobilization without tissue resection also lessens the risk of disturbing the septum's further growth and consequently altering facial features.

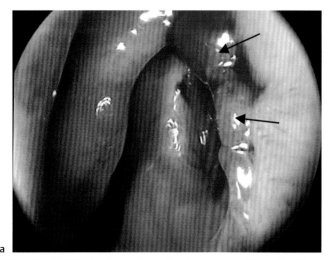
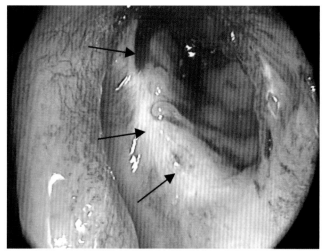

Fig. 11.24 (**a**) The lacrimal ostium after 4 weeks in an 18-month-old patient with granulations on the anterior lip of the ostium (*black arrows*). (**b**) The lacrimal ostium after removal of these granulations. The posterior region of primary intention healing without granulation tissue is marked with *black arrows*. The patient continued to heal well and was asymptomatic at follow-up.

◆ Rationale for the Insertion of O'Donoghue Tubes[20]

O'Donoghue tubes are placed after endoscopic DCR if the common canaliculus is tight and this is done in an attempt to dilate the common canaliculus opening into the lacrimal sac. The tubes are not placed in an attempt to keep the sac open as the sac is so widely marsupialized with lacrimal and nasal mucosa apposition it would be unnecessary. The aim of the O'Donoghue tube is insertion to dilate the common canaliculus opening by placing silastic tubes for 4 weeks. Over many years of observing the Bowman's lacrimal probe entering the lacrimal sac, it was apparent that the mucosal fold that forms the valve of Rosenmüller can be tight and that this may contribute to symptoms in some patients. It did not make sense to create a large lacrimal ostium but fail to address a potential more proximal obstruction. We have recently done research into placement of tubes only in those patients in whom the common canaliculus was tightly gripping the Bowman probe and found that the success rate in patients with a loose common canaliculus did not change whether tubes were placed or not.[20] We do think it more likely in patients who on DCG do not have penetration of the dye into the sac but on scintigraphy have penetration of the radioisotope into the sac. We also found that in functional nasolacrimal obstruction, we have a lower threshold for placing tubes as these patients have a lower success rate and the common canaliculus may be contributing to this. The radioisotope has more time to slowly penetrate the valve than the dye does and may indicate a tight common canaliculus opening. In **Fig. 11.25** we present two examples of tight valves of Rosenmüller and it can clearly be seen how the mucosal fold grips the end of the probe.

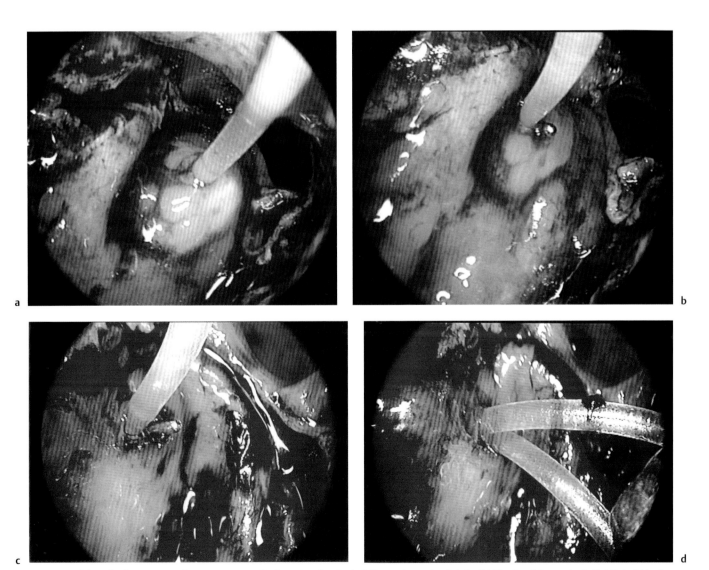

Fig. 11.25 (**a**) In the first patient, the common canaliculus grips the single O'Donoghue tube tightly. (**b**) The tip of the probe is tightly held by the valve. In the second patient, (**c**) the silastic tube and probe are tightly held by the valve and (**d**) the two tubes are seen to dilate the valve.

◆ Ancillary Procedures

Septoplasty was necessary in 47% of patients. This was done endoscopically through a Killian's incision. The area of obstructing septal deflection directly adjacent to the anterior end of the middle turbinate was removed while the anterior cartilage was kept intact. In 15% of patients, ESS was necessary for ongoing nonresponsive chronic sinusitis or nasal polyposis.

◆ Complications

Complications in powered endoscopic DCR are very rare. There were three cases of postoperative hemorrhage giving a complication rate of 1.9%. No other complications occurred. Serious complications can occur if the surgeon loses anatomical landmarks. These include damage to the orbit and orbital contents and damage to the anterior cranial fossa with a cerebrospinal fluid (CSF) leak. If the landmarks described above are kept in mind and the surgeon stays anterior to the insertion of the uncinate, penetration of the orbit is unlikely. Dissection posterior to the uncinate, however, will usually result in orbital fat exposure. Should this occur, it should be left alone and not manipulated in any way. As the bone is removed above the middle turbinate, the mucosa of the agger nasi cell will be exposed. The diamond bur should be kept in contact with the bone directly above the sac and bone removal should continue to the mucosal incision. If there is any doubt as to exactly which part of mucosa is sac wall and which is skin or agger nasi cell mucosa, a DCR light pipe* (Integra) is introduced into the sac and the sac transilluminated. If the surgeon stays in close proximity to the sac while removing the bone the likelihood of damage to the skull base with a subsequent CSF leak is very small.

◆ Key Points

It is beneficial when starting to do endoscopic DCRs that the sinus surgeon develops a close liaison with an ophthalmologist.[11] Both have expertise in different areas and the combination of this expertise helps in both the workup for surgery and during the surgical procedure. Our team consists of an ENT surgeon and an oculoplastic surgeon. We assess patients together in the lacrimal clinic. The oculoplastic surgeon helps with the assessment of other causes of epiphora such as blepharitis, entropion, ectropion, lid laxity, etc., and will be able to teach the sinus surgeon how to syringe and probe the lacrimal system. The sinus surgeon is able to endoscopically assess the nasal cavity, septum, and any ancillary sinus disease that may be present. At surgery the sinus surgeon has the endoscopic skills to deal with the septum and expose the lacrimal sac. The oculoplastic surgeon has the expertise in probing the lacrimal system and passing O'Donoghue tubes and dealing with lid laxity, entropion, or ectropion. Both surgeons should learn to be comfortable with all aspects of assessment and surgery and we routinely alternate our roles during surgery.

The key to success in powered endoscopic DCR is being able to picture the anatomy of the lacrimal sac as it will be encountered when the sac is approached from the nasal cavity. Understanding the anatomical relationships allows complete exposure of the sac and marsupialization of the sac into the lateral nasal wall. In addition, preservation of mucosa with fashioning of mucosal flaps allows the nasal and lacrimal mucosa to be opposed with first intention rather than second intention healing. This decreases the risk of granulation tissue and scar formation and gives a reliable and reproducible result.

References

1. Caldwell G. Two new operations for obstruction of the nasal duct, with preservation of the canaliculi, and with an incidental description of a new lacrymal probe. NY Med J. 1893;57:581–582
2. Toti A. Nuovo Metodo conservatore dicura radicale delle suppurazione croniche del sacco lacrimale (dacricistorhinostomia). Clin. Moderna (Firenza) 1904;10:385
3. Hartikainen J, Antila J, Varpula M, Puukka P, Seppä H, Grénman R. Prospective randomized comparison of endonasal endoscopic dacryocystorhinostomy and external dacryocystorhinostomy. Laryngoscope 1998;108(12):1861–1866
4. McDonogh M, Meiring JH. Endoscopic transnasal dacryocystorhinostomy. J Laryngol Otol 1989;103(6):585–587
5. Metson R. Endoscopic surgery for lacrimal obstruction. Otolaryngol Head Neck Surg 1991;104(4):473–479
6. Steadman M. Transnasal Dacryocystorhinostomy. Otolaryngol. Clin. of Nth. America 1985;6:107–111
7. Gonnering RS, Lyon DB, Fisher JC. Endoscopic laser-assisted lacrimal surgery. Am J Ophthalmol 1991;111(2):152–157
8. Massaro BM, Gonnering RS, Harris GJ. Endonasal laser dacryocystorhinostomy. A new approach to nasolacrimal duct obstruction. Arch Ophthalmol 1990;108(8):1172–1176
9. Woog JJ, Metson R, Puliafito CA. Holmium:YAG endonasal laser dacryocystorhinostomy. Am J Ophthalmol 1993;116(1):1–10
10. Linberg JV, Anderson RL, Bumsted RM, Barreras R. Study of intranasal ostium external dacryocystorhinostomy. Arch Ophthalmol 1982; 100(11):1758–1762
11. Wormald PJ, Nilssen E. Endoscopic DCR: the team approach. Hong Kong Journal of Ophthalmology 1998;1:71–74
12. Welham RAN, Wulc AE. Management of unsuccessful lacrimal surgery. Br J Ophthalmol 1987;71(2):152–157
13. Wormald PJ, Kew J, Van Hasselt A. Intranasal anatomy of the nasolacrimal sac in endoscopic dacryocystorhinostomy. Otolaryngol Head Neck Surg 2000;123(3):307–310
14. Wormald PJ. Powered endoscopic dacryocystorhinostomy. Laryngoscope 2002;112(1):69–72
15. Ünlü HH, Gövsa F, Mutlu C, Yücetürk AV, Senyilmaz Y. Anatomical guidelines for intranasal surgery of the lacrimal drainage system. Rhinology 1997;35(1):11–15
16. Rebeiz EE, Shapshay SM, Bowlds JH, Pankratov MM. Anatomic guidelines for dacryocystorhinostomy. Laryngoscope 1992;102(10):1181–1184
17. Wormald PJ, Tsirbas A. Investigation and endoscopic treatment for functional and anatomical obstruction of the nasolacrimal duct system. Clin Otolaryngol Allied Sci 2004;29(4):352–356
18. Tsirbas A, Wormald PJ. Endonasal dacryocystorhinostomy with mucosal flaps. Am J Ophthalmol 2003;135(1):76–83
19. Wormald PJ. Powered endoscopic dacryocystorhinostomy. Otolaryngol Clin North Am 2006;39:539–549
20. Callejas CA, Tewfik MA, Wormald PJ. Powered endoscopic dacryocystorhinostomy with selective stenting. Laryngoscope 2010;120(7): 1449–1452
21. Leibovitch I, Selva D, Tsirbas A, Greenrod E, Pater J, Wormald PJ. Paediatric endoscopic endonasal dacryocystorhinostomy in congenital nasolacrimal duct obstruction. Graefes Arch Clin Exp Ophthalmol 2006;244(10):1250–1254
22. Mann BS, Wormald PJ. Endoscopic assessment of the dacryocystorhinostomy ostium after endoscopic surgery. Laryngoscope 2006;116(7): 1172–1174
23. Tsirbas A, Davis G, Wormald PJ. Revision dacryocystorhinostomy: a comparison of endoscopic and external techniques. Am J Rhinol 2005; 19(3):322–325

12 Cerebrospinal Fluid Leak Closure

◆ Introduction

The traditional management of anterior skull base cerebrospinal fluid (CSF) leaks was via an anterior craniotomy and intracranial repair of the CSF leak. This was usually done by elevating the frontal lobes in the region of the suspected site of the leak and laying a sheet of fascia lata over this area. The success rate of this technique was around 70% but usually left the patient with some loss of smell. In addition, frontal lobe retraction is associated with the risk of postoperative epilepsy. In the late 1980s and early 1990s, endoscopic closure of CSF leaks was first reported. Since then, many published series have reported success rates of above 90%.[1–3] This high success rate and the very low associated morbidity are the major advantages of the endoscopic technique.[1] A variety of materials have been used to close these leaks.[3,4] Free mucosal grafts, pedicled mucosal grafts, fat, fascia, muscle, and synthetic materials such as hydroxyapatite have all been described with similar success rates.[3,4] In a recent review, Hegazy et al[3] felt that the type of material did not appear to make a significant difference to the success rate of the closure. Although this may indeed be the case in small CSF leaks, the purely on-lay technique may not be as suitable for larger leaks.[3,4] The techniques proposed in this chapter (the bath-plug closure and with or without naso-septal flap) have been used in a large series of patients and have been found to be reliable for both large and small leaks.[5,6] In our experience, if the on-lay technique alone is used for medium or large defects with a free flow of CSF, the graft tends to be pushed away from the skull base and hence from the dural defect and the flow of CSF resumes. Although the leak may be sealed at the end of the operation, coughing or straining in the postoperative period may raise the CSF pressure sufficiently to cause the leak to start again. An analogy of patching these high-flow CSF leaks with on-lay technique alone is trying to patch a plastic bag of water by applying a patch to the outside of bag.[5,6] The bath-plug technique allows the plug to be placed on the inside of the bag and uses the pressure from the water to increase the seal on the plug. The other technique presented (underlay alone or underlay and on-lay fascia grafting) and the indications for this technique also overcome this problem of the CSF pressure pushing the graft away from the skull base as the fascia is placed intracranially and the CSF pressure again helps create the seal. This chapter does not attempt to describe all the alternative techniques but concentrates on the bath-plug and underlay fascia techniques as we have considerable experience in a wide variety of situations with these techniques and have found them to be both versatile and reliable.[5,6]

◆ Etiology of Cerebrospinal Fluid Leaks

Anterior skull base CSF leaks can be divided into four broad categories according to their etiology. In a recent large series from our department, there was a fairly even spread between leaks caused from skull base trauma, spontaneous, meningoencephaloceles, and iatrogenic leaks.

Traumatic Cerebrospinal Fluid Leaks

Traumatic CSF leaks usually follow an anterior skull base fracture. The initial management is conservative as most of these leaks will cease within 10 days of the injury. However, leaks that persist longer than 10 days should be closed. One of the major causes of continued CSF leakage is rotation of a bony spicule that continues to hold the edges of the torn dura apart as demonstrated in a traumatic CSF leak of the sphenoid in **Fig. 12.1**. If the bone fragment is freely mobile then this should be removed at the time of closure of the leak (**Fig. 12.1**).

More common than traumatic CSF leaks of the sphenoid are those seen in the fovea ethmoidalis or at the fovea ethmoidalis–olfactory fossa junction (**Fig. 12.2**).

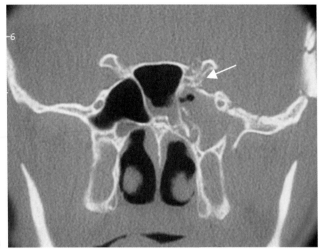

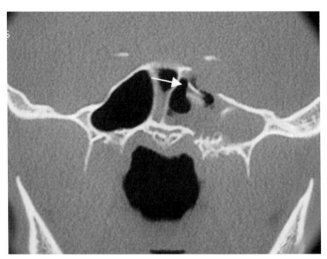

a   b

Fig. 12.1 CT scans of patient with a fracture through the clinoid (**a**) (*white arrow*) with a displaced bony fragment (**b**) (*white arrow*) and a CSF leak. Note the fluid level in the sphenoid.

Less frequent are fractures in the posterior table of the frontal sinus. Fortunately, these leaks at the base of skull fractures rarely need closure but if they persist, access is usually only possible with an endoscopic Grade 6 frontal drill-out procedure or an osteoplastic flap. The endoscopic frontal drill-out procedure allows most of the posterior table of the frontal sinus to be accessed and the CSF leak can be closed under direct visualization (**Fig. 12.3**). The reason that skull base fractures tend to heal spontaneously, as opposed to injuries created during ESS, is that although the dura is torn, there is usually no bony displacement so there is no prolapse of the torn dura preventing sealing. Where there is bony fragment displacement, surgical closure of the CSF leak should be done expeditiously and not watched expectantly. CSF leaks during ESS almost always have associated bony loss and dural prolapse so all are closed expeditiously without any conservative management prior to surgery.

Spontaneous Cerebrospinal Fluid Leaks

Spontaneous CSF leaks are usually seen either in the cribriform plate or lateral wall of the sphenoid sinus. Cribriform fossa leaks often result from a dilatation of the dural sheath around the olfactory fibers. A small prolapse of dura may result which may leak CSF (**Fig. 12.4**).

Spontaneous CSF leaks in the sphenoid sinus are usually seen in well-pneumatized sphenoid sinuses where the sinus pneumatizes into the sphenoid wing under the maxillary nerve. This brings this region of the sphenoid sinus in contact with the temporal lobe region of the middle cranial fossa with only thin bone separating the two. One theory as to why the skull base becomes eroded in this region is that arachnoid granulations in the floor of the middle cranial fossa often do not have a venous connection. When these arachnoid sacks fill with CSF and pulsate, they may gradually

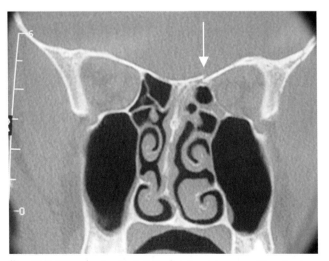

Fig. 12.2 CT scan of patient following head trauma with a fracture through the fovea ethmoidalis (*white arrow*) and with an associated CSF leak. Note the fluid level in the adjacent ethmoid sinus.

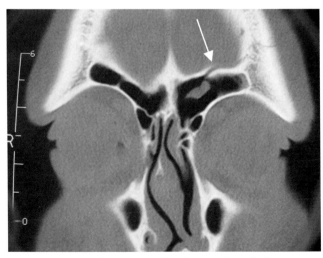

Fig. 12.3 CT scan of a patient with a fracture through the posterior table (*white arrow*) of the frontal sinus with an associated CSF leak.

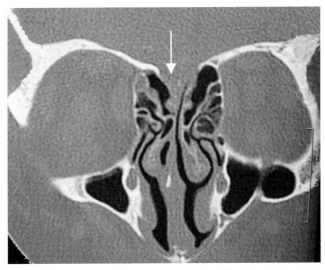

Fig. 12.4 A coronal CT illustrating a triangular dilatation of the cribriform plate around an olfactory neuron (confirmed at surgery).

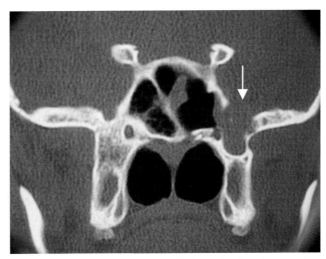

Fig. 12.5 Defect in left lateral wing of sphenoid with prolapse of dura through the defect.

erode the bone, eventually leading to a prolapse of dura and arachnoid into the sphenoid with an associated leak.[7–10] In addition, it is thought that a number of these patients may have undiagnosed benign raised intracranial pressure as part of the etiology. In **Fig. 12.5** a defect is seen in this lateral aspect of this well-pneumatized sphenoid with an associated opacity (prolapsing meninges and CSF).

Meningoencephaloceles with Associated Cerebrospinal Fluid Leaks

Meningoencephaloceles may either be spontaneous (congenital or acquired) or associated with a previous traumatic event. Congenital meningoencephaloceles usually present within the first few years of life. The meningoencephalocele consists of meninges and dura containing CSF with a variable amount of brain tissue prolapsing through the skull base defect into the nasal cavity or sinuses. The brain tissue

within the encephalocele is usually nonfunctional and is usually resected as the first step of the procedure. Posttraumatic meningoencephaloceles often have a funnel-shaped defect in the skull base and these need to be recognized during the repair process as this affects the ability of the surgeon to properly visualize the edges of the bony skull base defect as well as the intracranial cavity. The funnel-shaped bony defect is caused by the intracranial contents protruding through the defect and pushing the edges of the bony defect downward into the nasal cavity/sinuses (**Fig. 12.6**).

Iatrogenic Cerebrospinal Fluid Leaks

Iatrogenic leaks will frequently be seen on the lateral wall of the olfactory fossa and fovea ethmoidalis. The lateral wall of the olfactory fossa forms the medial limit of the dissection of the frontal recess. It can be very thin, varying from 0.1 to 1 mm

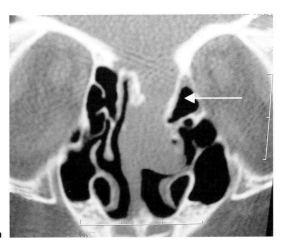

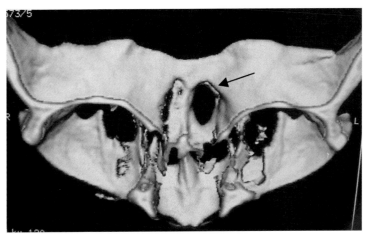

a   b

Fig. 12.6 (**a**) The CT scan shows the beveling of the edges of the meningoencephalocele (*white arrow*). (**b**) Three-dimensional reconstruction also illustrates the funnel shape of the skull base defect through which the meningoencephalocele protrudes (*black arrow*).

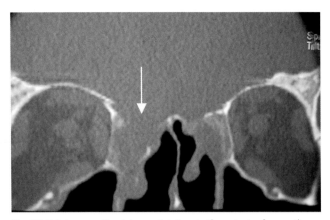

Fig. 12.7 Intraoperative iatrogenic injury to the anterior fovea ethmoidalis (*white arrow*) on the right side.

in thickness, and is perforated by the anterior ethmoidal artery. Damage to this lateral wall of the olfactory fossa may occur if the dissecting instruments are turned medially during surgery in this region. Laceration of the anterior ethmoidal artery with bleeding may prompt the use of diathermy in an attempt to obtain hemostasis. Unipolar diathermy, if used to cauterize a bleeding vessel, may burn through the bone and dura, causing a CSF leak. The remaining skull base (fovea ethmoidalis) may be damaged if the surgeon loses orientation and fails to recognize that the dissection has reached the skull base. If cells are assumed to be present on the skull base, an attempt to remove these "cells" may damage the skull base with an associated CSF leak (**Fig. 12.7**). Generally, these leaks are readily apparent at the time of surgery and can be fixed with the bath-plug technique described.

◆ Preoperative Assessment

This is performed if the patient presents with a suspected CSF leak. Intraoperative CSF leaks should be dealt with at the time of the surgery. The most reliable method of confirming a CSF leak is to test the clear watery secretions from the nose for β2 transferrin (β2 transferrin is only present in CSF).[4,5,7,11] Once the CSF leak has been confirmed, the site of the leak is sought by performing a high-resolution, fine-cut CT scan of the sinuses.[5,11] On this scan dehiscences of the anterior skull base are sought. Depending on the suspected cause, different areas in the anterior skull base are thoroughly scrutinized for bony defects. An additional clue may be the presence of fluid in the sinuses indicating that the leak is in the region of the opacified sinuses. Patients with spontaneous CSF leaks without evidence of any bony dehiscences on CT scan and without any opacification of any sinuses should have the cribriform plate region carefully examined intraoperatively for the CSF leak as it has been our experience that this is the most likely source of the leak (**Fig. 12.4**).

If the site of the leak is not apparent on the CT scan, a high-resolution T2-weighted MRI scan may allow visualization of fluid within the sinuses and if the patient is leaking at the time of the MRI, it may allow identification of the site

of the leak.[5,11] All patients with suspected meningoceles or meningoencephaloceles should have a preoperative MRI. This allows brain tissue within the meningoencephalocele to be identified and the opinion of the neurosurgeon should be sought whether the resection of this tissue transnasally is considered reasonable and safe (**Fig. 12.8**).

Although in the past there have been other investigations used to identify CSF leaks, the above investigations are the only ones recommended. Intrathecal contrast does not improve the sensitivity of the detection of the site of a CSF leak. Intrathecal radioisotope may confirm the presence of CSF in the nasal cavity, but does not add additional information to that obtained by a positive β2 transferrin test.[3] If the site of the leak is not able to be determined with the above investigations, the patient is taken to theatre and intrathecal fluorescein is injected into the CSF space and the site of the leak sought while the patient is under general anesthetic.[5,11,12]

◆ Surgical Technique

Broad-spectrum intravenous antibiotics are given with induction of anesthesia.

Intrathecal Fluorescein

Most patients undergoing elective CSF leak repair will have intrathecal fluorescein injected before surgery.[4,5,11,12] Patients who have a CSF leak during surgery will have the leak repaired at the time of the surgery without the placement of fluorescein intrathecally. All our patients preoperatively sign a separate consent form designed specifically to explain the risks of the administration of intrathecal fluorescein. The most common side effects are paresthesias and tingling in the hands and feet and convulsions. These side effects were reported when significantly higher concentrations of fluorescein were used and have not been seen in our series or other very large patient series.[4–6,11–15] In elective CSF leak closure, the lumbar drain is placed while the patient is awake. Ten milliliters of CSF are removed from the intrathecal space. A 90- to 130-pound person will have 0.2 mL of 5% fluorescein mixed with the 10 mL of CSF administered, whereas patients 130 pounds and above are administered 0.25 mL of 5% fluorescein mixed with the 10 mL of CSF.[4,5,11,12] The fluorescein-stained CSF is reinjected through a filter into the intrathecal space at a rate of 1 mL per minute. This is done while the patient is awake so that any possible side effects can be identified. Once the fluorescein-stained CSF has been reinjected, the patient is kept in the theatre recovery area for 1 to 2 hours in the head down position to allow for the fluorescein to enter the cranial cavity and mix with the CSF around the brain. If there is a significant flow of CSF at this time, the appearance of fluorescein within the CSF is fairly rapid (within 20 minutes) but may take significantly longer in low-flow CSF leaks or where there is a relative paucity of CSF within the system. Once the patient is anesthetized, they are placed in the head down position during preparation of the patient's nose with local anesthetic solution. This draping

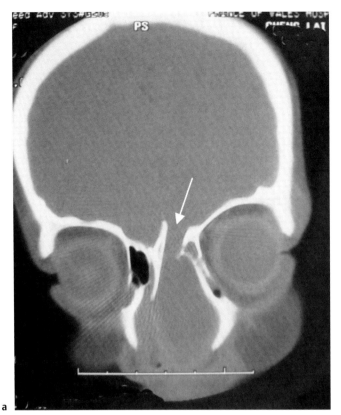

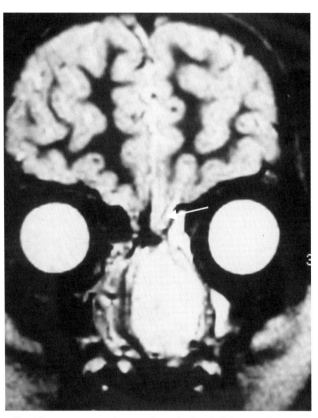

Fig. 12.8 (**a**) CT scan showing the skull base defect of a congenital me-ningoencephalocele (*white arrow*), whereas (**b**) is a T2-weighted MRI showing a large CSF-filled sac filling the nasal cavity with an associated stalk of brain tissue prolapsing through the skull base defect (*white arrow*). This meningoencephalocele was managed endoscopically.

and setup of the theatre equipment usually takes about 10 to 20 minutes, allowing additional time for the fluorescein to penetrate the intracranial cavity.

Intrathecal fluorescein can be invaluable for locating those difficult to find CSF leaks. Fluorescein can help iden-tify the site of a small CSF leak or a leak that is intermittent or that has recently stopped leaking (usually just prior to the surgery). If a blue-light filter is used on the light source, even the smallest quantities of fluorescein can be visual-ized intraoperatively and the leak can then be closed.[5,6] If, at this stage, the leak is still not visible, the patient should be placed in the head down position and a forced inspira-tion maneuver (Valsalva-like) performed by the anesthetist. This should be repeated a number of times while the sur-geon examines the most likely sites for the CSF leak. If no leak is seen, the patient should be placed head down and ventilated for a further 30 minutes before the nasal cavity and sinuses are re-examined for fluorescein-stained CSF.[6] Again, the blue light filter can be very useful. If the site of the leak is still not apparent, manipulation of the CSF space is attempted. The lumbar drain is attached to an arterial pressure monitor with a three-way tap. The CSF pressure is measured (normal 0 to 15 mm water). Twenty milliliters of Ringers lactate is injected into the intrathecal space through the lumbar drain and the pressure remeasured. After 40 mL have been injected, the head down forced inspiration ma-neuver is repeated with the blue light filter to see if the leak is visible. The Ringers lactate aliquots can be repeated but

the intrathecal pressure must be measured after each ali-quot to ensure that it does not go over 30 mm of water. In our series, one patient required 120 mL of Ringers before the leak became apparent.[6]

A cornerstone of this procedure is the identification of the site of the CSF leak. The leak cannot be closed if the site cannot be identified.

Another major advantage of the fluorescein-stained CSF is the ability of the surgeon to test if the CSF leak closure is watertight once the leak has been repaired.[5] After the repair has been performed as described below, the patient is placed head down and the forced inspiration maneuver repeated. The smallest leak of CSF can be easily seen as the CSF is a bright yellow/green color.

Bath-Plug Technique for Cerebrospinal Fluid Leak Repair

This technique forms the mainstay for the closure of CSF leaks with over 90% of our patients undergoing this tech-nique. Once the site of the CSF leak has been identified, the dural defect is enlarged until the bony rim of the skull base can be clearly seen. As the dural defect is enlarged, a strong flow of fluorescein-stained CSF is usually apparent. It is im-portant to remove the prolapsed dura and meninges and not to attempt repair of a dural or meningeal defect without identifying the surrounding bone being exposed as the dura

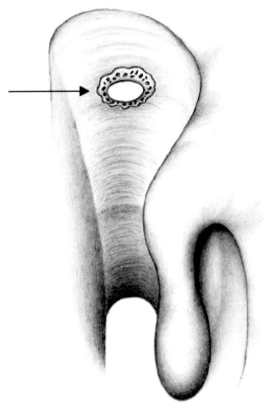

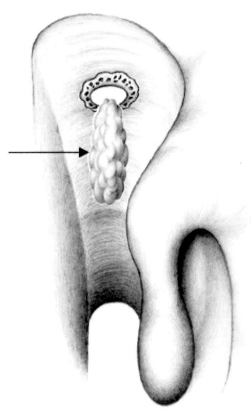

Fig. 12.9 The bony margins of the defect in the skull base are identified, prolapsing dura removed, and the mucosa circumferentially stripped away from edge of defect for about 5 mm (*black arrow*).

Fig. 12.10 Demonstration of the fat plug (*black arrow*) relative to the size of the defect. Note that the fat plug is the same diameter as the defect.

and meninges provide no support for the tissue used to repair the defect. The bone of the skull base is solid and if the repair is based around this solid support, a good result is more likely. On occasion, the bone of the skull base may be fractured and unstable. If small pieces of bone are visible, these should be removed before repair. Large pieces of bone should be left in place and the dura opened to the edge of these large pieces. If large bony fragments are present, the bath-plug technique is still suitable but the graft needs support as the suture is pulled after intracranial placement of the graft. Once the bony rim of the defect has been identified, the nasal mucosa around the defect is stripped away for at least 5 mm. This allows the free mucosal graft to stick to the bone and ultimately a better seal is achieved (**Fig. 12.9**).

The skull base defect is measured using a curette. For example, the defect may be two curettes wide and three long. If a 3-mm curette is used, the defect would be 6 by 9 mm. A 6 × 9 mm fat graft is then harvested from the earlobe. If the defect is larger than 12 mm, fat is obtained either from the region of the greater trochanter of the thigh or from the abdomen. If possible, the earlobe is the preferred region for obtaining the fat graft as the fat globules are tightly knitted and easy to work with. However, if there have been multiple piercings of the earlobe, or the defect is large, then the greater trochanter region is preferred as the fat globules in this region are again more fibrous and tightly knitted than the fat from the abdomen. The fat plug should be the same diameter as the defect

(otherwise there will be difficulty introducing it through the defect) and about 1.5 to 2 cm long (**Fig. 12.10**).

A 4-0 Vicryl suture (Ethicon; Somerville, NJ) is knotted through the one end of the fat plug and the suture passed down the length of the fat plug (**Fig. 12.11**).

A free mucosal graft is harvested from the lateral nasal wall (usually on the opposite side to that which has the CSF leak). The mucosa is taken from the lateral nasal wall anterior to the middle turbinate and is usually about 3 × 3 cm (larger if the defect is large). The fat plug is placed below the defect and the malleable frontal sinus probe (Integra ; Plainsboro, NJ) is used to gently introduce the fat plug through the defect. The malleable frontal sinus probe does not have a ball-tip on the end which aids the introduction of the fat plug. If a probe with a ball-tip is used, the fat tends to stick to the ball and, as the probe is pulled back after introducing fat intracranially, fat is pulled with the probe and this results in difficulty introducing the fat plug intracranially.[5] The important part of this technique is to introduce only a very small amount of fat through the defect with each maneuver. If a large amount of fat is introduced through the defect with one maneuver, significant pressure may be required and the probe can slip a significant distance into the intracranial cavity with the potential to injure intracranial structures.[5] If small amounts of fat are introduced with each maneuver then greater safety is achieved as the probe does not need to enter the intracranial cavity by more than a few millimeters with each maneuver[4,5] (**Fig. 12.12**).

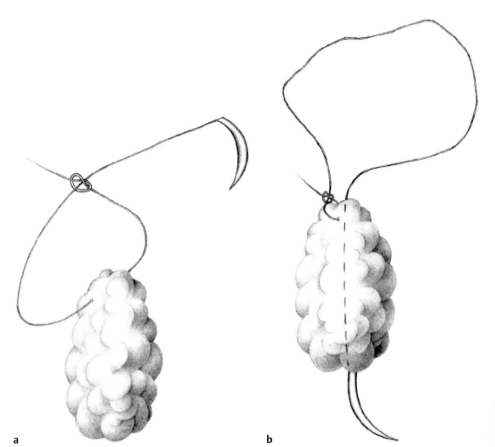

a   b

Fig. 12.11 The 4-0 Vicryl suture is knotted at the one end of the fat plug before being passed along the length of the fat plug.

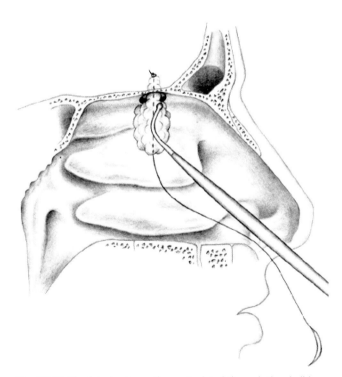

Fig. 12.12 The fat plug is gently manipulated through the skull base defect into the intracranial cavity. Only a small piece of fat is introduced with each maneuver.

Consideration needs to be given to the possibility that there may be a vessel present in the region where the fat plug is introduced. This likelihood is increased with repair of meningoencephaloceles as vessels are present that supply blood to the prolapsed brain and dura. In addition, the brain tissue that prolapses into the defect is often adherent to the edges of the defect, decreasing the amount of intracranial space available for introduction of the fat plug. In these situations, the technique of placing one layer of fascia lata intracranial and the second layer as an on-lay or closed with a pedicled septal flap is preferred. However, if the fat plug is manipulated gently into the intracranial cavity the likelihood of damage of intracranial structures is very small. In our large series, no such injuries occurred.

Once the fat plug has been safely introduced through the defect, the plug is stabilized with the probe and the Vicryl suture is gently pulled. This expands the fat plug on the intracranial side of the defect and allows the CSF pressure to increase the seal of the fat in the defect (much like the water pressure of the bath sealing the bath plug in the drain) (**Fig. 12.13**).

The seal is tested by placing the patient head down and asking the anesthetist to perform a forced inspiration (Valsalva) maneuver. No fluorescein-stained CSF should be seen. This maneuver further pushes the fat plug into the defect and a little prolapse of fat through the defect is normal. The patient is placed head up (15 degrees) and the free mucosal graft is slid up the Vicryl suture until it covers the defect. Ensure that the graft is correctly orientated with the mucosal surface facing the nasal cavity (**Fig. 12.14**).

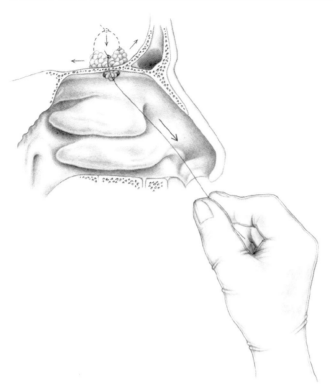

Fig. 12.13 The Vicryl suture is gently pulled while the fat graft is supported. This expands the fat graft on the intracranial surface and pulls the fat into the defect giving a solid seal of the defect.

Fibrin glue is applied and the Vicryl suture is cut. Gelfoam (Pfizer; Kalamazoo, MI) is placed over the free mucosal graft and fibrin glue reapplied. A number of layers can be placed in this manner. No other nasal packing is used.

Special Situations

Meningoencephaloceles with a Cerebrospinal Fluid Leak (see video)

The meninges and protruding brain tissue are resected up to the skull base. This is normally done with a powered microdebrider or coblater. If significant brain tissue is seen on the MRI prolapsing into the nasal cavity or sinuses, a neurosurgical consultation should be sought regarding the safety of resection of the brain tissue. After resection, the dural edges are cauterized with a suction bipolar forceps to ensure hemostasis. Exposure of the bony limits of the skull base defect is important as proper closure of the defect cannot be achieved by placing grafts against prolapsed dura and such a repair is doomed to failure. Once the bone of the skull base defect is clearly exposed and surrounding mucosa on the nasal surface gently removed from the edges of the bony defect, the prolapsing brain tissue can be addressed. The brain tissue is shrunk using the suction bipolar until the stump of remaining brain tissue lies within the intracranial cavity. At this point an assessment needs to be made as to whether the edges of the prolapsed brain tissue are in contact with the edges of the skull base defect and whether it is adhesive to the dura around the defect. This is often the case

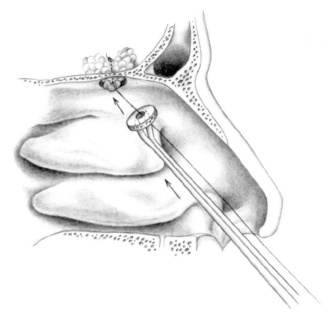

Fig. 12.14 The free mucosal graft is slid up the Vicryl suture to cover the slightly protruding fat plug and skull base defect.

and in these patients a fat plug graft is not suitable because there is insufficient space on the intracranial surface of the defect to place the fat plug. This is especially true in defects larger than 5 mm as greater amounts of brain tissue tend to prolapse into the larger defects with a greater chance of this prolapsed brain becoming adherent to the dura around the defect. The first step is to use the suction bipolar forceps to shrink the brain tissue adherent to the edges of the defect. Any blood vessels visualized are cauterized with the suction bipolar. The malleable suction Freer elevator from the Frontal Sinus Malleable Set* or from the Skull Base Set* (Integra) is bent to the appropriate angle and the brain tissue gently mobilized from the dural edges around the defect to create sufficient space circumferentially around the bony defect. The fascia lata graft is measured to be about 20 mm larger than the defect's diameter so that there is at least 5 mm of graft to be slid into this space between brain and dura around the whole circumference of the defect. In some instances the two-surgeon approach can be useful. The second surgeon can gently push the prolapsing brain tissue intracranially to allow the graft to be placed. The CSF and brain tissue then seals this graft into place and in most cases no further fluorescein-stained CSF should be visible (**Fig. 12.15**).

For large skull base defects (> 2 cm), either a second layer of fascia lata is placed on the nasal surface or a pedicled septal flap is rotated to close the defect followed by fibrin glue. In smaller defects, a free mucosal graft with the mucosa harvested from the middle turbinate or floor of the nose is placed over this intracranial graft followed by fibrin glue. Defects from the posterior wall of the frontal sinus up to the anterior face of the pituitary and from lamina papyracea to lamina papyracea have been successfully closed using this two-layer fascia lata or septal flap approach. When large defects are closed, the fibrin glue is covered by Gelfoam and then a nasal pack is placed in the nose for 5 days. No lumbar drain is used in large defects as this is likely to result in air being

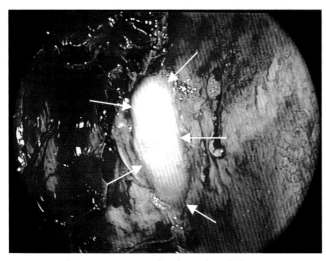

Fig. 12.15 This patient presented with a right-sided spontaneous CSF leak and at surgery a 1.5 cm × 8 mm defect was found in the olfactory fossa. The brain was adherent to the dura around the defect and needed to be carefully mobilized before the fascia lata graft was placed. This photo shows the fascial graft in place as an underlay (*white arrows* mark the limits of the defect). No fluorescein can be seen and a solid seal has been achieved. This graft was covered with a free mucosal graft and fibrin glue and Gelfoam. No nasal pack was placed.

sucked into the intracranial cavity rather than improving the chances of a seal. **Fig. 12.16** illustrates the postoperative view of the skull base after a large defect was closed with the two-layered fascia lata technique.

Some authors have recommended the use of bone or cartilage in the repair of large skull base defects but we have found this to be unnecessary. If cartilage or bone is introduced intracranially, it pushes the fat plug or fascia away from the

dura and bony rim of the defect and does not allow for a solid seal. In patients in whom we placed bone or cartilage in an attempt to provide a solid reconstruction of the skull base, these were removed intraoperatively because the defect could not be adequately sealed and CSF continued to leak. In patients with a large skull base defect postsurgery and with factors that can potentially cause postoperative intracranial hypertension, solid reconstruction of the skull base is considered. In these patients, a strip of titanium mesh is cut that is a few millimeters longer than the width of the skull base defect. A fascia lata in-lay graft is used to cover the brain. The titanium mesh is then positioned from one orbital roof to the other, resting on the orbital roofs and hence reconstructing the skull base. Fascia lata is then placed as an underlay over the titanium overlapping the defect edges. Finally, a pedicled septal flap is placed over this construction to achieve the final seal of the skull base. This has worked very well even in patients who are due to undergo further radiotherapy as part of the ongoing management. The repair is supported with BIPP ribbon gauze pack for a week. We have had two patients who have undergone large defect reconstructions of their skull base and have subsequently developed an encephaloceles over years of follow-up. We prefer to use titanium mesh to reconstruct the skull base as bone and cartilage can become sequestra and behave like a foreign body.

Defects in the Lateral Wall of a Very Pneumatized Sphenoid Sinus: The Transpterygopalatine Fossa Approach (see video)

In this series, there were four patients who had a defect in the lateral wall of a very pneumatized sphenoid sinus. All presented with meningoceles or meningoencephaloceles with associated CSF leaks (**Fig. 12.17**).

In three of the four patients, multiple previous attempts at closure had been made at other institutions usually by attempting to obliterate the sphenoid with fat. These had failed and the patients were referred to our department for closure. In order to close these leaks, adequate exposure of

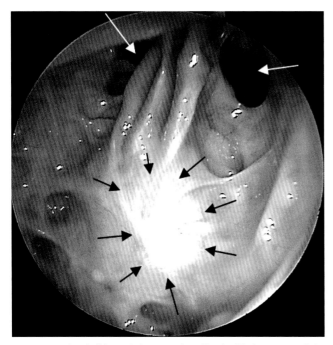

Fig. 12.16 The skull base defect is outlined by the *black arrows* and the frontal sinus ostia by the *white arrows*. Note the remucosalization of the region of the defect.

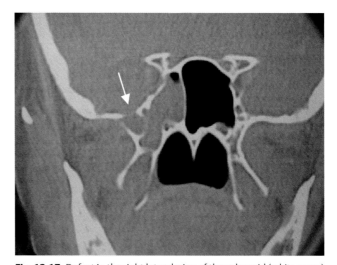

Fig. 12.17 Defect in the right lateral wing of the sphenoid (*white arrow*) with CSF-filled sphenoid sinus.

the lateral wall of the sphenoid is required. This is achieved by removal of the posterior wall of the maxillary sinus, and removal of the contents of the medial region of pterygopalatine fossa with preservation of the maxillary nerve. The Vidian nerve and pterygopalatine ganglion may need to be sacrificed during this exposure. The posterior wall of the pterygopalatine fossa (which is also the anterior wall of the sphenoid) is removed and direct access through the pterygopalatine fossa is achieved. This will usually involve division of the sphenopalatine artery and other branches of the maxillary artery. Division of such a large artery is preceded by cauterization with the suction bipolar forceps* (Integra) otherwise significant bleeding may result. The posterior wall of the pterygopalatine fossa is thick and is resected with the high-speed skull base diamond bur. Care is taken not to injure the maxillary nerve as it traverses the pterygopalatine fossa. Once direct access is achieved in this manner, the meningocele or meningoencephalocele is dealt with in the same manner as described above.

◆ Postoperative Care

The patient is given broad-spectrum antibiotics for 5 days postoperatively. Saline nasal wash is started the next day after the operation. The patient is instructed not to blow the nose for at least 2 to 3 weeks postoperatively. The lumbar drain is only opened if the patient leaks CSF. Drainage should be kept at 5 to 10 mL per hour. If the lumbar drain drains more than 5 to 10 mL per hour, it is raised above the shoulder to slow the drainage. If the lumbar drain is still in place, after 24 hours, it is removed and the patient is slowly mobilized over the following 24 hours and then discharged.

◆ Results

To date, 39 patients have been managed with this technique.[4,5] If these patients are divided into the four broad categories, there were seven traumatic CSF leaks, eight spontaneous CSF leaks, 12 meningoencephaloceles, and 12 iatrogenic CSF leaks. The average age was 40 years and the male to female ratio was 1.2:1.

Table 12.1 summarizes the site, size, and success of the closure of the bath-plug technique.

Eight of the iatrogenic CSF leaks were referred to our department from outside institutions for closure. Thirty-six of the 39 leaks were closed at the first operation giving a primary success rate of closure of 93%. The mean follow-up time for all patients was 28 months (STD = 23) ranging from 14 months to 95 months. The three patients who failed surgery were revised and all are currently successfully closed. Two of these patients had CSF leaks in the lateral wall of the sphenoid sinus and both had undergone multiple previous attempts at closure before referral to our department.[4,5] These patients were examined for evidence of raised intracranial pressure and in one patient there was mild left papilledema. This patient probably has mild

idiopathic interventricular hypertension and is currently being monitored to ensure no other problems develop. The third patient had a previous cranialization of the frontal sinus and developed a CSF leak in the posterior wall of the cranialized frontal sinus. Access was achieved by a modified endoscopic Lothrop procedure but the leak was high and lateral in the frontal sinus and there was difficulty with the placement of the fat plug. The patient started leaking within 48 hours of the repair and was taken back to theatre where the fat plug was found to be partially extruded. A new fat plug was placed and closure was successful.

The technique and results of the closure of large skull base defects after the endoscopic removal of large sections of the skull base to provide access to the intracranial cavity for tumor removal are not included in the above results but discussed in the later chapters on skull base surgery. For non–skull base surgery–related defects, we have found that two layers of fascia lata (with one placed intracranially and the other on the nasal surface of the skull base or in association with a pedicled septal flap) in combination with fibrin glue, Gelfoam, and nasal packing gives a reliable closure. The one leak we have had in this patient group was the first patient operated upon in whom we closed a large 3 × 3 cm defect with fat and fibrin glue alone.

◆ Key Points

The CSF leak cannot be closed if it cannot be identified. There were five patients in this series in whom a fine-cut CT scan and an MRI scan could not identify the site of the leak preoperatively. Intrathecal fluorescein was placed in all elective CSF leak closures, including those in whom the radiological investigations indicated the likely site of the leak. This is an off-label usage of fluorescein so all patients had counseling regarding the potential complications of its usage and signed a separate consent form for its use.[4,5,11,12] In four patients, the blue-light filter and manipulation of the CSF space were needed before the site of the leak could be identified. Although placement of a lumbar drain and the off-label use of fluorescein are controversial, we have found this to be very useful in some patients in whom there was difficulty identifying the site of the CSF leak. In addition, the staining of the fluorescein allows the surgeon to carefully evaluate the security of the seal of the CSF leak by testing the leak by raising the intracranial pressure and looking for any evidence of fluorescein-stained CSF. Finally, the lumbar drain is kept in for 24 hours in case the patient starts to leak postoperatively.

The introduction of a fat plug into the intracranial space has the potential risk of damage to intracranial vascular structures. The risk of such vessels being in the region of the CSF leak is higher in patients who have a meningoencephalocele, especially if the brain is adherent to the dura around the skull base defect. We have modified our technique in these cases to use a two-layer closure (small defects fascia and mucosa and large defects two layers of fascia) or an underlay fascia lata graft with a nasal pedicled rotated septal flap. If there is concern regarding vessels in the region of the defect,

Table 12.1 Summary of patients treated with the bath-plug closure for CSF leak repair

Number	Site	Size (mm)	Follow-up (months)	Second closure required	Successful
Traumatic CSF leaks					
1	Lateral wall of sphenoid	4 × 3	28	No	Yes
2	Around carotid in sphenoid with bony fragment	4 × 3	5	No	Yes
3	Posterior table of frontal sinus	3 × 3	6	No	Yes
4	Cribriform plate	6 × 4	5	No	Yes
5	Ethmoid	3 × 3	26	No	Yes
6	Sphenoid	7 × 5	26	No	Yes
7	Sphenoid	6 × 6	18	No	Yes
Iatrogenic CSF leaks					
1	Posterior ethmoid in association with skull base dehiscence from previous trauma	3 × 2	15	No	Yes
2	Posterior wall of frontal sinus. Sinus previous cranialized with mucocele formation	6 × 4	28	**Yes**	Yes
3	Posterior ethmoids	4 × 3	32	No	Yes
4	Posterior ethmoids after resection of adenocarcinoma; previous CSF leak at same spot with previous resection of adenocarcinoma	4 × 5	12	No	Yes
5	Posterior ethmoids	6 × 4	4	No	Yes
6	Posterior ethmoids	5 × 5	12	No	Yes
7	Adjacent to anterior ethmoidal artery	3 × 3	74	No	Yes
8	Sphenoid after intracranial meningioma removal	3 × 3	15	No	Yes
9	Post craniofacial surgery in anterior ethmoids	3 × 3	20	No	Yes
10	Post adenocarcinoma resection anterior ethmoid	2 × 3	12	No	Yes
11	Post adenocarcinoma resection anterior ethmoid	3 × 3	10	No	Yes
12	Ethmoid roof (appeared to have an abnormally thin fovea ethmoidalis on both sides and had primary surgery at another institution)	16 × 12	16	No	Yes
Spontaneous CSF leaks					
1	Cribriform plate	6 × 3	11	No	Yes
2	Cribriform plate	2 × 1	12	No	Yes
3	Cribriform plate	3 × 2	38	No	Yes
4	Lateral wall of sphenoid	6 × 4	7	No	Yes
5	Cribriform plate	5 × 5	64	No	Yes
6	Roof of sphenoid	12 × 8	70	No	Yes
7	Posterior ethmoid	8 × 6	68	No	Yes
8	Sphenoid	1 × 2	8	No	Yes
Meningoencephaloceles associated with a CSF leak					
1	Sphenoid meningocele on lateral wall of very pneumatized sphenoid; two previous attempted closures failed; mild intracranial hypertension	8 × 6	5	**Yes**	Yes
2	Cribriform plate meningoencephalocele	10 × 8	58	No	Yes
3	Meningoencephalocele found 2 years after cribriform plate trauma as a neonate	12 × 10	8	No	Yes
4	Sphenoid meningocele in lateral wall of very pneumatized sphenoid	8 × 6	7	No	Yes
5	Frontal sinus meningoencephalocele	6 × 4	28	No	Yes
6	Cribriform plate meningocele	3 × 3	11	No	Yes
7	Cribriform plate meningoencephalocele	4 × 4	30	No	Yes
8	Sphenoid meningoencephalocele on the lateral wall of a very pneumatized sphenoid	4 × 4	26	No	Yes
9	Anterior ethmoid meningoencephalocele	13 × 8	62	No	Yes
10	Cribriform plate meningoencephalocele	14 × 8	75	No	Yes
11	Posterior cribriform plate meningoencephalocele after craniofacial surgery 2 years previously	12 × 9	30	No	Yes
12	Sphenoid meningocele on the lateral wall of a very pneumatized sphenoid sinus	8 × 8	6	Yes	Yes
Totals					
39		5.9 × 4.5	23.5	3	39

appropriate radiological investigations should be performed. The advent of radiological software that is able to reconstruct the vasculature of the skull base without the need to perform an angiogram makes this a relatively simple investigation to perform. If doubt exists about the resection of brain tissue, neurosurgical opinion should be sought. Finally, the manipulation of the fat plug through the defect should be very gentle and the probe should not be introduced more than a few millimeters intracranially with each maneuver. This will minimize the risk of intracranial damage. In this series of patients, no such complication occurred and from postoperative observation of the patients there was no need to perform any postoperative radiological investigations.

References

1. Marshall AH, Jones NS, Robertson IJA. CSF rhinorrhoea: the place of endoscopic sinus surgery. Br J Neurosurg 2001;15(1):8–12
2. Hughes RGM, Jones NS, Robertson IJ. The endoscopic treatment of cerebrospinal fluid rhinorrhoea: the Nottingham experience. J Laryngol Otol 1997;111(2):125–128
3. Hegazy HM, Carrau RL, Snyderman CH, Kassam A, Zweig J. Transnasal endoscopic repair of cerebrospinal fluid rhinorrhea: a meta-analysis. Laryngoscope 2000;110(7):1166–1172
4. Bolger WE, McLaughlin K. Cranial bone grafts in cerebrospinal fluid leak and encephalocele repair: a preliminary report. Am J Rhinol 2003;17(3):153–158
5. Wormald PJ, McDonogh M. 'Bath-plug' technique for the endoscopic management of cerebrospinal fluid leaks. J Laryngol Otol 1997;111(11):1042–1046
6. Wormald PJ, McDonogh M. The bath-plug closure of anterior skull base cerebrospinal fluid leaks. Am J Rhinol 2003;17(5):299–305
7. Casiano RR, Jassir D. Endoscopic cerebrospinal fluid rhinorrhea repair: is a lumbar drain necessary? Otolaryngol Head Neck Surg 1999;121(6):745–750
8. Badia L, Loughran S, Lund V. Primary spontaneous cerebrospinal fluid rhinorrhea and obesity. Am J Rhinol 2001;15(2):117–119
9. Ommaya AK, Di Chiro G, Baldwin M, Pennybacker JB. Non-traumatic cerebrospinal fluid rhinorrhoea. J Neurol Neurosurg Psychiatry 1968;31(3):214–225
10. Har-El G. What is "spontaneous" cerebrospinal fluid rhinorrhea? Classification of cerebrospinal fluid leaks. Ann Otol Rhinol Laryngol 1999;108(4):323–326
11. Gacek RR. Arachnoid granulation cerebrospinal fluid otorrhea. Ann Otol Rhinol Laryngol 1990;99(11):854–862
12. Mattox DE, Kennedy DW. Endoscopic management of cerebrospinal fluid leaks and cephaloceles. Laryngoscope 1990;100(8):857–862
13. Syms CA III, Syms MJ, Murphy TP, Massey SO. Cerebrospinal fluid fistulae in a canine model. Otolaryngol Head Neck Surg 1997;117(5):542–546
14. Mao VH, Keane WM, Atkins JP, et al. Endoscopic repair of cerebrospinal fluid rhinorrhea. Otolaryngol Head Neck Surg 2000;122(1):56–60
15. Zweig JL, Carrau RL, Celin SE, et al. Endoscopic repair of cerebrospinal fluid leaks to the sinonasal tract: predictors of success. Otolaryngol Head Neck Surg 2000;123(3):195–201

13 Endoscopic Pituitary Tumor Surgery

◆ Introduction

Pituitary tumors are commonly benign pituitary adenomas and only rarely are pituitary carcinomas or posterior pituitary neoplasias diagnosed.[1] Pituitary adenomas present most commonly in the third and fourth decades.[1] Their clinical presentation depends on whether the tumor is secreting (less common) or nonsecreting (more common).[1] Secreting adenomas present with the endocrine manifestations of the hormone secreted.[1,2] The most common is a prolactin-secreting tumor, followed by growth hormone, ACTH, follicle-stimulating hormone, and luteinizing hormone.[1,2] Nonsecreting adenomas usually present due to their mass effects. Symptoms may include headache, hypopituitarism, visual loss and visual field defects (most commonly bilateral hemianopia), and cranial nerve defects.

MRI is the radiologic investigation of choice for pathologic tumor evaluation and used to define involvement of surrounding structures. Pituitary adenomas are divided, for clinical purposes, into microadenomas (<1.0 cm in diameter) and macroadenomas (>1.0 cm in diameter). Microadenomas are often difficult to see on MRI, but the normal anterior pituitary gland will usually be visible with a gadolinium-enhanced T1-weighted image allowing the microadenoma to be identified. In patients who have macroadenomas, the normal anterior pituitary will usually not be visualized. There are a number of grading systems available, but the most commonly used is based on extrasellar extension of the tumor (**Table 13.1**).[3]

In recent years, the surgical approach to the pituitary fossa has been either transeptal or transethmoid.[4,5] The transeptal approach is performed through either a sublabial incision or through a hemitransfixion incision. Once the septal flaps have been raised and the anterior face of the sphenoid removed, the Cushing speculum is inserted. The microscope is swung into place and the anterior face of the pituitary fossa visualized. The sphenoid rostrum is removed and the intersinus septum identified and removed. The advantage of this technique is that the surgeon can now use an instrument in each hand to proceed with the surgery. The disadvantages of this technique are the morbidity associated with a sublabial incision and dissection and the incidence of septal perforations, adhesions, and postoperative sinusitis. In addition, the surgeon cannot visualize lateral or superior extensions of the tumor.

Recently, a number of surgeons have advocated a transnasal approach where the sphenoid sinus and the pituitary fossa are approached transnasally with lateralization of the middle turbinate and resection of the superior turbinate and anterior face of the sphenoid.[5–9] The Cushing speculum is introduced through the nares and into the sphenoidotomy and opened.[6,7] Opening of the speculum tends to further fracture the middle turbinate laterally as well as fracture the septum toward the opposite nasal cavity. Once the speculum is in place, the microscope is again brought in by the surgeon and the anterior face of the pituitary fossa resected with the surgeon using an instrument in each hand.[6,7] The advantages of this technique are the lack of any incisions around the face but the disadvantage is the fracture or displacement of the septum and middle turbinate. Additionally, and most importantly, the surgeon cannot visualize tumor extensions laterally or superiorly. When the speculum is opened, it fractures the septum laterally. The septum is usually unstable and will often result in a septal deviation postoperatively. The middle turbinate may remain displaced and may cause obstruction of the sinus ostia, although this would be unusual.

The major reason for developing endoscopic pituitary tumor resection techniques is to minimize intranasal complications and to provide superior visualization. The endoscopic view is panoramic when compared to the microscopic view and this helps with identification of critical anatomical landmarks within the sphenoid. In addition, angled endoscopes allow tumor that extends outside the sella to be seen and this improves the surgeon's ability to achieve complete tumor resection.[8,9] Tumor remnants in the recesses of the sella which would not have been seen with the microscope may be visualized with an endoscope (**Fig. 13.1**). If complete tumor resection is achieved there is less likelihood of recurrence.

Table 13.1 Wilson grading system for pituitary adenomas based on extrasellar extension[3]

Stage 0	No suprasellar extension
Stage A	Extension into suprasellar cistern only
Stage B	Extension into anterior recess of the third ventricle
Stage C	Obliteration of anterior recess and deformation of floor of third ventricle
Stage D	Intradural extension into anterior, middle, or posterior fossa
Stage E	Extradural invasion into cavernous sinus

◆ Preoperative Assessment

The standard radiological evaluation prior to endoscopic resection of a pituitary tumor is a standard CT scan of the sinuses and MRI scan of the brain. These two modalities allow assessment of the nose, sinuses, and the pituitary tumor. The MRI scan requested is performed according to the image guidance protocol for our computer-aided surgical (CAS) guidance system.

Image guidance during surgery adds to the safety of the procedure by confirming the positions of the optic nerves and carotid arteries. In addition, during tumor resection, image guidance is used to confirm the limits of the pituitary fossa and the position of the internal carotid arteries within the cavernous sinuses, which may add to the safety of the procedure. In the preoperative evaluation of the radiology, special attention needs to be paid to the course of the internal carotid arteries. Normally, the carotid arteries enter the base of the sphenoid sinus and turn vertically to ascend to the base of the pituitary gland where they move posteriorly and slightly medially before turning back on themselves, forming the internal carotid siphon lateral to the pituitary gland in the cavernous sinus. They then travel anteriorly and can usually be seen on the lateral nasal wall before turning

vertically and posteriorly to run lateral to the optic nerve into the middle cranial fossa (**Fig. 13.2**).

The most important assessment that should be performed prior to pituitary surgery is to evaluate the position of the carotids on the lateral wall and their relationship with the tumor and the anterior face of the sphenoid. If the tumor wraps around the carotid in the lateral wall, this can cause displacement of the carotid, pushing the carotid up against the anterior wall of the sphenoid (**Fig. 13.3**). In the axial MRI scan we can see the right carotid abuts the anterior wall of the sphenoid and that tumor envelopes the carotid. In **Fig. 13.4**, the Kerrison approaches the anterior face of the carotid to open up the sphenoid to allow visualization of the tumor when inadvertently with this maneuver the carotid is opened (**Fig. 13.5**). Fortunately, a muscle patch and stent were placed and the patient suffered no adverse outcome. The management of a carotid bleed is presented in Chapter 22.

In some patients, the carotid may turn medially as it moves anteriorly after the siphon and in so doing covers the anterior face of the pituitary fossa limiting the access to the gland (**Fig. 13.6**). In such a patient, care needs to be exercised so that the carotid is not injured as the dura is opened for access to the pituitary tumor (**Fig. 13.6**).

◆ Surgical Technique

Macroadenoma

Patients are catheterized prior to surgery. This allows manipulation of fluid balance during surgery and allows the patient's postoperative urine output to be monitored. This is important in identifying and managing diabetes insipidus due to disturbance in antidiuretic hormone regulation. This may result from the manipulation of the pituitary stalk (relatively

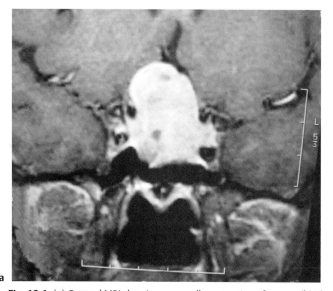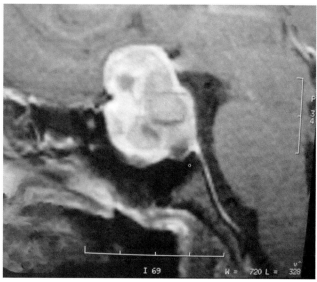

Fig. 13.1 (a) Coronal MRI showing suprasellar extension of tumor. (b) The same tumor is shown in the parasagittal plane in MRI. Angled telescopes can be very helpful to visualize extensions above the sella as shown in these two MRI scans.

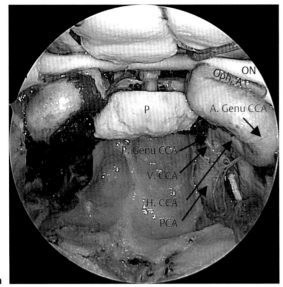
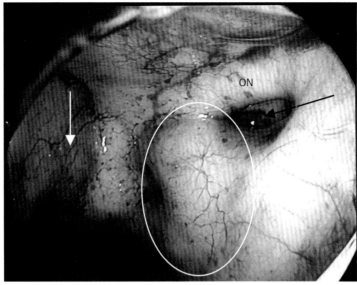

Fig. 13.2 (**a**) Cadaveric dissection image after removal of bone from the lateral wall of the sphenoid. The paraclival carotid artery (*PCA*) enters the base of the sphenoid sinus and then runs in a vertical direction. At approximately the level of V2 (maxillary division of the trigeminal nerve) the carotid enters the cavernous sinus and becomes the intercavernous carotid artery (*CCA*). Once the artery enters the cavernous sinus it ascends for a short distance called the vertical portion of the cavernous carotid artery (*V.CCA*), before turning anterior forming the posterior genu of the CCA (*P.Genu CCA*). This posterior genu is usually at the level of the floor of the sella. The artery then runs anteriorly as the horizontal portion of the CCA (*H.CCA*) before reaching the anterior genu of the CCA (*A. Genu CCA*). After the anterior genu the artery becomes extracavernous, exiting the roof of the cavernous to form the clinoidal segment of the ICA. This clinoidal segment is at the base of the optic strut (lateral opticocartoid recess before exiting intracranially to form the cisternal segment of the ICA. In (**b**) the *solid white arrow* indicates the beginning of the siphon where the vertical portion of the artery is reflected anteriorly to form an anterior genu before exiting the cavernous sinus into the anterior cranial fossa behind the optic nerve (*ON*). The portion of this artery usually seen in the lateral sphenoid wall is indicated by the *white oval*. The optico-carotid recess is marked with a *black arrow*.

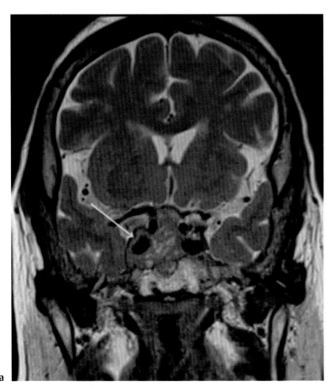
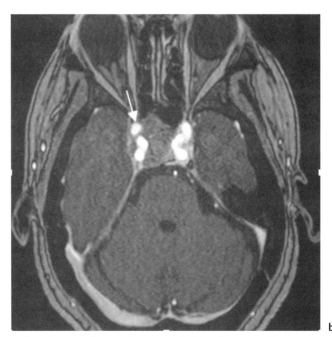

Fig. 13.3 (**a**) In this coronal MRI scan, the pituitary tumor can be seen encircling the carotid artery (*green arrow*). (**b**) In the MRI axial scan, note how the carotid abuts the anterior face of the sphenoid (*white arrow*).

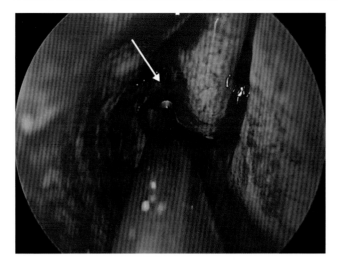

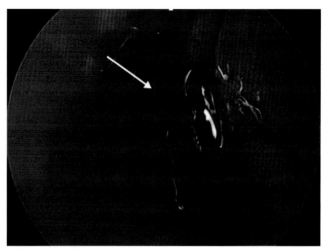

Fig. 13.4 The Kerrison approached the upper lateral aspect of the anterior face of the sphenoid with a view to widening the approach for the resection of a tumor that wraps around the carotid in this region.

Fig. 13.5 The Kerrison is still in place (*black arrow*) while the bleeding is welling up from the defect in the carotid wall (*white arrow*).

common and usually transient) or from injury or dysfunction of the posterior pituitary gland during the procedure. Intravenous antibiotic prophylaxis is given—usually cephalosporin, gentamycin, and metronidazole. Standard preparation of the nose is performed with topical vasoconstriction and

infiltration. Any significant septal deviation is dealt with via either a Killian's or Freer (hemitransfixion) incision. Correction of any septal defect allows both nasal cavities to be used for access to the sphenoid during the surgery. If a significant septal deflection is not dealt with, significant trauma of that

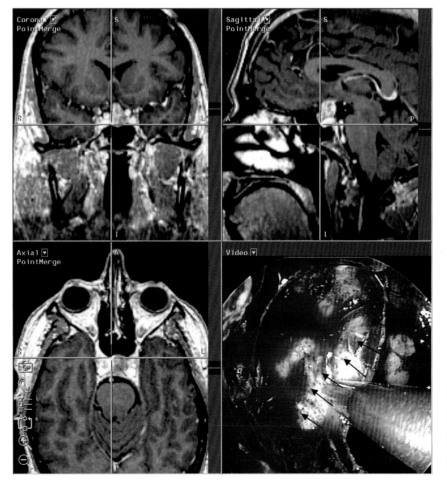

Fig. 13.6 This picture from our CAS system illustrates the course of the internal carotid arteries in all three planes as they approach the midline bilaterally with a small window between them through which the pituitary tumor can be accessed. The *black arrows* indicate on the endoscopic image the medial extent of the right carotid artery. The septation on the anterior face of the pituitary is almost in the midline.

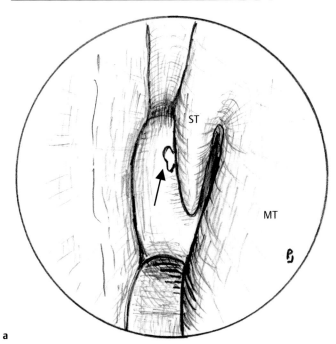

Fig. 13.7 (**a**) Endoscopic diagrammatic view of the left superior meatus and sphenoid ostium indicated with a *black arrow* and the superior turbinate (*ST*) and middle turbinate clearly visible. (**b**) Cadaveric dissection image of the left superior meatus and sphenoid ostium. The superior turbinate shares a common border with the middle turbinate, with the antero-superior border of the superior turbinate attaching to the middle turbinate.

nasal cavity may occur. During surgery instruments are often passed through the nasal cavity without endoscopic visualization. Difficulty in passing instruments in such a blinded manner can be due to septal deflection and may slow the surgery significantly.

The endoscope and microdebrider are passed medial to the middle turbinate and the superior turbinate and the sphenoid ostium is identified (**Fig. 13.7**).

The next step is to remove bilaterally the lower two-thirds of the superior turbinate and expose the natural ostium of the sphenoid sinus (**Fig. 13.8**). In order to protect the vascular pedicle of the septal flap, a horizontal incision from the lower edge of the sphenoid ostium is made onto the septum angulating superiorly. This allows a suction Freer to be used to roll this pedicle inferiorly and in this rolled mucosa will lie the postnasal artery which is the major blood supply of the

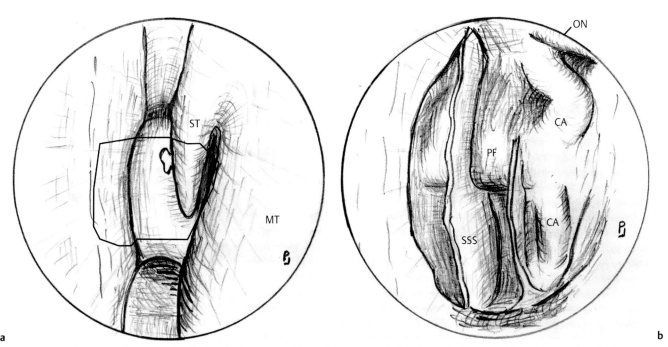

Fig. 13.8 (**a**) The area to be resected including the lower two-thirds of the superior turbinate, posterior ethmoids, and large sphenoidotomy are shaded. (**b**) After resection, the carotid artery (*CA*), optic nerve (*ON*), pituitary fossa (*PF*), and sphenoid sinus septum (*SSS*) are seen.

septal flap. In patients who end up with large defects in the diaphragm or with exposed carotid arteries, repair with the septal flap is needed. If this pedicle is not raised and a standard opening of the sphenoid performed, the pedicle will be destroyed as the anterior face of the sphenoid is lowered sufficiently to allow adequate endoscopic approach to the pituitary. After preservation of the pedicle, the sphenoid ostium is enlarged inferiorly until a straight instrument is passed easily under the floor of the pituitary fossa. This is done bilaterally. The posterior 1 cm of the septum is removed with the cutting bur and back-biting forceps and the sphenoid sinus septum visualized. This is important as a Kerrison punch will be placed in the left nostril and will be used to remove the bone of the right side of the pituitary fossa and vice versa for the right nostril. The sphenoidotomies are enlarged up to the lateral wall of the sphenoid. The access provided should allow passage of an instrument below the pituitary fossa and laterally onto the internal carotid artery and optic nerve eminences (**Fig. 13.8**). The next step is to remove the sphenoid mucosa starting on the sphenoid septum in the larger of the two sinuses. The mucosa is removed from medial to lateral over the entire pituitary fossa and left pedicled in the lateral inferior aspect of the sphenoid. This is covered with a strip of Surgicel (Ethicon; Somerville, NJ) to prevent it from been suctioned during the remainder of the surgery. The sphenoid sinus septum is removed flush with the pituitary fossa (**Fig. 13.9**). If the anterior wall of the pituitary fossa is thick, the drill is used to thin this down until it is soft. Most patients with macroadenomas will have a soft anterior face of the pituitary as the pressure exerted by the expanding tumor thins the bone. However, patients who have a microadenoma may have thick bone forming the anterior face of the pituitary.

The key to endoscopic pituitary surgery is to have full access to the pituitary fossa from both sides of the nose. This allows two surgeons to work off the video monitor at the same time. Our team consists of a neurosurgeon (with endoscopic interest and skill) and a sinus surgeon. The roles of these surgeons are interchangeable, with both surgeons able to perform all parts of the procedure. Having two surgeons allows an endoscope with camera attached and two instruments to be used at all times during the procedure. If significant bleeding occurs, a blood-free field can be maintained by one of the surgeons using a high volume suction. The thin bone of the anterior face of the pituitary is fractured and removed with Kerrison's punch (**Fig. 13.10** and **Fig. 13.11**). Wide opening of the anterior face of the pituitary is achieved with bone removal from one cavernous sinus to the other. Care is taken with the superior bone removal as a fold of dura occurs below the tuberculum sella and in this region it is closely attached to the bone. If the Kerrison's punch is not kept solidly in contact with the undersurface of the bone, this dural fold can be caught by the punch and a cerebrospinal fluid (CSF) leak can result.

In most cases, the dura is not cauterized as this tends to shrink the dura. If, however, cautery is felt to be needed for visible blood vessels on the surface of the dura, a suction bipolar* (Integra) is used to cauterize the dura before a number 11 scalpel blade on a number 7 BP handle is used to create a U-shaped incision into the dura (**Fig. 13.12**). We prefer the U-shaped incision to the cruciate incision as the dural corners of the cruciate incision partially block the view into the sella during surgery. The U-shaped incision allows an unobstructed view of the diaphragm and the

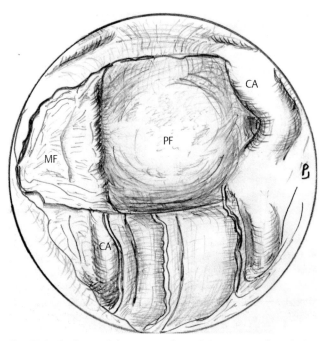

Fig. 13.9 The bone of the anterior face of the pituitary fossa (*PF*) is widely removed. The mucosal flap (*MF*) has been laid aside and the bone of the pituitary fossa (*PF*) exposed from one cavernous sinus to the other.

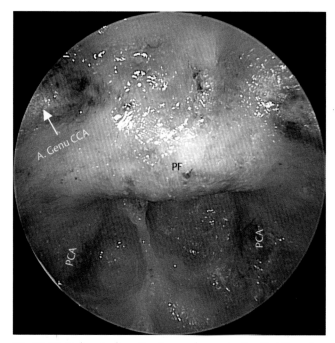

Fig. 13.10 Cadaveric dissection image demonstrating that the sphenoid sinus septum has been removed flush with the pituitary fossa (*PF*). *PCA*, paraclival carotid artery; *A. Genu CCA*, anterior genu of the intracavernous carotid artery.

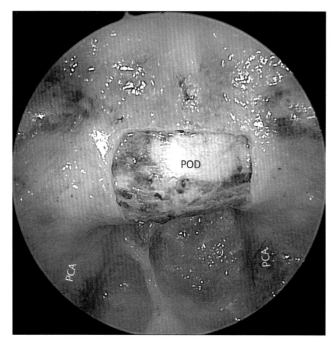

Fig. 13.11 Cadaveric dissection of the sphenoid sinus with bone removal over the pituitary fossa exposing the periosteal layer of dura (*POD*).

lateral walls and lateral and superior recesses of the sella where residual tumor may be missed if a clear view is not obtained. In addition, the dura can be used to help seal any small leaks on the anterior edge of the diaphragm by rolling the dura into the pituitary fossa over the leak.

In patients with a macroadenoma, tumor under pressure will often ooze through these dural incisions. A Deckers or skull base Blakesley forceps (Integra) is used to remove a sample of tumor for histology. Malleable suction ring curettes* (Integra skull base set) and standard pituitary ring curettes are used to first clear the tumor along the floor of the pituitary fossa until the posterior wall of the pituitary fossa is seen (**Fig. 13.13**).

Attention is then turned to tumor sited laterally on the cavernous sinuses. The ring curette is gently scrapped along the cavernous sinus and tumor removed using the suction on the ring curette. The curette can be felt rolling over the carotid artery. Finally, the tumor on the pituitary fossa diaphragm is removed. Care should be taken to visualize the diaphragm as it descends with the tumor removal. In patients who have a significant suprasellar tumor extension, a 30-degree endoscope can be used to visualize this suprasellar extension and to remove it under direct vision. This use of angled endoscopes is the great advantage of the endoscopic approach. It allows tumor that traditionally cannot be visualized with the standard microscopic approach to be seen and removed under vision. In addition, the malleable skull base set* (Integra) has malleable suction ring curettes that can be bent so that even a large suprasellar component can be reached from below. **Fig. 13.14** shows a patient with a large suprasellar extension. In this patient the tumor was removed from below. As the tumor was debulked from below so the suprasellar component descended into the pituitary fossa. This is especially true for tumors with a broad-based suprasellar extension. Tumors with a dumbbell-shaped extension or narrow neck may have ruptured through the diaphragm

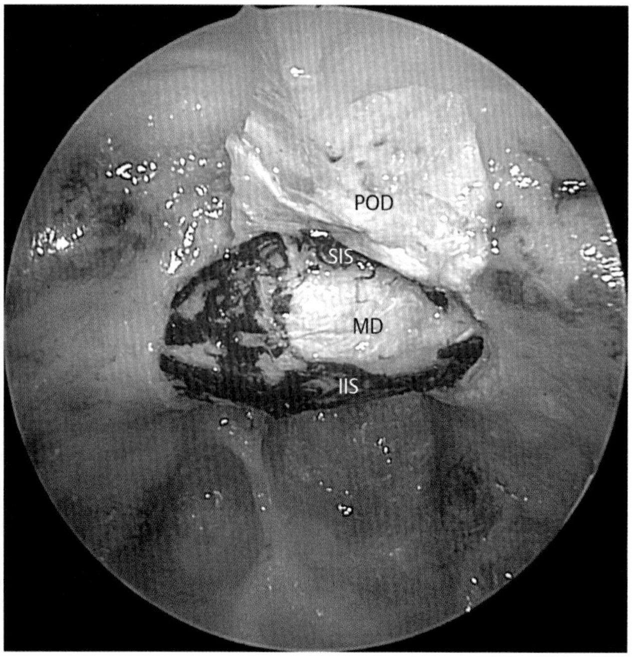

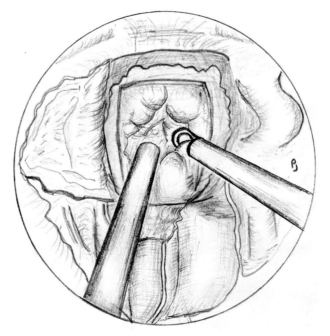

Fig. 13.12 Cadaveric dissection illustrating the U-shaped incision performed into the dura. In this dissection just the periosteal layer of dura (*POD*) has been reflected, exposing the superior (*SIS*) and inferior intercavernous dural sinus (*IIS*). These sinuses run between the periosteal layer of dura and the meningeal layer of dura (*MD*).

Fig. 13.13 The first surgeon is using the ring curette to remove tumor from the lower half of the pituitary fossa while the second surgeon is holding the endoscope and a second suction to keep the surgical field clear or to retract the dura so that the first surgeon may obtain a better view of the lateral walls and diaphragm region.

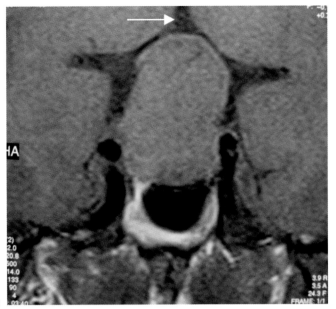
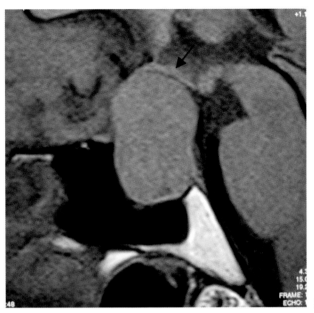

Fig. 13.14 The large suprasellar extension is seen with extension of the into the third and lateral ventricles (*white arrow*). Note the broad-based extension in both (**a**) and (**b**) and the superior compression of the pituitary gland in (**b**) (*black arrow*).

and be better approached with an extended pituitary approach (**Fig. 13.15**).

The other significant advantage of the two-surgeon approach is the ability of one surgeon to hold the diaphragm up while the other surgeon removes tumor that may otherwise be left unresected in the angle between the diaphragm and cavernous sinus (**Fig. 13.16**). In our experience, this is the most common area for residual tumor and this area is not usually visible with the microscope as it sits above the level of the anterior bony opening made in the pituitary fossa. In addition, the diaphragm may obliterate this angle as it descends. Gently holding the diaphragm up with a Freer elevator helps to keep this angle open and

allows the other surgeon to gently remove any residual tumor (**Fig. 13.16**).

In order to remove any microscopic or small pieces of tumor that may still be adherent to one of the walls of the sella, a small neuropattie is placed into the sella and wiped around the sella (**Fig. 13.17**). This also absorbs blood clots and allows clear visualization of the diaphragm and lateral walls and floor of the sella (**Fig. 13.17**). The 30-degree endoscope is usually placed within the sella cavity and rotated so that anterosuperior and anterolateral recesses can be clearly seen. In **Fig. 13.17b**, the white arrow indicates anterolateral residual tumor that was missed by a solely microscopic hypophysectomy for a growth hormone–secreting tumor.

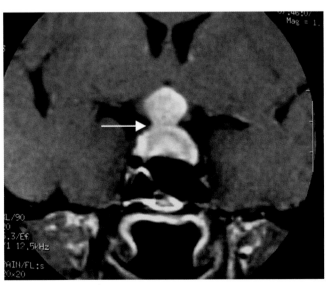
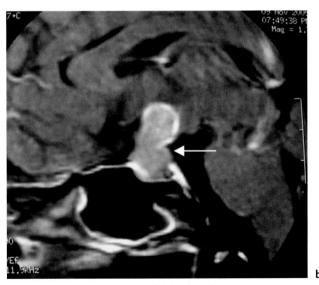

Fig. 13.15 Dumbbell suprasellar extension in in the coronal plane in (**a**) and parasagittal in (**b**). The neck is marked with a *white arrow*.

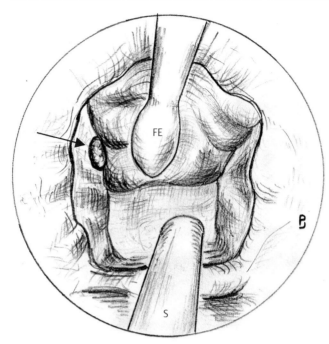

Fig. 13.16 The Freer elevator (*FE*) is being held up by one surgeon while the second surgeon visualizes the residual tumor (*RT*) (*arrow*) in the angle between the cavernous sinus and diaphragm and removes it.

This residual tumor could be clearly seen with the angled endoscope and was removed and the growth hormone levels have remained low to normal in the postoperative period. This case illustrates one of the most important advantages of the endoscopic approach to resection of both macro- and microadenomas.

Once the tumor has been completely removed, Gelfoam paste (Gelfoam powder mixed with saline to form a paste

[Pfizer; Kalamazoo, MI]) is placed within the pituitary fossa. The preserved dural flap and sphenoid mucosa are positioned over the anterior face of the sella and fibrin glue applied to the surface (**Fig. 13.18**).

The middle turbinates are repositioned in their correct orientation and the operation is complete. No packing is placed within the sphenoid or the nasal cavity. If the patient has a CSF leak from the diaphragm, then the hole in the diaphragm is identified and a conically shaped fat graft is placed into the defect and gently pushed through the hole with the malleable probe* (Integra skull base set) until the leak is completely sealed. This plug forms a dumbbell with some of the fat through the defect but with most of the fat still in the sella. The rest of the sella is filled with fat and a fascia lata graft is placed over the fat with the edges of the graft tucked under the dura of the opening into the sella. The dura and sphenoid mucosa is placed over this facia and fibrin glue applied (**Fig. 13.19**). This region is covered with Gelfoam and the sphenoid sinus is packed with bismuth iodoform paraffin paste (BIPP)-impregnated ribbon gauze or antibiotic-soaked ribbon gauze. The gauze allows pressure to be placed on the fascia during the healing period. The ribbon gauze is trailed into the nasal cavity and is removed after 5 days in the outpatient department. No additional nasal packing is used. If the CSF leak was profuse, a lumbar drain is inserted postoperatively for 2 to 3 days to ensure the pressure is taken off the fat plug during healing.

Microadenoma Resection

The image guidance scan for these patients is an MRI scan. This helps with the intraoperative localization of the microadenoma and ensures that the correct portion of the gland is removed. Essentially the same approach is used for microadenomas as is used for macroadenomas up to the point where

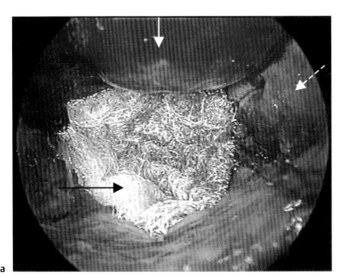

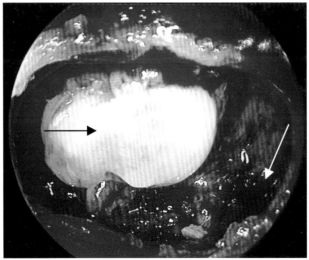

Fig. 13.17 (**a**) A neuropattie (*black arrow*) placed against the posterior wall of the sella. The diaphragm (*white solid arrow*), cavernous sinus (*white broken arrow*), and floor of the sella can all be clearly seen. (**b**) A hypophysectomy had been performed by a microscopic approach 3 weeks previously and although the growth hormone

levels initially dropped, they rose to high levels in the third week. The patient underwent an endoscopic exploration and residual tumor was seen in the lateral anterior region (*white arrow*) and removal of this has resulted in a cure for the patient. The diaphragm can be clearly seen (*black arrow*).

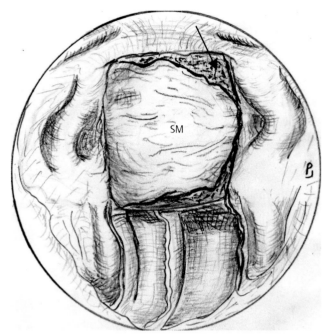

Fig. 13.18 The dural flap is positioned over the Gelfoam paste and then the sphenoid mucosal (*SM*) flap is placed over the dura to cover the anterior face of the sella. Fibrin glue is applied.

the dura is incised. After opening the dura, incisions are made over the region of the microadenoma. Using blunt dissection, this region of the gland is explored. Usually the tumor is soft and a different consistency from the rest of the gland and, in most cases, can be dissected from the gland. However, some microadenomas are unable to be differentiated from

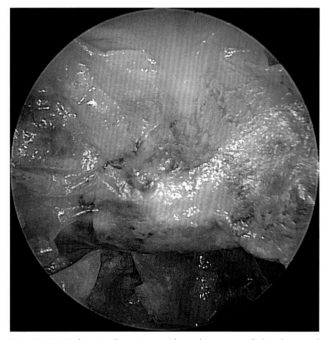

Fig. 13.19 Cadaveric dissection with replacement of the dura and sphenoid sinus mucosa at the end of the pituitary procedure.

normal gland and the gland may need to be sliced in multiple places before the tumor is found. Care should be taken to avoid confusing the posterior pituitary gland with tumor as it is softer and often a paler color than the anterior pituitary gland.

Cavernous Sinus Invasion

Pituitary tumors may invade the cavernous sinus to various degrees. The classification of tumor invasion that we use is by Knosp et al[10] (**Fig. 13.20**).

Grades 1 and 2 are treated no differently to a standard pituitary dissection as described above. Grade 3 has tumor lateral to the carotid. It is important to plot out the carotid artery and to see where the tumor has entered the cavernous sinus. Normally tumor enters the sinus above the horizontal portion of the intracavernous portion of the carotid (**Fig. 13.21**). If invasion is extensive there may be an inferior component that wraps underneath this part of the carotid. In general, tumor from nonsecreting adenomas that does not come away easily are not extensively looked for or followed into the cavernous sinus. A more conservative approach is adopted in these nonsecreting tumors, as well as in elderly patients. However, in secreting tumors, these extensions are actively chased in an attempt to remove all tumors so that an endocrinological cure can be achieved. Tumor can be followed into the cavernous sinus from the pituitary fossa. In some instances, this is broad-based but in other patients it may have a narrow neck and form a dumbbell through this dural opening. The tumor in the cavernous sinus will obliterate the venous sinusoids and following the tumor into the cavernous sinus does not normally result in a significant increase in bleeding. This dissection is done with a 30-degree scope angled laterally and usually placed within the pituitary fossa for this dissection. Angled and malleable ring curettes are used to remove the tumor. In some instances, the third nerve may be visible in the lateral wall of the cavernous sinus. Suction on the third nerve will almost always result in a neuropraxia with postoperative palsy. However, when this has happened to us, the palsy has fully recovered after 3 months. Tumor extensions under the carotid artery and into the cavernous can also be followed in this manner and removed. In patients who have secreting tumor lateral and anterior to the carotid, an additional incision is made lateral to the carotid directly into the cavernous sinus. This allows dissection into the cavernous with a direct access into the cavernous sinus from an anterior approach. Remember that the sixth cranial nerve traverses the cavernous sinus and may be at risk if the dissection is taken below the anterior genu of the carotid as this nerve hugs the inferior anterior border of this genu (**Fig. 13.21**).

Extended Pituitary Dissection

This approach is used for pituitary tumors that extend anterior to the tuberculum sella or that extend significantly into the suprasellar region with disruption of the diaphragm. Additionally, this approach is used for tuberculum sella

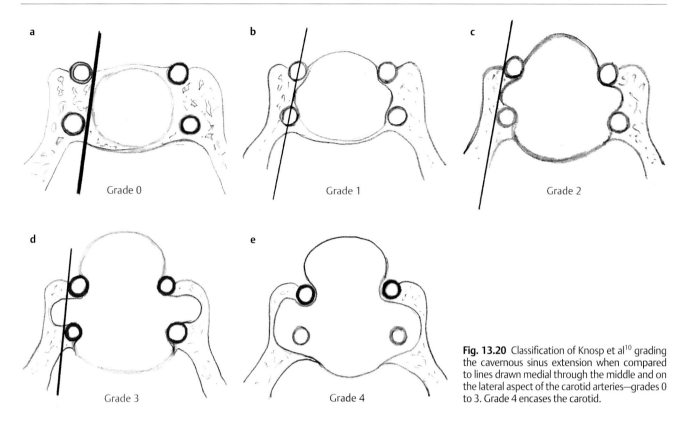

a

Grade 0

b

Grade 1

c

Grade 2

d

Grade 3

e

Grade 4

Fig. 13.20 Classification of Knosp et al[10] grading the cavernous sinus extension when compared to lines drawn medial through the middle and on the lateral aspect of the carotid arteries—grades 0 to 3. Grade 4 encases the carotid.

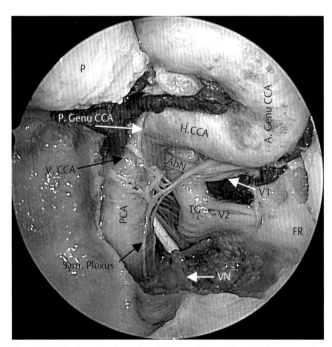

Fig. 13.21 Cadaveric dissection (photo taken with a 70-degree endoscope) of the lateral sphenoid wall demonstrating the different portions of the intracavernous carotid artery (*CCA*). *P*, pituitary; *A. Genu CCA*, anterior genu of the intracavernous carotid artery; *H. CCA*, horizontal portion of the intracavernous carotid artery; *P. Genu CCA*, posterior genu of the intracavernous carotid artery; *V. CCA*, vertical portion of the intracavernous carotid artery; *PCA*, paraclival carotid artery; *Sym*. Plexus, sympathetic plexus; *TG*, trigeminal ganglion; *V2*, maxillary division of the trigeminal nerve; *FR*, foramen rotundum; *VN*, vidian nerve; *AbN*, abducens nerve.

tumors such as meningiomas that push the pituitary inferiorly and ride over the tuberculum sella onto the planum sphenoidale. Pituitary tumors that disrupt the diaphragm are suspected when the tumor has a significant dumbbell shape or if extension occurs into or beyond the third ventricle. The exposure for this approach involves removing the bone above the pituitary fossa and on the planum sphenoidale. Once dural exposure of the pituitary is achieved, the bone overlying the tuberculum sella is removed. Both optic nerves are identified and the bone removed from between them. The bone between the optic nerve and anterior superior portion of the carotid anterior genu is called the medial opticocarotid recess (medial OCR) (**Fig. 13.22**). Between these two medial OCRs is the narrowest part of the access into the subchiasmatic cistern and care should be taken to remove as much of this bone as possible to widen surgical access. However, be aware that the two structures bordering this bone are the optic nerve and carotid artery so great care should be taken with this bone removal. Should the medial OCRs not be removed, then surgeons can have difficulty manipulating instruments through this narrow access and may compromise the resection of the tumor. Once the dura is exposed between the optic nerves, the dissection progresses onto the planum sphenoidale (**Fig. 13.23**). Bone is removed up to the anterior face of the sphenoid sinus. The dural exposure widens over this area giving an hourglass exposure. The dura is incised with an 11-blade in the midline and the subchiasmatic cistern inspected (**Fig. 13.24**). The superior hypophyseal artery should be seen with both optic nerves and suprasellar extension of the tumor. In patients with a

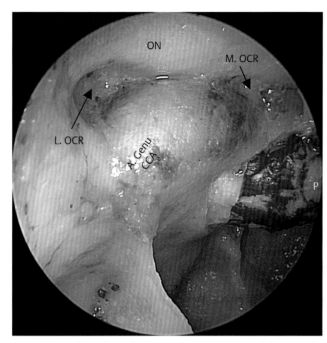

Fig. 13.22 In this cadaver dissection, the anterior genu of the carotid is seen with the optic nerve (*ON*) running above it and creating the lateral opticocarotid recess (*L.OCR*). Between the optic nerve as it exits the sphenoid and the carotid as it enters, the anterior cranial fossa is the medial opticocarotid recess (*M. OCR*). *P*, pituitary gland.

prefixed optic chiasm, displacement of the optic chiasm is limited which severely limits surgical access into the region above the optic chiasm as the optic nerves and chiasm form the anterior limit and the lower they are fixed the more the surgeons are forced to work around them. If this can be detected preoperatively this is a relative contraindication to the extended pituitary approach.

All patients who have an extended approach to their pituitary performed required an underlay fascia lata graft with or without fat and an onlay pedicled vascularized septal flap placed over the defect to ensure solid closure. The subchiasmatic cistern is a high CSF flow region and needs to be managed with best possible closure techniques (**Fig. 13.24**).

◆ Postoperative Care

Patients are monitored in high dependency overnight with routine neurological observations and hourly monitoring of urine output. If the urine output is greater than 250 mL per hour for more than 2 hours an endocrinologist should be consulted and desmopressin may be given. Cortisol is usually not given in the perioperative period but levels are monitored by the endocrinologists and augmentation prescribed if necessary. If the procedure was uncomplicated, the patient is mobilized the following day and discharged when the endocrinologists are satisfied with their hormone status.

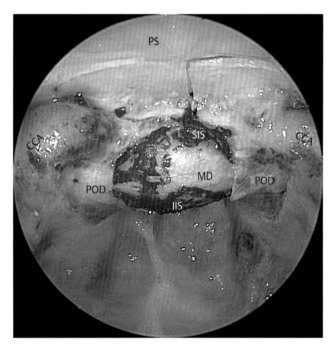

Fig. 13.23 Cadaveric dissection with further bone exposure between the intracavernous carotid arteries (*CCA*) and optic nerves. A portion of the planum sphenoidale (*PS*) has been removed allowing for wider exposure of the periosteal layer of dura (*POD*). *SIS*, superior intercavernous sinus; *IIS*, inferior intercavernous sinus; *MD*, meningeal layer of dura.

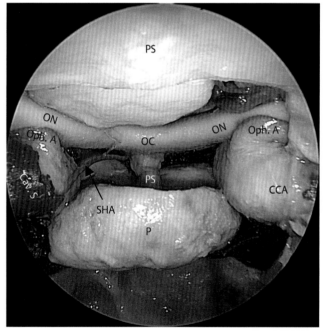

Fig. 13.24 Cadaveric dissection with view into the subchiasmatic cistern. *PS*, planum sphenoidale; *ON*, optic nerve; *OC*, optic chiasm; *Oph. A*, ophthalmic artery; *CCA*, intracavernous carotid artery; *SHA*, superior hypophyseal artery; *PS*, pituitary stalk; *P*, pituitary.

◆ Results[11]

Although we have reported on our first 32 consecutive and unselected patients who underwent an entirely endoscopic resection of their pituitary tumors utilizing the technique described, this number in now in the hundreds. In this report, five patients had secretory microadenomas. In the macroadenoma group, there were six patients with extensive suprasellar and/or parasellar extensions. Postoperative imaging showed residual tumor in four patients with tumor located lateral to the carotid artery in three of these patients.[11] In the microadenoma group all patients have normalized their hormone status. Six CSF leaks were seen during surgery and repaired. Two patients developed CSF leaks postoperatively and one patient who had a very fibrous tumor developed a leak after revision surgery and required two returns to theatre before closure of the leak was achieved. No other complications were seen. In the remaining 22 patients, complete removal of the macroadenoma was achieved and verified with postoperative MRI scanning.[11] Five patients have required continued treatment for diabetes insipidus and eight patients have required ongoing hormonal replacement therapy. These results are compatible with the published results of most international centers.[12,13] In an analysis of our most recent case series (unpublished), our CSF leak rate is now less than 5% and the tumor recurrence rate in macroadenomas is less than 15%. The cure rate for hormone secretory tumors is greater than 85%.

◆ Key Points

The two major advantages of this technique are the minimal trauma involved in accessing the pituitary gland with bilateral sphenoidotomies and in some cases septoplasty being the only surgery necessary for the approach to the pituitary. In addition, there is considerable advantage in the use of angled telescopes in the pituitary fossa during the resection of the tumor. This allows for tumor that may remain unseen with the traditional microscopic approaches to be resected under direct vision (see **Fig. 13.17**). It also allows the descending diaphragm to be held up so that any residual tumor remaining in the angle between the diaphragm and the cavernous sinus can be visualized with a 30-degree angled telescope and to be removed under vision.

Patients with extensive invasion of the cavernous sinus have their tumors aggressively chased if these tumors are secretory. Nonsecretory tumors in the cavernous sinus are followed as long as the tumor continues to come away easily without putting the patient at risk.

Patients with an anterior or significant superior extension of their tumor may have an extended approach to the pituitary performed. This patient group requires septal flap closure of the defect.

The technique does require two surgeons working together off the video monitor and our team consists of a neurosurgeon and an otolaryngologist. Both surgeons have developed the skills to do all parts of the surgery and this maintains the skill level and enthusiasm for the different aspects of the operation.

References

1. Otori N, Haruna S, Kamio M, Ohashi G, Moriyama H. Endoscopic transethmosphenoidal approach for pituitary tumors with image guidance. Am J Rhinol 2001;15(6):381–386

2. Sawers HA, Robb OJ, Walmsley D, Strachan FM, Shaw J, Bevan JS. An audit of the diagnostic usefulness of PRL and TSH responses to domperidone and high resolution magnetic resonance imaging of the pituitary in the evaluation of hyperprolactinaemia. Clin Endocrinol (Oxf) 1997;46(3):321–326

3. Wilson CB. A decade of pituitary microsurgery. The Herbert Olivecrona lecture. J Neurosurg 1984;61(5):814–833

4. de Divitiis E, Cappabianca P. Microscopic and endoscopic transsphenoidal surgery. Neurosurgery 2002;51(6):1527–1529, author reply 1529–1530

5. Thomas RF, Monacci WT, Mair EA. Endoscopic image-guided transethmoid pituitary surgery. Otolaryngol Head Neck Surg 2002;127(5):409–416

6. Mason RB, Nieman LK, Doppman JL, Oldfield EH. Selective excision of adenomas originating in or extending into the pituitary stalk with preservation of pituitary function. J Neurosurg 1997;87(3):343–351

7. Aust MR, McCaffrey TV, Atkinson J. Transnasal endoscopic approach to the sella turcica. Am J Rhinol 1998;12(4):283–287

8. Shah S, Har-El G. Diabetes insipidus after pituitary surgery: incidence after traditional versus endoscopic transsphenoidal approaches. Am J Rhinol 2001;15(6):377–379

9. Cooke RS, Jones RA. Experience with the direct transnasal transsphenoidal approach to the pituitary fossa. Br J Neurosurg 1994;8(2):193–196

10. Knosp E, Steiner E, Kitz K, Matula C. Pituitary adenomas with invasion of the cavernous sinus space: a magnetic resonance imaging classification compared with surgical findings. Neurosurgery 1993;33(4):610–617, discussion 617–618

11. Uren B, Vrodos M, Wormald PJ. Fully endoscopic transsphenoidal resection of pituitary tumors: technique and results. Technique and Results Am J Rhinol 2007;21(4):510–514

12. Cappabianca P, Cavallo LM, Colao A, et al. Endoscopic endonasal transsphenoidal approach: outcome analysis of 100 consecutive procedures. Minim Invasive Neurosurg 2002;45(4):193–200

13. Kabil MS, Eby JB, Shahinian HK. Fully endoscopic endonasal vs. transseptal transsphenoidal pituitary surgery. Minim Invasive Neurosurg 2005;48(6):348–354

14 Endoscopic Orbital Decompression for Exophthalmos, Acute Orbital Hemorrhage, and Orbital Subperiosteal Abscess

◆ Introduction

Endoscopic orbital decompression plays an important role in the management of patients with Graves' orbitopathy, in patients with acute orbital hemorrhage with proptosis, and for the drainage of orbital subperiosteal abscesses.

◆ Graves' Disease

Exophthalmos in Graves' disease is thought to result from the deposition of immune complexes in the extraocular muscles and fat, which in turn leads to edema and fibrosis.[1] The resultant increase in intraorbital pressure pushes the globe forward, causing proptosis. If this proptosis becomes severe enough, the eyelids cannot close properly and chemosis with or without exposure keratitis of the cornea may occur. In addition, the crowding of the orbital apex by the significantly enlarged extraocular muscles places pressure on the optic nerve. In a small minority of patients, stretching of the optic nerve by increasing proptosis may play a role the development of optic neuropathy and visual loss. Visual loss is uncommon in Graves' disease, occurring in only 2–7% of patients.[2,3] If medical treatment (high-dose steroids with or without low-dose radiotherapy) fails, surgical decompression of the eye is indicated.[4] Although this has in the past been performed via external procedures, excellent reduction of proptosis is now possible with endoscopic techniques.[5,6] **Fig. 14.1** shows the extraocular muscle enlargement commonly seen in patients with Graves' disease and visual loss.

Preoperative diplopia is seen in up to 30% of patients with Graves' disease. If **Fig. 14.1** is reviewed, it can be seen that the extensive muscle enlargement limits globe movement in the extremes of gaze which in turn will cause diplopia. After decompression, significant medial and inferior prolapse of orbital tissue occurs and diplopia can be seen in up to 30% of patients who did not have preoperative diplopia.

Decompression of the lateral wall is thought to balance this intraorbital tissue displacement with resultant less likelihood of postoperative diplopia.[7] Although orbital decompression results in significant reduction in proptosis, the patient's eyes may still have a staring appearance due to fibrosis and shortening of the levator palpebrae muscle. This results in increased sclera show and although there may have been significant reduction of proptosis, the cosmetic appearance would still not be ideal. A release of the levator muscles can be performed which can reduce or eliminate the scleral show.

◆ Intraorbital Hemorrhage

Intraorbital hemorrhage is fortunately a rare occurrence and usually occurs during ESS as a result of injury to the anterior ethmoidal artery. The damaged artery retracts into the orbit and continues to bleed within the orbital contents with increasing intraorbital pressure. This pressure results in progressive proptosis with stretching or compression of the optic nerve. This, combined with impairment of arterial blood flow to the retina from increasing intraorbital pressure, can result in progressive visual loss. Color vision is reduced before visual acuity is lost. If impending visual loss is suspected, the patient should be tested for loss of red color discrimination and tested for a relative afferent pupil defect. Color vision is tested by showing the patient a picture with red in it and asking them to name the colors in the picture. Once visual acuity is lost, the time before irreversible blindness occurs is variable but can be as short as 40 minutes if blood flow to the retina is lost. It is therefore important that, if intraorbital hemorrhage occurs, the surgeon immediately takes appropriate steps to reduce intraorbital pressure and restore blood flow to the retina and optic nerve. Other than progressive proptosis, subconjunctival and periorbital hemorrhage may also be visible. If the proposed globe is palpated,

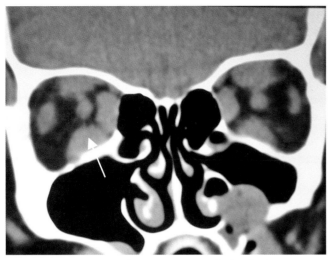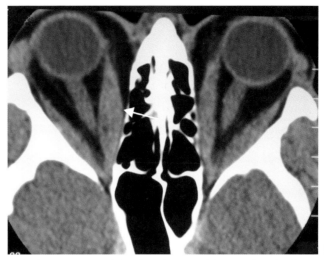

Fig. 14.1 Extraocular muscle enlargement marked with *white arrow* in coronal soft tissue CT scan (**a**) and axial CT scan (**b**). Note the orbital apex crowding.

it is hard and resists direct pressure. If the optic fundus can be visualized, the retinal arterial circulation may be seen to be intermittent or pulsatile.

If an intraorbital hemorrhage is recognized intraoperatively and the patient is still on the operating table, an orbital decompression should be performed as described below. If the patient is in recovery area or on the ward, and significant proptosis and visual loss is noticed, then the following steps should be taken:

◆ Sit the patient up in bed
◆ Remove any nasal packing
◆ Infiltrate the lateral canthus with local anesthetic and perform a lateral canthotomy and cantholysis

These are important steps with which to buy time, thus allowing the patient to be taken back to theatre for reexploration and orbital decompression.

Surgical Technique of Lateral Canthotomy and Cantholysis

Local anaesthetic (lidocaine 2% with 1:80,000 adrenaline) is placed in the lateral canthal region. A sharp scissors is used to make a horizontal incision through skin and soft tissue at the lateral junction of the eyelids onto the bone of the orbital rim (**Fig. 14.2**).

The eyelid is drawn outward with forceps exposing the tendon attaching the inferior tarsal plate to the bone (**Fig. 14.3**) and the scissors are turned vertically and this tendon cut (**Fig. 14.3**).

Orbital fat should be seen as this tendon is cut and the eyelid should be able to be laid on the cheek without tension (**Fig. 14.4**). This reduces the intraorbital pressure and should allow reperfusion of the optic nerve and retina. However, it may be insufficient and is used only to buy time and allow

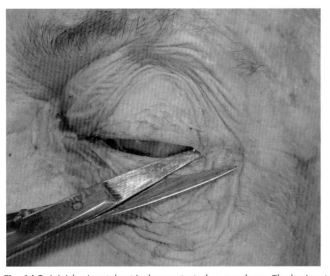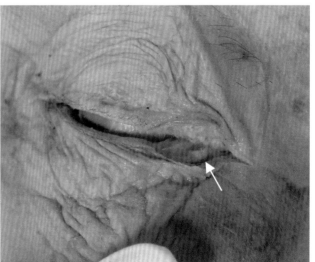

Fig. 14.2 (**a**) A horizontal cut is demonstrated on a cadaver. The horizontal cut is made onto the orbital rim through the lateral canthus. (**b**) Pulling the eyelid down reveals the lateral canthal tendon (*white arrow*).

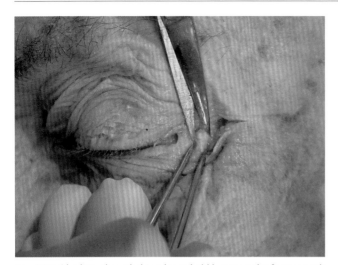

Fig. 14.3 The lateral canthal tendon is held between the forceps with the scissors held vertically to cut the tendon.

the patient to return to theatre for a formal decompression of the orbit.

No stitches are placed in this wound and a dressing is placed over the wound. The wound and the lateral canthal tendon can be sutured after 24 to 48 hours. The lateral canthal tendon is sutured to the orbital periosteum. As the incision is in the crease formed by the eyelids, scarring is uncommon.

Surgical Technique for Endoscopic Orbital Decompression[5]

After standard preparation and infiltration of the nasal cavity and lateral nasal wall, an uncinectomy is performed. The natural ostium of the maxillary sinus is identified and enlarged into the area of the posterior fontanelle with straight through-biting Blakesley forceps and the microdebrider.[5] It is essential to create the largest possible antrostomy as this

gives access to the floor of the orbit and, after the decompression, prevents obstruction of the ostium if significant prolapse of fat occurs. If the antrostomy is small, blockage of the antrostomy and resultant sinusitis may develop.

An axillary flap is performed and the frontal recess cleared of cells with identification of the frontal ostium. A total sphenoethmoidectomy is performed with identification of the sphenoid sinus ostium.[5] This ostium is enlarged into the posterior ethmoids, allowing entry into the sphenoid through the posterior ethmoids. The skull base is identified and cleared so that the entire lamina papyracea is able to be viewed (**Fig. 14.5**).

The hard bone of the frontal process of the maxilla is palpated with a Freer elevator and the soft lacrimal bone identified (in much the same way as is done for endoscopic DCR; **Fig. 14.6**). This soft lacrimal bone may be left and the junction of the lacrimal bone and lamina papyracea identified. If there is doubt about the lacrimal bone, this may be flaked off and the lacrimal sac palpated to accurately identify the lacrimal sac. The blunt end of the Freer elevator is then gently pushed through the lamina papyracea and the thin bone forming the lamina papyracea flaked off.[5] Great care must be taken to preserve the orbital periosteum at this early stage as a tear of the orbital periosteum with prolapse of orbital fat can obscure the remaining lamina papyracea and make its removal more difficult (**Fig. 14.7**). Care should also be taken not to remove the bony lamina papyracea for at least 1.5 cm below the frontal ostium. This bone is left in place to prevent prolapse of orbital fat obstructing the outflow tract of the frontal sinus. If chronic frontal sinusitis results after endoscopic orbital decompression this can be difficult to treat. The remaining bone of the lamina papyracea is removed up to the skull base and posterior as far

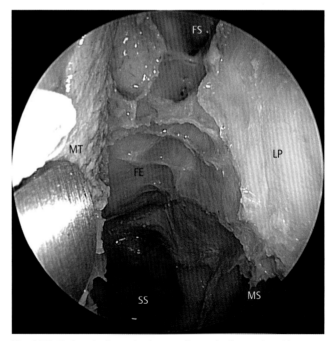

Fig. 14.5 Cadaveric dissection image of a total sphenoethmoidectomy with complete removal of the ethmoid air cells and exposure of the fovea ethmoidalis (*FE*), lamina papyracea (*LP*), sphenoid sinus (*SS*), maxillary sinus (*MS*), and frontal sinus (*FS*). *MT*, middle turbinate.

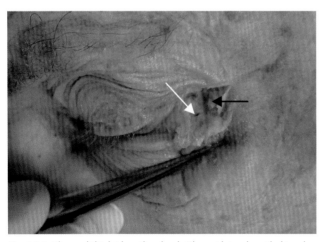

Fig. 14.4 The eyelid is laid on the cheek. The cut lateral canthal tendon is marked with a *black arrow* and the orbital fat with a *white arrow*.

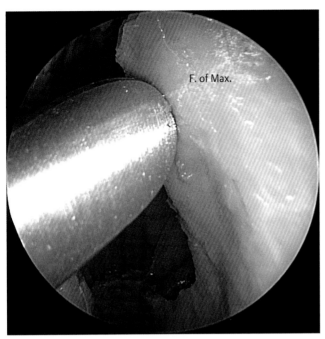

Fig. 14.6 Cadaveric image of the palpation of the left frontal process with a Freer elevator.

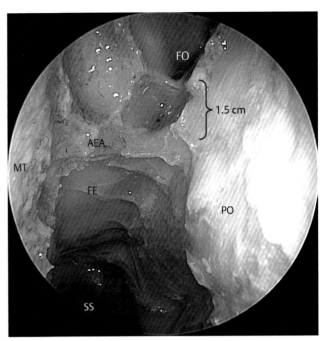

Fig. 14.7 Cadaveric dissection demonstrating the removal of the lamina papyracea and exposure of the periorbita (*PO*). Care has been taken not to tear the periorbita and prevent the prolapse of orbital fat. A 1.5-cm margin of bone below the frontal ostium (*FO*) is preserved to prevent frontal sinus obstruction by fat. *SS*, sphenoid sinus; *FE*, fovea ethmoidalis; *AEA*, anterior ethmoidal artery; *MT*, middle turbinate.

as the sphenoid sinus. Orbital periosteum is then removed (**Fig. 14.8**). This may be sufficient for orbital decompression for intraorbital hemorrhage or for a small reduction in proptosis from exophthalmos from Graves' disease (around 2 mm).[5–11] If a greater amount of decompression and globe retrogression is required, further decompression can be achieved by removal of the posterior half of the orbital floor.[5,11] The bone thickens

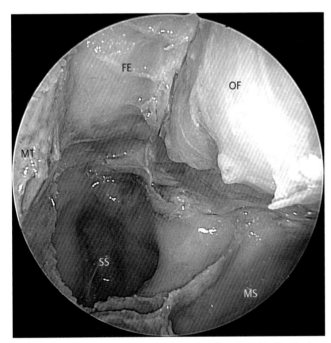

Fig. 14.8 Cadaveric dissection clearly shows that the orbital periorbita has been removed exposing orbital fat (*OF*). *MT*, middle turbinate; *FE*, fovea ethmoidalis; *SS*, sphenoid sinus; *MS*, maxillary sinus.

at the transition from medial orbital wall to floor of the orbit. Angled curettes and Blakesley forceps are used to fracture this bone and remove it. The infraorbital nerve is identified as it runs along the floor of the orbit (roof of the maxillary sinus). The posterior floor of the orbit is removed up to the infraorbital nerve (**Fig. 14.9**). Only the posterior half of the orbital floor can be accessed through the maxillary antrostomy. This is a technical problem as access to the anterior half of the orbital floor is usually not possible through the antrostomy with currently available instrumentation.[5,11] The average amount of globe retrogression with the removal of both the medial wall and floor of the orbit is 5 mm.[5–11] The orbital periosteum is either incised in a series of horizontal incisions or removed entirely. Retention of a median strip of orbital periosteum may reduce the incidence of postoperative diplopia but this is not my practice to retain this strip. If still greater regression of the globe is necessary, then the anterior part of the orbital floor and lateral orbital wall is approached through a subciliary incision. The conjunctiva is incised and further dissection identifies the lower lid fat pads. The orbital rim is identified and orbital periosteum elevated. The remaining anterior floor of the orbit is removed both medial and lateral to the infraorbital nerve. This is done with Kerrison forward- and backward-biting punches. This dissection is continued onto the lateral orbital wall and the lateral orbital wall removed with a diamond drill. This lateral decompression balances to some extent the orbital fat prolapse and may result in less postoperative diplopia. It certainly increases the amount of orbital regression that can be achieved and, in our series, this three-walled decompression averaged 5–7 mm.

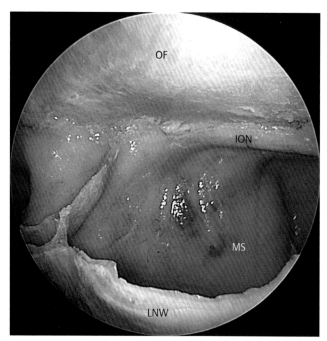

Fig. 14.9 Cadaveric dissection image taken with a 70-degree endoscope of the left maxillary sinus (*MS*). The floor of the orbit has been removed up to the infraorbital nerve (*ION*) through an enlarged maxillary antrostomy. *OF*, orbital fat; *LNW*, lateral nasal wall.

Results of Orbital Decompression for Graves' Disease

The degree of regression of proptosis in the 16 orbits decompressed was 5.4 mm.[5] If only the medial wall and floor were operated on, the average globe regression was 5.75 mm. In four orbits, only the medial orbital wall was removed with an average globe regression of 1.75 mm. In six orbits, a three-wall decompression was performed with an average regression of the globe of 6.5 mm. These results are slightly different from those results we published recently as we have added three subsequent patients who underwent bilateral three wall orbital decompression.[5] Of the 16 orbits done, one patient with complete long-standing visual loss had no improvement in vision. All other patients had normal vision preoperatively and no patient had worsening of vision in the postoperative period.[5] Two patients who did not have preoperative diplopia developed postoperative diplopia. In both of these patients, their diplopia was transient and lasted between 1 and 3 months before fully resolving. Four patients had preoperative diplopia which continued postoperatively and required extraocular muscle surgery for correction.

◆ Orbital Decompression for Subperiosteal Abscess

Patients presenting with orbital complications of sinusitis commonly have a degree of cellulitis and edema (chemosis) around the eye with associated proptosis. There may also be some restriction of eye movement. Patients typically give a history of nasal obstruction, purulent rhinorrhea, and facial pressure or pain. Endoscopy reveals an inflamed and edematous nasal mucosa usually with the presence of pus in the middle meatus (**Fig. 14.10**).

If a subperiosteal abscess is suspected, a CT scan of the sinuses with contrast will reveal the classic presentation of a mass located on the lamina papyracea or in relation to the floor of the frontal sinus. The rim of the mass will enhance with the contrast as seen in **Fig. 14.11**. In addition, the proptosis will be visible on the axial scans.

The surgeon should consider their endoscopy experience and skill level before deciding if a patient with a subperiosteal abscess should be managed endoscopically or through an external approach. The external approach is quick, easy, and the abscess can usually be rapidly and safely drained. If the surgeon is skilled and experienced in ESS, endoscopic drainage of the subperiosteal abscess can be performed. The difficulty with this procedure is the significant vascularity that is associated with acute sinusitis. If a mucosal surface is touched with an instrument or endoscope, it will usually bleed and if the surgeon is inexperienced they may lose orientation and complications may occur. Frequent packing with decongestant-soaked neuropatties throughout the procedure helps to minimize the bleeding but will not control it entirely. In a patient with acute sinusitis, the anesthetist needs to optimize the patient's hemodynamic parameters to create the optimal surgical field (Chapter 2). If the anesthetist is inexperienced with creating optimal conditions for sinus surgery patients, as may be the case on an emergency operating surgery lists, this may lead to more troublesome bleeding.

The surgical approach is to perform an uncinectomy and enlarge the maxillary ostium to a moderate degree. Uncinectomy alone without antrostomy carries the risk of postoperative closure of the maxillary sinus as the inflammation and edema predisposes to scarring and adhesion formation. Clearance of the frontal recess depends on whether the frontal sinus is thought to be the origin of the subperiosteal abscess. If the

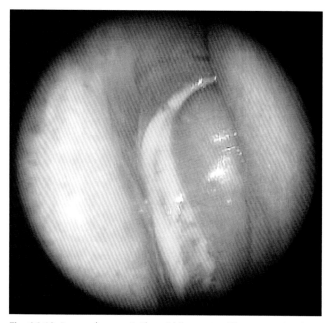

Fig. 14.10 Pus can be seen in the middle meatus. The mucosa is edematous with obliteration of the space between the middle turbinate and lateral nasal wall.

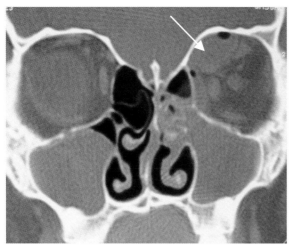
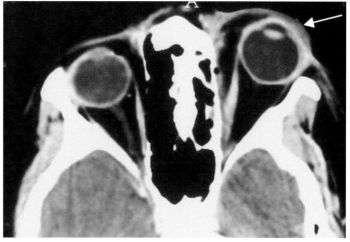

Fig. 14.11 (**a**) Subperiosteal abscess (*white arrow*) seen associated with the roof of the left orbit in coronal CT scan. (**b**) Proptosis (*white arrow*) of left globe visible on the axial soft tissue scan.

abscess is located adjacent to the ethmoidal sinuses (the most common location), then the frontal recess should be left alone and no surgery performed in this region. Clearance of the bulla ethmoidalis and posterior ethmoids is performed with identification of the lamina papyracea. The lamina papyracea over the subperiosteal abscess is widely exposed and removed. If the abscess is related to the floor of the frontal sinus, it can still be drained endoscopically. A mini-trephine is usually placed in the frontal sinus before dissection of the frontal recess. This aids in identification of the frontal sinus outflow track (the pathway along which the instruments will be passed to remove the cells of the frontal recess). The frontal recess is cleared and the frontal ostium identified. The lamina papyracea directly behind the lacrimal sac is removed and, using a curette, the orbital periosteum (which is mobile) is kept intact and gently pushed laterally while the curette advances into the subperiosteal abscess. The abscess is drained. Palpation of the globe with the abscess open will aid the drainage of the abscess.

A malleable suction Freer elevator or frontal sinus suction* (Integra) is introduced into the cavity and any fibrin within the cavity removed. A narrow triangulated corrugated Penrose drain is slid into the abscess cavity and left in place. This ensures that pus does not reaccumulate in the abscess cavity. It is shortened the next day and removed the second day after surgery. Endoscopic drainage of subperiosteal abscesses remains highly effective but it must be emphasized that the surgeon should be an experienced sinus surgeon.

◆ **Key Points**

Orbital decompression for exophthalmos from Graves' disease is an effective method for reduction of proptosis for cosmetic proptosis, eye complications from exposure of the cornea, and for visual loss. The amount of regression of proptosis is related to the number of walls decompressed at the time of surgery. Three-walled decompression may give a more balanced decompression with less likelihood of postoperative diplopia. However, this still has to be conclusively demonstrated.

Intraorbital hemorrhage should be managed with lateral canthotomy and cantholysis (if the patient has left the operating suite) followed by orbital decompression with removal of the medial orbital wall. Orbital decompression can be performed without canthotomy and cantholysis if the complication is noticed intraoperatively.

Endoscopic decompression of a subperiosteal abscess should only be performed by very experienced endoscopic sinus surgeons as the surgical field can be very bloody and this can increase the degree of difficulty significantly and complications are more likely. If the surgeon is not experienced, then the abscess should be drained via an external incision.

References

1. Konishi J, Herman MM, Kriss JP. Binding of thyroglobulin and thyroglobulin-antithyroglobulin immune complex to extraocular muscle membrane. Endocrinology 1974;95(2):434–446

2. Warren JD, Spector JG, Burde R. Long-term follow-up and recent observations on 305 cases of orbital decompression for dysthyroid orbitopathy. Laryngoscope 1989;99(1):35–40

3. Garrity JA, Fatourechi V, Bergstralh EJ, et al. Results of transantral orbital decompression in 428 patients with severe Graves' ophthalmopathy. Am J Ophthalmol 1993;116(5):533–547

4. Asaria RHY, Koay B, Elston JS, Bates GEM. Endoscopic orbital decompression for thyroid eye disease. Eye (Lond) 1998;12(Pt 6):990–995

5. Wee DTH, Carney AS, Thorpe M, Wormald PJ. Endoscopic orbital decompression for Graves' ophthalmopathy. J Laryngol Otol 2002;116(1):6–9

6. Lund VJ, Larkin G, Fells P, Adams G. Orbital decompression for thyroid eye disease: a comparison of external and endoscopic techniques. J Laryngol Otol 1997;111(11):1051–1055

7. Kennedy DW, Goodstein ML, Miller NR, Zinreich SJ. Endoscopic transnasal orbital decompression. Arch Otolaryngol Head Neck Surg 1990;116(3):275–282

8. Metson R, Dallow RL, Shore JW. Endoscopic orbital decompression. Laryngoscope 1994;104(8 Pt 1):950–957

9. Metson R, Shore JW, Gliklich RE, Dallow RL. Endoscopic orbital decompression under local anesthesia. Otolaryngol Head Neck Surg 1995;113(6):661–667

10. Neugebauer A, Nishino K, Neugebauer P, Konen W, Michel O. Effects of bilateral orbital decompression by an endoscopic endonasal approach in dysthyroid orbitopathy. Br J Ophthalmol 1996;80(1):58–62

11. Koay B, Bates G, Elston J. Endoscopic orbital decompression for dysthyroid eye disease. J Laryngol Otol 1997;111(10):946–949

15 Endoscopic Optic Nerve Decompression

◆ Introduction

The most common indication for endoscopic optic nerve decompression is traumatic optic neuropathy.[1] Currently it is thought that about 5% of severe head injuries will have a concomitant injury to the optic nerve, optic tract, or optic cortex.[1-3] However, if the literature is reviewed, there are only a limited number of patients who have undergone this procedure.[4] Major brain injury occurs in 40–72% of patients with traumatic optic neuropathy[5] and the management of this injury obviously takes precedence. This may result in the optic nerve injury only being diagnosed sometime after the original injury. Some authors feel that early diagnosis and treatment of traumatic optic neuropathy may be of greater benefit to the patient[6,7] and advocate diagnosis of the optic nerve deficit by the presence of an absolute or relative afferent pupillary defect supported by disc edema and congestion of the vessels.[6] These findings, in combination with the CT scan, possibly an MRI scan, and visual evoked potentials, may provide sufficient evidence to undertake optic nerve decompression.[6,7] However, the patient management protocol suggested in this chapter is more conservative as there is still considerable debate as to the value of both high-dose steroid treatment and surgical optic nerve decompression.[3-5,7] Currently, there are no properly conducted randomized controlled trials comparing high-dose steroid therapy, surgical decompression, and observation.[8] In a meta-analysis of all published cases in the literature, Cook et al concluded that treatment in the form of high-dose steroids or surgery or both was better than no treatment.[4] Tandon et al evaluated the role of steroids with and without surgery in a large study of 111 patients who were placed in two groups: one group of patients had high-dose steroids and if they failed to improve underwent an optic nerve decompression whereas the second group had steroids alone.[1] This study showed that the patient group treated with steroids and surgery had significantly better outcomes than the patient group treated with steroids alone.[1] Sofferman, in a study on an animal model of traumatic optic neuropathy, showed that injury to the optic nerve results in a progressive loss of myelin but with preservation of axons so that in theory the progression of the injury may be reversed with steroid or surgical decompression.[7]

Traumatic optic neuropathy is thought to result from two distinct injuries to the nerve. The primary injury results from either a direct contusive force on the optic canal and nerve or as a result of elastic deformation of the sphenoid with a transfer of force into the intracanalicular optic nerve disrupting the axons and blood vessels.[5] This primary injury may result in compression of the nerve by bony fragments or in hemorrhage into the nerve sheath. If this injury is not treated a secondary injury may occur. As the nerve swells in its dural sheath and bony canal, compression of the blood supply to the nerve occurs with resultant ischemia and continued axon loss.[5,7] Our department has adopted a conservative approach to traumatic neuropathy with all patients undergoing high-dose steroid treatment first before being offered surgical intervention. The exception is when bony fragments are seen to impinge on the optic nerve.

◆ Medical Therapy for Traumatic Optic Nerve Injury

Currently, mega-dose intravenous methylprednisolone is used following the spinal cord injury management protocol. Methylprednisolone 30 mg/kg IV loading dose is given followed by an infusion of 5.4 mg/kg/hr thereafter.[4] The patient's visual acuity is monitored hourly and surgical intervention is considered if the patient meets any of the criterion listed below:

a. Fracture of optic canal on CT scan with vision < 6/60
b. Fracture of the optic canal with vision > 6/60 but the patient's vision deteriorates on steroids

c. Vision is < 6/60 (or there is a deterioration of vision) after 48 hours of steroid treatment with probable canal injury (indicated by the presence of fluid levels in the posterior ethmoids and sphenoid and/or the presence of fractures of the ethmoids, orbital apex, and sphenoid)

◆ Surgical Technique for Traumatic Optic Neuropathy

The standard preparation of the nose is performed with decongestion and infiltration. An uncinectomy with exposure of the maxillary ostium is performed. An axillary flap is performed and the agger nasi cell removed. This improves access to the skull base. The fovea ethmoidalis is exposed in the region above the bulla ethmoidalis. If there is disruption of the cells of the frontal recess or reason to suggest that the frontal recess is obstructed, then this will

be cleared; otherwise, the cells in the frontal recess are left untouched. In some patients with severe sinus fractures, the entire skull base may be mobile. In the patient presented in **Fig. 15.1** the entire posterior skull base was mobile.

In most patients, the posterior ethmoid cells will be full of blood and when this is combined with mobility of the lamina papyracea and skull base, the surgeon can become disorientated. Therefore, this surgery should only be undertaken by very experienced endoscopic sinus surgeons. A posterior ethmoidectomy and sphenoidotomy should be performed as described in Chapter 8. In the posterior ethmoids, the posterior lamina papyracea and fovea ethmoidalis should be identified (**Fig. 15.2**). If significant disruption of the posterior ethmoids and lamina papyracea has occurred, then a large middle meatal antrostomy provides an extra reference point and lessens the likelihood of surgeon disorientation (**Fig. 15.2**). The natural ostium of the sphenoid sinus should be identified and the anterior face of the sphenoid

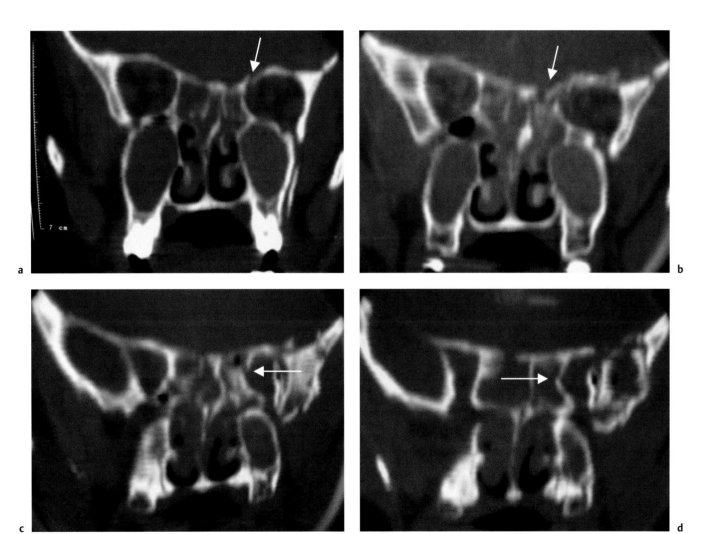

Fig. 15.1 (**a–d**) Sequential coronal CTs from posterior ethmoids (**a**) to sphenoid sinus (**d**). The *white arrows* indicate fractures and note the blood in the ethmoids and sphenoids. (**b**) In addition, the *white arrow* indicates the loose segment of skull base. The scans are of relative poor quality due to patient movement from confusion from an associated head injury.

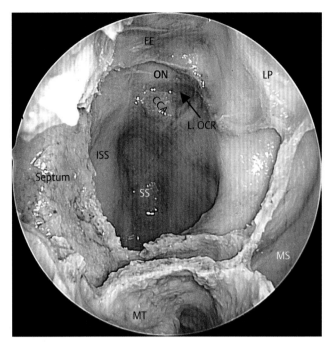

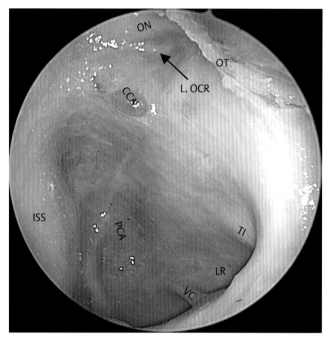

Fig. 15.2 Cadaveric dissection image taken of the left sphenoid sinus demonstrating the fovea ethmoidalis (*FE*) and lamina papyracea (*LP*). *ON*, optic nerve; *CCA*, anterior genu of the intracavernous carotid artery; *L. OCR*, lateral opticocarotid recess; *ISS*, sphenoid intersinus septum; *SS*, sphenoid sinus, *MS*, maxillary sinus; *MT*, middle turbinate.

Fig. 15.3 Cadaveric dissection image taken of the left sphenoid sinus through a maximal sphenoidotomy. The vidian canal (*VC*) and trigeminal impression (*TI*) for the maxillary division of the trigeminal nerve can be clearly seen. If the sphenoid sinus is well pneumatized then the lateral recess (*LR*) can be seen, a depression in the lateral sphenoid wall between the VC and the TI. The lateral opticocarotid recess can be seen. This depression corresponds to pneumatization of the optic strut (the bony bridge that separates the optic canal from the superior orbital fissure). Further pneumatization into the optic strut may result in a pneumatized anterior clinoid process which will place the optic nerve on a mesentery. The optic tubercle (*OT*) is the bone located at the junction of the orbital apex and the sphenoid sinus. *ISS*, intersinus septum; *ON*, optic nerve; *CCA*, anterior genu of the intracavernous carotid artery; *PCA*, paraclival carotid artery.

widely opened. It is important for the surgeon to be fully aware of the anatomy of the lateral wall of the sphenoid (**Fig. 15.3**). If available, computer-aided surgery (CAS) navigation system may help in patients where there has been significant anatomical disruption.

The anterior face of the sphenoid needs to be taken as high as possible so that the roof of the sphenoid and the posterior ethmoids is continuous.[3,9,10] The sphenoid should be inspected and the optic nerve, carotid artery, and pituitary fossa identified.[9,10] If there has been significant disruption of the orbital apex or the lateral wall of the sphenoid, then identification of these basic structures can be difficult (**Fig. 15.4**). In these cases, image guidance may help.

The thick bone overlying the junction of the orbital apex and sphenoid sinus is known as the optic tubercle. This bone is normally too thick to flake off and an irrigated diamond bur (the 15-degree 3.2-mm diamond skull base bur or the 2.5-mm 25-degree DCR diamond bur from Medtronic ENT) is used to thin this bone down until it is almost transparent[9,10] (**Fig. 15.4**).

A blunt Freer elevator is pushed through the lamina papyracea about 1.5 cm anterior to the junction of the posterior ethmoids air cell(s) and the sphenoid (**Fig. 15.4**). Care should be taken to keep the orbital periosteum intact while this is done; otherwise, prolapse of orbital fat can severely obstruct the dissection of the optic nerve. The bone of the posterior orbital apex is flaked off the underlying orbital periosteum[9,10] (**Fig. 15.4**).

Once the bone over the orbital apex is removed, the bone of the optic canal is approached. This bone is usually quite thin and can, in a large proportion of patients, be simply flaked off the underlying nerve (**Fig. 15.5**). However, in some cases,

the bone over the nerve can be too thick and will need to be thinned with a diamond bur prior to removal. Once the bone is thin enough to be flaked off the underlying nerve, only suitably designed instruments should be used. Any instrument that has a thick working end is unsuitable. If the back of the instrument indents the nerve as the edge of the instrument is used to engage the edge of the optic canal bone, it should not be used. Suitable instruments include the Beale elevator and the House curette, both from the ear tray[9] (**Fig. 15.5**).

Once all the bone has been cleared off the optic canal and the underlying optic nerve sheath is clearly visible, the sheath should be incised[9,10] (**Fig. 15.6**). The location of the ophthalmic artery should be kept in mind. The ophthalmic artery usually runs in the posteroinferior quadrant of the nerve. However, in a small proportion of patients, this artery can migrate around the lower edge of the nerve and potentially into the surgical field[8] (**Fig. 15.7**). However, if the nerve is incised in the upper medial quadrant, the risk to this artery should be minimal.[9,11] A sharp sickle knife* (single-use disposable DCR mini-sickle knife [Integra] is the most suitable) is used to incise the sheath of the optic nerve. Usually the pressure from the swollen optic nerve will cause the sheath to split as it is incised. The underlying pressure will often cause the nerve to protrude through the incision.

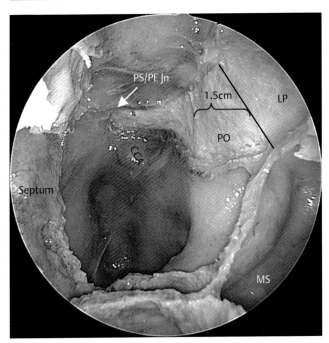

Fig. 15.4 Cadaveric dissection image of the left sphenoid sinus. The anterior face of the sphenoid has been removed so that the roof of the sphenoid and posterior ethmoids is continuous. A diamond bur has been used to allow the removal of bone at the junction of the orbital apex and sphenoid sinus (the optic tubercle). The lamina papyracea (*LP*) has been removed 1.5 cm from the junction of the posterior ethmoids with the sphenoid sinus, exposing periorbita (*PO*).

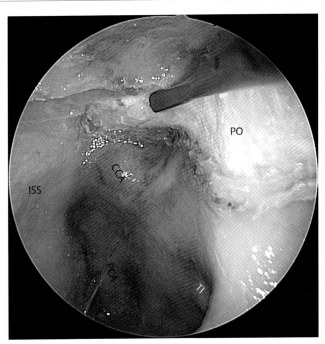

Fig. 15.5 The thin bone overlying the orbital apex and optic nerve is gently flaked off. *PO*, periorbita; *CCA*, anterior genu of the intracavernous carotid artery; *PCA*, paraclival carotid artery; *ISS*, intersinus septum; *TI*, trigeminal impression.

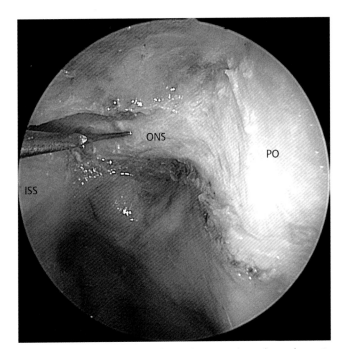

Fig. 15.6 The optic nerve sheath (*ONS*) is incised to release the optic nerve. *PO*, periorbita; *ISS*, intersinus septum.

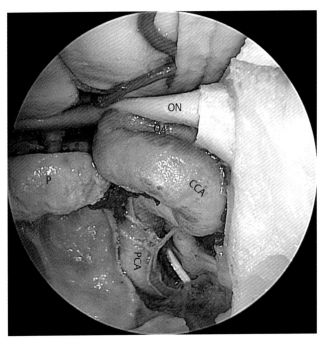

Fig. 15.7 Cadaveric dissection image taken of the left optic nerve and ophthalmic artery. The optic sheath has been removed to expose the contents within. The ophthalmic artery (*OA*) can be seen branching from the carotid artery at the lower medial quadrant of the optic nerve (*ON*). Therefore, incision in the upper medial quadrant poses little risk to the artery. *P*, pituitary gland; *PCA*, paraclival carotid artery; *CCA*, anterior genu of the intracavernous carotid artery.

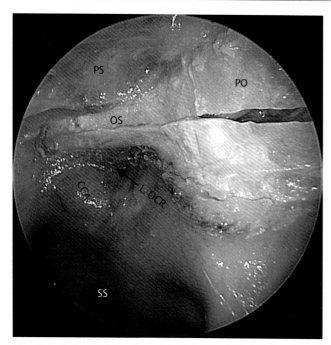

Fig. 15.8 Cadaveric dissection of the lateral wall of the left sphenoid sinus. The optic sheath and periorbita (*PO*) of the orbital apex has been incised. *PS*, planum sphenoidale; *CCA*, anterior genu of the intracavernous carotid artery; *L. OCR*, lateral opticocarotid recess; *OS*, optic sheath.

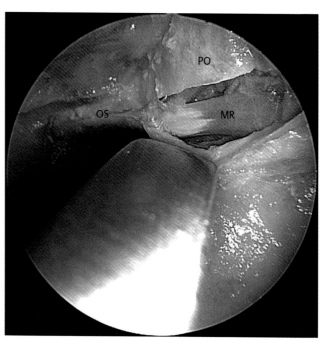

Fig. 15.9 Cadaveric dissection demonstrating the medial rectus muscle (*MR*) at the orbital apex. *PO*, periorbita; *OS*, optic sheath.

This incision is continued onto the orbital periosteum of the posterior orbital apex with resultant protrusion of orbital fat (**Fig. 15.8**). The orbital fat covering this area of the medial rectus muscle is thin and care should be taken to avoid injuring this muscle (**Fig. 15.9**). Potentially such an incision can create a cerebrospinal fluid (CSF) leak but to date none has been seen after this incision. This may be due to the fact that the nerve has swollen and any potential CSF space has been obliterated. No packs are placed on the nerve or in the sinuses.

◆ Results of Optic Nerve Decompression for Traumatic Optic Neuropathy

Blunt Injury

Four patients presented with traumatic optic neuropathy after blunt trauma (usually a motor vehicle accident). Visible trauma to the frontal bone was seen with fractures involving the posterior ethmoids and sphenoid. Blood was seen in posterior ethmoids and sphenoid in all patients.

Two patients had an obvious fracture through the bony optic canal (**Fig. 15.10**).

All patients were operated on after failed medical therapy (high-dose intravenous steroids) for the optic neuropathy and all underwent surgery within 5 days of the original injury. Two patients with hematomas around the orbital apex (**Fig. 15.1**) improved from light perception preoperatively to 6/9 vision. The third patient improved from light perception to 6/60 vision, and the fourth patient improved from no light perception to 6/60 vision. Three of these patients were left with limited visual field defects.

Sharp Injury to the Optic Nerve

Two patients suffered optic neuropathy after a penetrating knife wound and both had no light perception after the initial injury. One patient underwent surgery 8 days after the injury and the second patient 12 days after the injury. Preoperative medical therapy was significantly delayed due to patients presenting to a rural hospital before referral to our hospital. Preoperative CT and MRI suggested the optic nerve was intact and in one case an obvious injury to the optic canal was seen. At surgery in one patient a bony fragment was seen to significantly indent the nerve. This was removed and the optic nerve decompressed and sheath was slit but the patient showed no postoperative improvement in vision. The other patient also showed no improvement after surgery. It is not known if the mechanism of injury after such a localized insult is different or whether the delayed presentation may have also contributed to the lack of improvement after surgery.

◆ Results of Optic Nerve Decompression for Pseudotumor of the Orbital Apex and for Tumors Compressing the Optic Canal

Four patients presented with compressive lesions of the orbital apex or optic canal with progressive visual loss. One patient had a pseudotumor of the orbital apex that extended

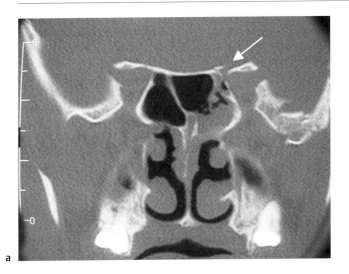

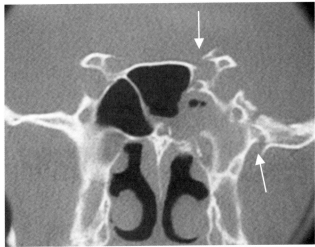

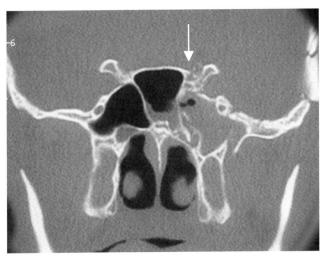

Fig. 15.10 (**a–c**) Sequential coronal CTs through the sphenoid sinus from one of the patients who presented with significant fractures through the optic nerve canal, around the carotid artery, and in the lateral aspects of the sphenoid (*white arrows*).

significantly into the bony optic nerve canal. This patient presented with progressive visual loss and underwent decompression of the posterior orbit and optic canal. Postoperatively she regained normal vision that slowly deteriorated over a period of months. The surgery was revised and the annulus of Zinn was divided. This again improved her vision to 6/18 without further deterioration (**Fig. 15.11**).

The second patient presented with an 8-month progressive visual loss and at presentation could only see hand movements. He had a fairly extensive compressive lesion

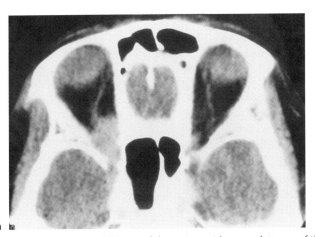

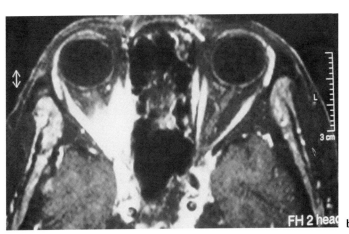

Fig. 15.11 (**a**) CT and (**b**) MRI of the patient with a pseudotumor of the orbital apex.

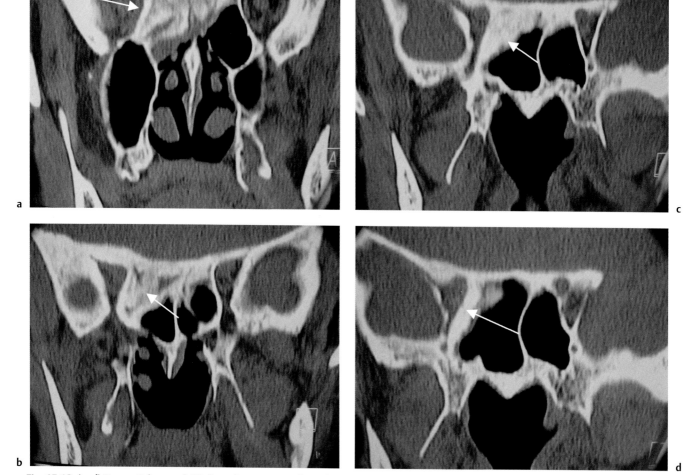

Fig. 15.12 (a–d) Sequential coronal CTs from the posterior ethmoids to the sphenoid. The compressive lesion on the orbital apex and optic canal is indicated by the *white arrows*.

of his orbital apex and optic canal. After decompression, his vision remained stable but did not improve (**Fig. 15.12**). Patients with long-term visual loss may not respond as well as patients who present with more rapid visual loss due to optic nerve decompression.

Two patients with compressive lesions (lateral sphenoid wing meningioma and an encircling fibrous dysplasia) both had significant visual acuity and visual field loss and both had their vision return to normal after decompression.

◆ Key Points

Optic nerve decompression is a highly complex procedure and should only be undertaken by endoscopic sinus surgeons with significant experience and skill. Potentially, injury to the skull base with a resultant CSF leak may occur and an associated injury to the internal carotid artery may also be present (see in **Fig. 15.10**).[12] Injudicious manipulation of bony fragments may have catastrophic consequences for the patient. Patients should be given a trial of medical

therapy before surgery is contemplated unless there is an obvious bony fragment impinging on the optic nerve.[4] Results from the small case series presented in this chapter and from larger studies in the literature[1–4,10] suggest that patients should be operated upon if medical therapy fails to improve the vision within 24 to 48 hours. Significant delays again would seem to lessen the potential for success of the surgery.[5,7] Great care should be taken in exposing the optic nerve especially when flaking the bone from the nerve. Injudicious use of inappropriate instruments has the potential to worsen the vision and this should be kept in mind during the procedure.[12] In the hands of an experienced endoscopic sinus surgeon this procedure is a relatively safe operation with low morbidity and has the potential to improve and, in some cases, restore lost vision especially after blunt trauma.

References

1. Tandon DA, Thakar A, Mahapatra AK, Ghosh P. Trans-ethmoidal optic nerve decompression. Clin Otolaryngol Allied Sci 1994;19(2):98–104

2. Kountakis SE, Maillard AA, El-Harazi SM, Longhini L, Urso RG. Endoscopic optic nerve decompression for traumatic blindness. Otolaryngol Head Neck Surg 2000;123(1 Pt 1):34–37

3. Kuppersmith RB, Alford EL, Patrinely JR, Lee AG, Parke RB, Holds JB. Combined transconjunctival/intranasal endoscopic approach to the optic canal in traumatic optic neuropathy. Laryngoscope 1997;107(3): 311–315

4. Cook MW, Levin LA, Joseph MP, Pinczower EF. Traumatic optic neuropathy. A meta-analysis. Arch Otolaryngol Head Neck Surg 1996;122(4): 389–392

5. Steinsapir KD, Goldberg RA. Traumatic optic neuropathy. Surv Ophthalmol 1994;38(6):487–518

6. Lübben B, Stoll W, Grenzebach U. Optic nerve decompression in the comatose and conscious patients after trauma. Laryngoscope 2001;111(2): 320–328

7. Sofferman RA. Harris P. Mosher Award thesis. The recovery potential of the optic nerve. Laryngoscope 1995; 105(7 Pt 3, Suppl 72):1–38

8. Steinsapir KD, Seiff SR, Goldberg RA. Traumatic optic neuropathy: where do we stand? Ophthal Plast Reconstr Surg 2002;18(3):232–234

9. Luxenberger W, Stammberger H, Jebeles JA, Walch C. Endoscopic optic nerve decompression: the Graz experience. Laryngoscope 1998;108(6): 873–882

10. Chow JM, Stankiewicz JA. Powered instrumentation in orbital and optic nerve decompression. Otolaryngol Clin North Am 1997;30(3): 467–478

11. Chou PI, Sadun AA, Lee H. Vasculature and morphometry of the optic canal and intracanalicular optic nerve. J Neuroophthalmol 1995;15(3): 186–190

12. Metson R, Pletcher SD. Endoscopic orbital and optic nerve decompression. Otolaryngol Clin North Am 2006;39(3):551–561, ix

16 Endoscopic Removal of Tumors Involving the Maxillary Sinus, Pterygopalatine Fossa, and Infratemporal Fossa

◆ Introduction

As ESS has progressed over the last 20 years, new techniques have been introduced to aid with the resection of tumors in regions that traditionally have been difficult to access.[1] In general, the approaches described in this chapter are more suitable for benign tumors but as techniques and adjuvant therapy develop, these techniques will be increasingly applied to the resection of malignant tumors.

To assess the endoscopic resectability of a tumor, both CT and MRI scans are required.[2–4] Using both these modalities, the surgeon can determine if sinuses that are opacified on the CT scan contain retained secretions or tumor.[2,3] Being able to accurately define the extent of the tumor means that the resection can then be carefully planned. Endoscopic resection of the medial maxilla is useful to access the anterior, posterior, and lateral walls of the maxillary sinus.[3,5,6]

◆ Surgical Techniques for Access to the Maxillary Sinus, Pterygopalatine Fossa, and Infratemporal Fossa

Prelacrimal Approach and Canine Fossa Trephination for Access to the Maxillary Sinus

Tumors that involve the medial wall, anterior floor, anterior wall, or anterolateral wall of the maxillary sinus cannot be accessed through a maxillary antrostomy regardless of how large this is made. It is necessary in these patients to provide an alternative route of access. Although this can be achieved through an inferior meatal puncture, placement of a 4-mm microdebrider blade through the inferior meatal antrostomy tends to destabilize the inferior turbinate as the blade is moved within the maxillary sinus. This is because the nasal vestibule provides a fulcrum around which the blade is rotated, causing significant disruption of the second

fulcrum which is the inferior meatal port. In addition, this route does not give access to the anterior and medial compartments of the maxillary sinus. The best access to the anterior and retrolacrimal regions is provided by the prelacrimal approach. The first step is to perform a large middle meatal antrostomy. Then an incision is made from the antrostomy along the insertion of the inferior turbinate to the lateral nasal wall, above the head of the inferior turbinate down onto the piriform aperture (**Fig. 16.1**). This incision should be onto bone. A malleable suction Freer is used to raise the mucosa over the head of the middle turbinate, exposing the vertical bone of the turbinate creating a medial turbinate mucosal flap (**Fig. 16.2**). The bony piriform aperture is identified and the 4-mm osteotome used to create several osteotomies encompassing the edge of the piriform aperture bone (**Fig. 16.3**). The bone over the head of the inferior turbinate is removed with further osteotomies progressing posteriorly until the nasolacrimal duct is exposed (**Fig. 16.4**). The duct is swept laterally out of its bony covering, exposing the bone posterior to the duct. Further osteotomies allow removal of this bone (**Fig. 16.5**) and leave the nasolacrimal duct running freely in the air from the sac to the inferior turbinate valve of Hasner (**Fig. 16.6**). If needed, further bone from the junction of the anterior and medial walls of the maxillary sinus can be removed with a Hajek Koefler punch. Vision should be unimpeded from the nose onto the anterior wall of the maxillary sinus. Tumors such as inverting papillomas that take origin from the anterior wall can be directly approached and dissected and their bony origin drilled away. Once the surgery is complete, the inferior turbinate mucosal flap is repositioned and held with a suture to reconstruct the anatomy with preservation of the nasolacrimal duct (**Fig. 16.7**). If the tumor is more posteriorly based, either on the medial wall, floor, or lateral wall, a canine fossa trephine can be performed for access. Canine fossa trephine is described in Chapter 5. In the canine fossa approach, there is only a single fulcrum around which the blade rotates, providing good access to the medial and lateral walls, and the floor of the maxillary sinus (**Fig. 16.8**). However, canine fossa trephine is not suitable for

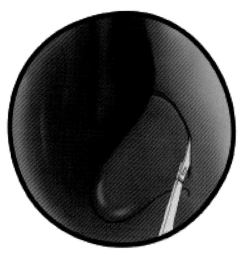

Fig. 16.1 Incision is made from the middle meatal antrostomy at the junction of the inferior turbinate to the lateral nasal wall and curved over the anterior end of the inferior turbinate onto the piriform aperture.

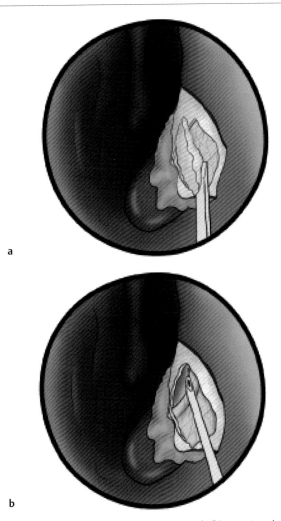

a

b

Fig. 16.4 (**a**) Bone is mobilized and removed, (**b**) exposing the naso-lacrimal duct.

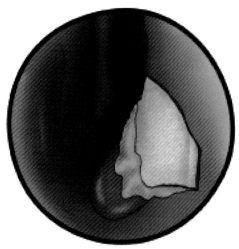

Fig. 16.2 A Freer elevator is used to mobilize the flap in the subperiosteal plane exposing the head of the inferior turbinate.

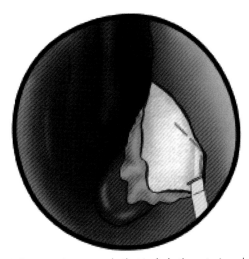

Fig. 16.3 Osteotomies are made that include the anterior edge of the piriform aperture and continue over the head of the inferior turbinate.

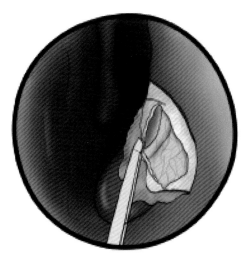

Fig. 16.5 The nasolacrimal duct is mobilized within its bony canal and ostomies are performed on the bone posterior to the duct and this bone removed.

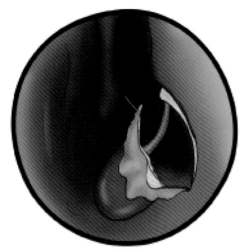

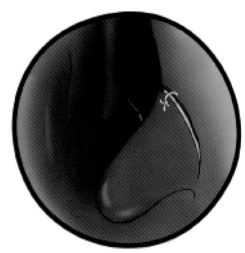

Fig. 16.6 The nasolacrimal duct is now free and runs from the lacrimal sac area to the inferior turbinate. A large window has been created anterior to the nasolacrimal duct, allowing access to the anterior wall of the maxillary sinus.

Fig. 16.7 Once tumor removal is complete, the mucosal flap is repositioned recreating the normal anatomy of the inferior turbinate and lateral nasal wall. The flap is secured with a suture.

tumors originating from or with extensive attachment to the anterior wall of the maxillary sinus as the trephine will be placed through tumor attachment.

Endoscopic Medial Maxillectomy for Access to the Anterior Wall of the Maxillary Sinus and Infratemporal Fossa[5,6]

The nasal cavity is prepared by placing cocaine- and adrenaline-soaked neuropatties in the nasal cavity. The lateral nasal wall and septum are infiltrated with 2% lidocaine and 1:80,000 adrenaline. A pterygopalatine fossa block is placed via the greater palatine canal using 2 mL of lidocaine and adrenaline (see Chapter 2). This helps to reduce bleeding during the dissection of medial wall of the maxilla and pterygopalatine fossa.

The first step in endoscopic medial maxillectomy is to remove the uncinate process and perform a large middle meatal antrostomy (**Fig. 16.9**). The maxillary antrum is enlarged posteriorly up to the posterior wall of the maxillary sinus (**Fig. 16.10**). This provides visualization of the medial orbital wall and allows removal of the residual medial maxilla without endangering the orbit. Most large tumors of the maxillary sinus and/or pterygopalatine fossa will involve the posterior ethmoids and sphenoid. In these patients, an axillary flap is performed and the frontal recess dissected with exposure of the frontal ostium. The bulla ethmoidalis is removed and a posterior ethmoidectomy and sphenoidotomy is performed. The skull base is clearly identified. Any tumor

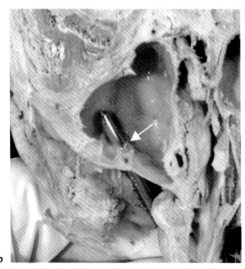

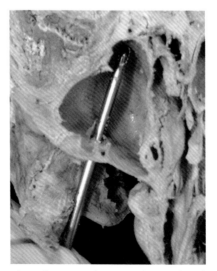

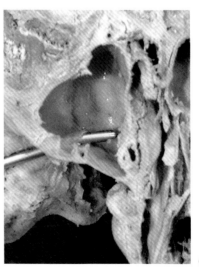

a,b   c

Fig. 16.8 (**a–c**) An axially cut right maxillary sinus of a cadaver illustrating the access that can be achieved within the maxillary sinus (lateral, floor, and medial) through a canine fossa trephine. The *white arrow* indicates the trephination port in the anterior face of the maxillary sinus.

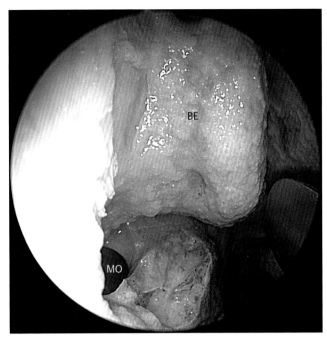

Fig. 16.9 Cadaveric image following a right sided uncinectomy. *BE*, bulla ethmoidalis; *MO*, maxillary ostium.

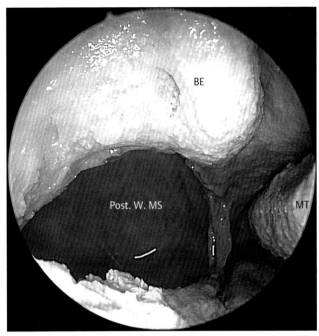

Fig. 16.10 Maxillary ostium enlargement to the posterior wall of the maxillary sinus. *Post. W. MS*, posterior wall of the maxillary sinus; *BE*, bulla ethmoidalis.

extension into the anterior and posterior ethmoids can be assessed and if necessary biopsies or frozen sections of the mucosa from these regions can be sent for examination. This helps ensure complete tumor clearance.

To perform the medial maxillectomy, the inferior turbinate is medialized. A Tilley packing forceps is used to crush the turbinate just distal to the junction of the anterior end of the turbinate and the lateral nasal wall.[5] If there is a large intranasal component of a soft nonvascular tumor, the tumor

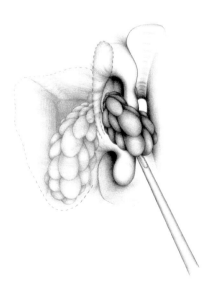

Fig. 16.11 Inverting papilloma originating in the maxillary sinus is partially debulked with a microdebrider in order to establish the region of origin of the tumor.

is debulked (**Fig. 16.11**). If the tumor is very vascular or firm, then it can be pushed superiorly or partially debulked. Because of the posterior location of angiofibroma, debulking is usually not necessary.

Turbinectomy scissors are used to cut along the crushed region of the inferior turbinate up to the point where the turbinate inserts into the lateral nasal wall (**Fig. 16.12**). A scalpel is used to make mucosal incisions from just below the inferior turbinate, placing the incisions so that after medial maxillectomy the mucosa can be rolled back over the raw bone of the residual medial maxillary wall at the junction of the floor of the nose and the sinus[5] (**Fig. 16.12**). A sharp osteotome is used to cut the bone at the junction of the medial maxillary wall and nasal floor (**Fig. 16.12**). The posterior vertical cut needs to enter the maxillary sinus adjacent to the posterior wall of the maxillary sinus and into the large antrostomy[5] (**Fig. 16.12**).

Once the bone forming the medial maxillary wall is mobilized, the nasolacrimal duct will tether the bone anteriorly and the duct will be visualized (**Fig. 16.13**). The duct should be transected with a scalpel (**Fig. 16.13**). At the end of the operation, the dacryocystorhinostomy (DCR) spear knife* (Medtronic ENT) is used to open the lower half of the sac creating anterior and posterior flaps that are then rolled out.[5–7] This prevents postoperative stenosis of the sac.[5,6] The edges of the resected portion of the maxilla are trimmed with the microdebrider. If a 70-degree telescope is used, the entire maxillary sinus should be able to be visualized[5] (**Fig. 16.14**). This includes the anterior wall and floor of the maxillary sinus (**Figs. 16.14** and **16.15**). Tumor can now be removed from the maxillary sinus under direct visualization. If additional access is required and the tumor does not attach to the

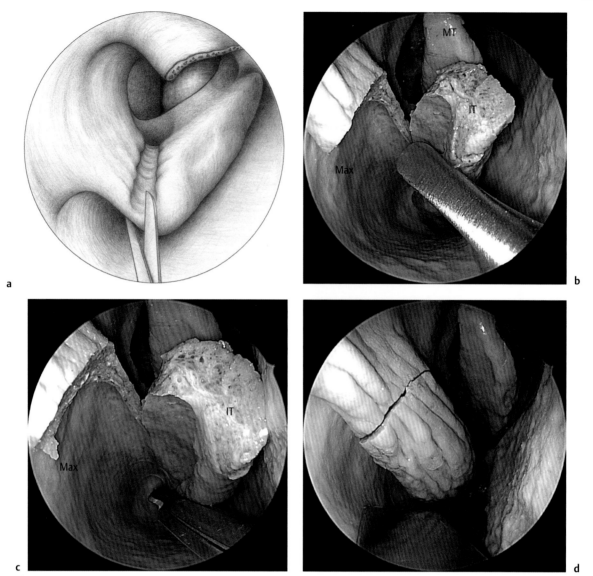

Fig. 16.12 (**a**) The inferior turbinate is crushed and cut up to the insertion of the turbinate on the medial wall of the maxilla. (**b**) Cadaveric image demonstrating the inferior turbinate (*IT*) has been cut up to the insertion on the medial wall of the maxilla (*Max*). *MT*, middle turbinate. (**c**) This incision is continued along the floor of the nose to the posterior region of the inferior turbinate. (**d**) A sharp chisel is used to cut the bone under the mucosal incisions following the mucosal incision.

anterior wall of the maxillary sinus, a canine fossa puncture can be performed. This allows instruments or an endoscope to be introduced through the anterior wall of the maxillary sinus, which can be useful to access areas within the sinus that may be otherwise difficult to access. Malleable suction dissectors* (both curette and Freer elevator; Integra) are also very useful as these instruments can be bent to the required angle for dissection in difficult areas such as the anterior wall or anterolateral region of the maxillary sinus.

If the anterior face of the maxillary sinus cannot be well seen or if better access to the anterior face is required for a tumor that attaches extensively to the anterior face of the maxillary sinus, further resection of the anteromedial wall and frontal process of the maxilla can be performed (**Fig. 16.16**). This is similar to what is done using a prelacrimal approach (Chapter 5) except here the inferior turbinate

has already being resected with the medial maxillectomy. In such cases, a canine fossa trephine is not thought to be suitable due to the small risk of seeding the tumor into the soft tissues of the cheek. Although seeding is unlikely to occur, this risk is thought to be greater if the entry point into the maxillary sinus is through tumor rather than through normal mucosa.

If access is still difficult and the anterior wall of the maxillary sinus is not fully accessible, a transseptal route provides a better angle of approach to this region. This access is achieved by performing a hemitransfixion incision in the opposite nasal vestibule (**Fig. 16.17a**) and then removing a small horizontal area of cartilage and/or bone opposite the region of the anterior maxillary sinus (**Fig. 16.17b**). The instrument can then be passed through the hemitransfixion incision, through the cartilage window (**Fig. 16.17c**),

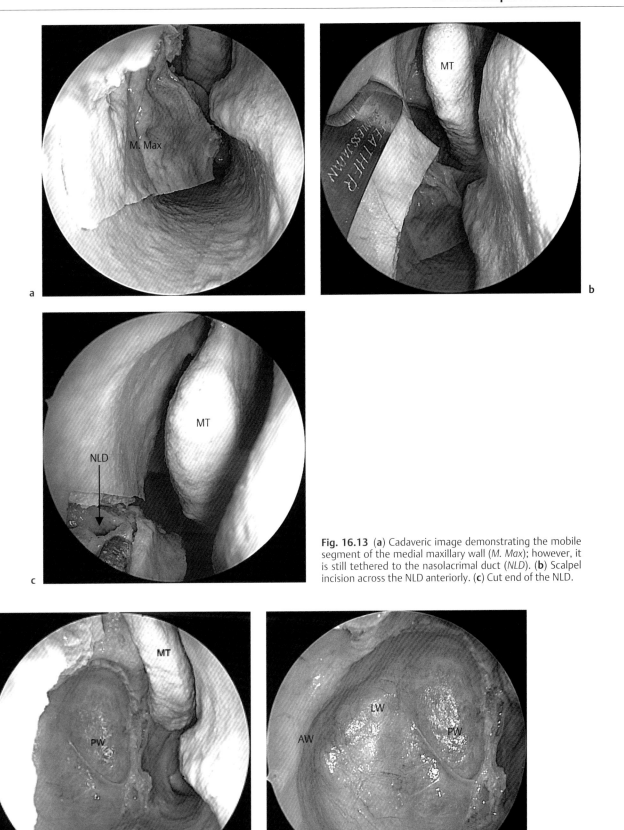

Fig. 16.13 (**a**) Cadaveric image demonstrating the mobile segment of the medial maxillary wall (*M. Max*); however, it is still tethered to the nasolacrimal duct (*NLD*). (**b**) Scalpel incision across the NLD anteriorly. (**c**) Cut end of the NLD.

Fig. 16.14 Cadaveric images demonstrating the exposure following a medial maxillectomy of the maxillary sinus taken with a (**a**) 0-degree and (**b**) 70-degree endoscope. *PW*, posterior wall; *LW*, lateral wall; *AW*, anterior wall; *MT*, middle turbinate.

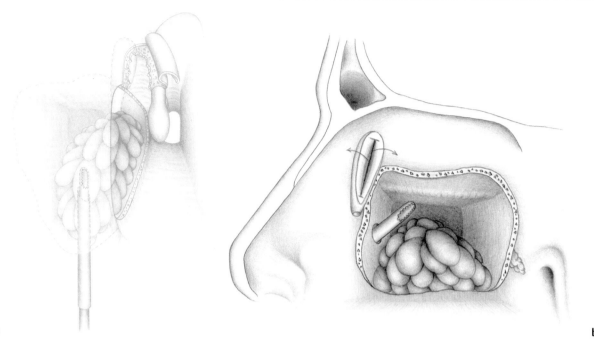

a

b

Fig. 16.15 (**a**) After endoscopic medial maxillectomy as viewed with a 0-degree endoscope. (**b**) The view of the maxillary sinus with a 70-degree endoscope. Note the microdebrider blade that has been placed through the canine fossa trephine.

and then through the horizontal mucosal incision in the opposite nasal cavity (**Fig. 16.17d**), giving greater access to the anterior wall of the maxillary sinus (**Fig. 16.18**). This approach significantly improves the angle of approach and usually allows complete access to the entire anterior maxillary wall (**Fig. 16.18**). This region is best approached using either a 60-degree microdebrider blade or a 70-degree diamond bur (Medtronic ENT).

Access to the Pterygopalatine Fossa

Access to the pterygopalatine fossa is achieved by removing the posterior wall of the maxillary sinus. In most cases a medial maxillectomy is unnecessary as most of the pterygopalatine fossa can be accessed through a large middle meatal antrostomy. If necessary, this antrostomy can be taken through the inferior turbinate to the floor of the nose

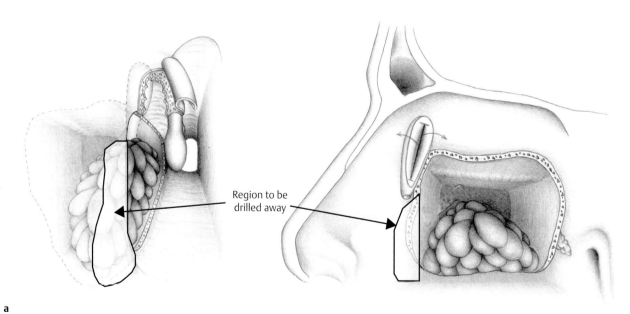

Region to be
drilled away

a

b

Fig. 16.16 (**a,b**) Region of the frontal process of the maxilla that should be drilled away if direct access to the anterior wall of the maxillary sinus is needed.

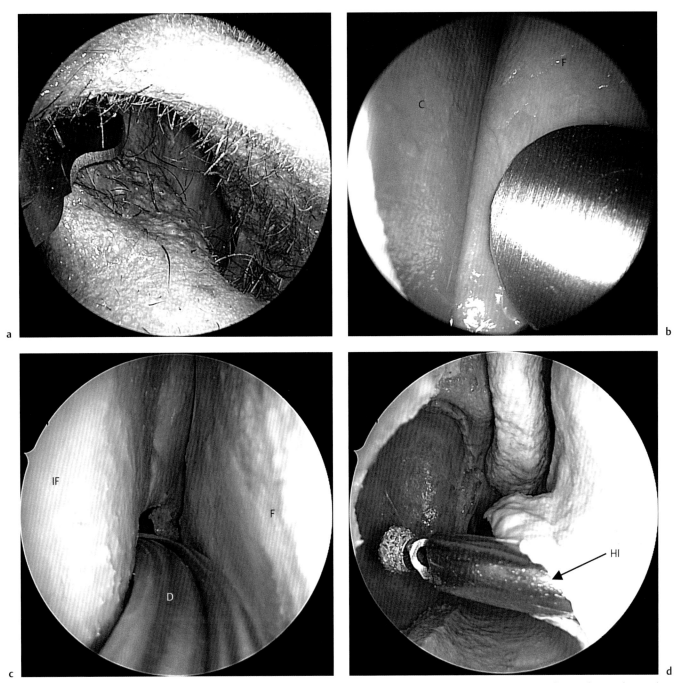

Fig. 16.17 (**a**) Cadaveric dissection image demonstrating a hemitransfixion incision anteriorly in the left nostril (contralateral side to the tumor dissection). (**b**) A mucoperichondrial flap is elevated. *C*, cartilage; *F*, flap. (**c**) A cartilaginous septal window has been removed and a vertical incision is performed through the mucoperichondrial flap on the ipsilateral side (*IF*). This allows the passage of a 70-degree diamond-tipped drill (*D*). (**d**) The endoscope has been placed within the right nasal cavity demonstrating the working tip of the drill passing into the right maxillary sinus through the left hemitransfixion incision and through the horizontal septal flap incision (*HI*).

by partial inferior turbinate resection. The mucosa from the posterior wall of the maxillary sinus is elevated and preserved. This exposes the bone and removal of this bone is necessary to expose the pterygopalatine fossa. In order to remove this bone, it is necessary to expose the sphenopalatine artery as described in Chapter 10. The artery is cauterized with suction bipolar forceps. A Hajek-Koeffler punch or 45-degree through-biting Blakesley forceps is used to remove the bone anterior to the sphenopalatine artery. The punch is introduced into the sphenopalatine foramen and the bone anterior to the foramen removed until the posterior wall of the maxillary sinus is reached (**Fig. 16.19**). Further removal of this bone can be done with either the punch or with a 45-degree through-biting Blakesley. Bone is removed until the contents of the pterygopalatine fossa are exposed (**Fig. 16.20**).

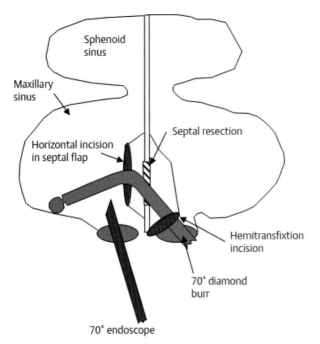

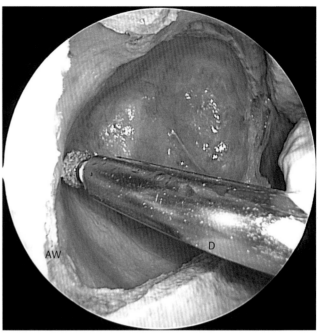

a

b

Fig. 16.18 (**a**) Illustration of the septal incisions necessary for the transeptal approach to achieve good access to the entire anterior wall of the maxillary sinus for tumors either originating from this region or with a significant anterior wall attachment. (**b**) Cadaveric image demonstrating the access to the anterior wall (*AW*) of the maxillary sinus with a 70-degree diamond drill (*D*).

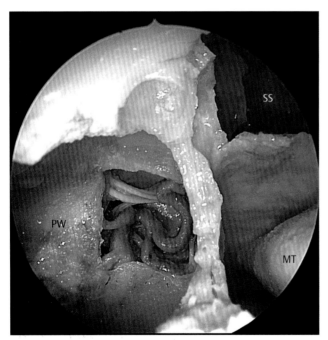

Fig. 16.19 Cadaveric dissection demonstrating the contents of the right pterygopalatine fossa as viewed through a large maxillary antrostomy. *PW*, posterior wall of maxillary sinus; *SS*, sphenoid sinus; *MT*, middle turbinate.

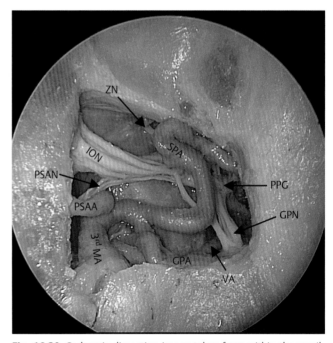

Fig. 16.20 Cadaveric dissection image taken from within the maxillary sinus on the right side. This image demonstrates the contents of the pterygopalatine fossa following fat removal. *PPG*, pterygopalatine ganglion; *GPN*, greater palatine nerve; *VA*, Vidian artery; *GPA*, greater palatine artery; *SPA*, sphenopalatine artery; *ZN*, zygomatic nerve; *ION*, infraorbital nerve; *PSAA*, posterior superior alveolar artery; *PSAN*, posterior superior alveolar nerve; *3rd MA*, third division of the maxillary artery.

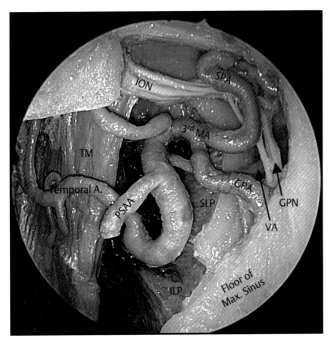

Fig. 16.21 Cadaveric dissection image following the removal of the lateral wall, floor, and posterior wall of the right maxillary sinus. This image reveals the temporalis muscle (*TM*) located directly behind the lateral wall of the maxillary sinus. The superior (*SLP*) and inferior (*ILP*) heads of the lateral pterygoid muscle can be seen where they attach and cover the superficial surface of the lateral pterygoid plates. *GPN*, greater palatine nerve; *VA*, Vidian artery; *GPA*, greater palatine artery; *SPA*, sphenopalatine artery; *ION*, infraorbital nerve; *PSAA*, posterior superior alveolar artery; *3rd MA*, third division of the maxillary artery.

Access to the Infratemporal Fossa

To access the infratemporal fossa, all of the bone of the posterior and lateral wall of the maxillary sinus needs to be removed. Most of the bone can be removed through the same nostril as the tumor using either the Hajek-Koeffler punch or through-biting Blakesley. For complete access, the bone should be removed from the roof to the floor of the maxillary sinus (**Fig. 16.21**).

Bone removal can continue until the anterior wall of the maxillary sinus is reached by inserting the punch or Blakesley forceps through the opposite nostril via a septal port. The septal port for the infratemporal fossa is very similar to that used to access the front wall of the maxillary sinus. This angle of approach allows the instruments to be advanced up to the anterior maxillary sinus wall as described under "Maxillary Sinus Access" earlier in this chapter.

◆ Endoscopic Anatomy

Endoscopic Anatomy of the Greater Palatine Canal and the Pterygopalatine Fossa

The greater palatine canal and the pterygopalatine fossa are continuous (**Figs. 16.22** and **16.23**). The pterygopalatine fossa is similar to an inverted cone and the bottom of this cone forms the greater palatine canal. The pterygopalatine fossa contains the distal branches of the maxillary artery namely the sphenopalatine artery and the greater palatine artery (**Fig. 16.20**). In addition, the Vidian nerve enters the posterior aspect of the fossa before moving laterally to end in the pterygopalatine ganglion, which is suspended from the maxillary nerve (**Fig. 16.20**). The pterygopalatine fossa narrows gradually as it opens laterally into the pterygomaxillary fissure before widening into the infratemporal fossa (**Figs. 16.22** and **16.23**).

The roof of the pterygopalatine fossa is formed by the greater wing of the sphenoid bone and the supraorbital fissure, foramen rotundum, and the maxillary nerve coursing from the foramen rotundum from medial to lateral across the roof of the fossa just below the orbital apex (**Figs. 16.22** and **16.23**). The medial wall is formed by the palatine bone, sphenopalatine foramen, and sphenopalatine artery (**Fig. 16.24**), whereas the floor is formed by the greater palatine canal and the lateral wall is formed by the pterygomaxillary fissure (**Figs. 16.20** and **16.22**). In **Fig. 16.25** the relationships between the foramina that enter the posterior wall of the pterygopalatine fossa namely the palatovaginal canal, the Vidian canal, and the foramen rotundum are demonstrated. In addition, the supraorbital fissure and pterygomaxillary fissure are seen (**Fig. 16.26**).

If the anatomy of this region is viewed endoscopically and each layer removed so that the underlying layer can be appreciated, a good understanding of the anatomy can be achieved. The first fact to be appreciated is that the pterygopalatine fossa forms a relatively small part of the total area behind the posterior wall of the maxillary sinus (**Fig. 16.19**). Secondly, the first structures to be encountered when entering the fossa are the blood vessels (**Fig. 16.20**). The neural structures all lie deep to this plexus of arteries (**Fig. 16.20**).

Further dissection in the roof to the fossa allows the maxillary nerve to be seen just below the orbit in the roof of the fossa. If this nerve is followed posteromedially the foramen rotundum can be seen (**Fig. 16.26**). If we now remove the major blood vessels from the fossa we can identify the Vidian nerve entering the fossa posteriorly (**Fig. 16.25**).

The Endoscopic Anatomy of the Supraorbital Fissure

The other relationship that is important to understand is how the pterygopalatine fossa and infratemporal fossa relate to the supraorbital fissure. It is through this fissure that tumors can extend from the infratemporal fossa and pterygopalatine fossa up toward the orbital apex. Additionally, tumors may follow the infraorbital nerve and maxillary nerve to enter the pterygopalatine fossa and move posteriorly toward the cavernous sinus and carotid artery. **Figure 16.26** shows the supraorbital fissure with the infraorbital nerve and zygomatic nerve running through it. Note how the medial part of the fissure communicates with the pterygopalatine fossa whereas the lateral part of the fissure communicates with the orbit.

As the orbital apex and sphenoid is approached, the inferior portion of the lamina papyracea thickens. The lateral wall of the fissure is formed by the medial wall of the middle

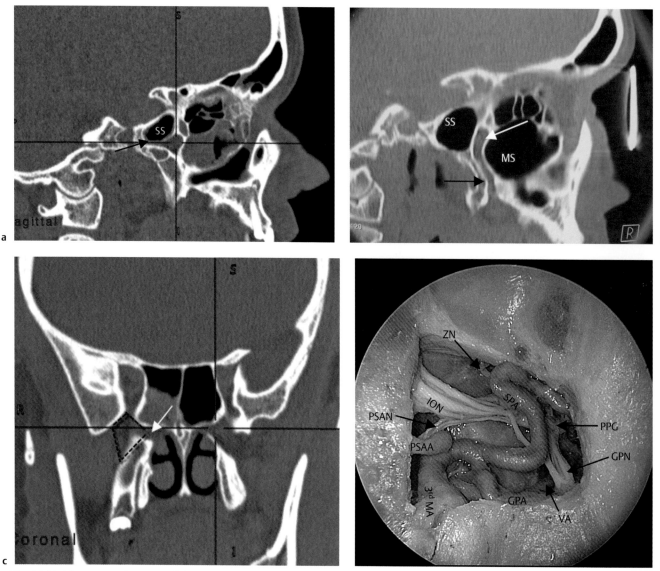

Fig. 16.22 (**a**) Parasagittal CT scan of the pterygopalatine fossa is cone shaped (*crosshairs*). The Vidian canal can be seen entering the posterior wall of the pterygopalatine fossa (*black arrow*). (**b**) The pterygopalatine fossa (*white arrow*) is seen to sit between the maxillary sinus (*MS*) and the sphenoid sinus (*SS*). The pterygopalatine fossa is continuous with the greater palatine canal (*black arrow*). Note how it narrows as it becomes the ptery-gomaxillary fissure before it expands into the infratemporal fossa. (**c**) In the coronal scan, the cone shape of the fossa is outlined by a *broken black line* and the sphenopalatine foramen is indicated with the *white arrow* and *cross-hairs*. (**d**) The contents of the pterygopalatine fossa are demonstrated on the right side following removal of the posterior wall of the maxillary sinus. *GPN*, greater palatine nerve; *VA*, Vidian artery; *GPA*, greater palatine artery; *SPA*, sphenopalatine artery; *ION*, infraorbital nerve; *PSAA*, posterior superior alveolar artery; *3rd MA*, third division of the maxillary artery.

cranial fossa. The infraorbital nerve can consistently be seen in the inferior aspect of the supraorbital fissure and it is around this structure that tumor can insinuate to reach the orbital apex and then expand into the space between the lateral sphenoid wall and middle cranial fossa (**Fig. 16.26**). Significant expansion can occur so that the tumor may reach the cavernous sinus and even the carotid artery.

In order to understand how the medial aspect of the supra-orbital fissure can be surgically accessed, **Figs. 16.27**, **16.28**, **16.29**, and **16.30** demonstrate the anatomy as it would be seen if this region were to be approached endoscopically. In **Fig. 16.24** note that the posterior wall of the maxillary sinus has been removed and a complete sphenoethmoidectomy

has been performed on the right side. In **Fig. 16.27** we can see the lateral wall of the sphenoid sinus. Note the land-marks of the lateral wall including the optic nerve, the ante-rior genu of the intracavernous carotid artery, the maxillary impression for the maxillary division of the trigeminal nerve, and the Vidian nerve in the floor of the sphenoid sinus. The optic nerve and the lateral opticocarotid recess can be seen. **Figure 16.28** is following the removal of the bone of the lat-eral sphenoid wall. The blue silicone shows the anterior genu of the intracavernous carotid is completely within the cav-ernous sinus. The anterior limit of this marks the beginning of the orbital apex, the supraorbital fissure. The occulomotor, trochlea, and ophthalmic division of the trigeminal nerve can

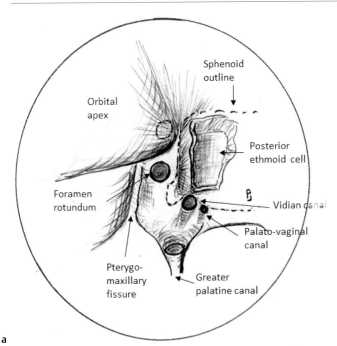

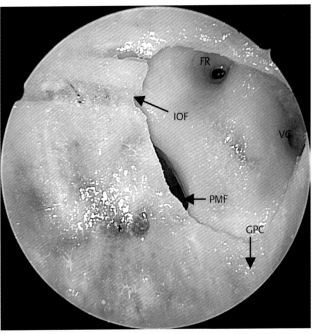

a

b

Fig. 16.23 (**a**) The relationships of the structures entering the posterior region, roof, and floor of the pterygopalatine fossa. The medial wall with the sphenopalatine foramen is not depicted. (**b**) This dry bone image has been taken with a 0-degree endoscope placed within the maxillary sinus. The posterior wall of the maxillary sinus has been removed in the region of the pterygopalatine fossa and we can visualize the pterygoid process and a number of important surrounding structures. The foramen rotundum (*FR*), Vidian canal (*VC*), and the infraorbital fissure (*IOF*) can be appreciated, along with the pterygomaxillary fissure (*PMF*). Note how the pterygomaxillary fissure and the infraorbital fissure are continuous with each other. *GPC*, greater palatine canal.

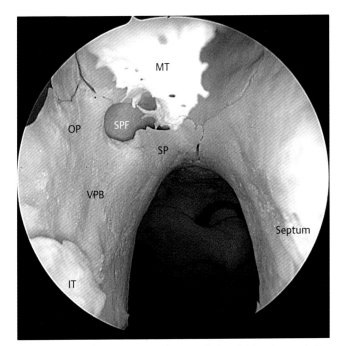

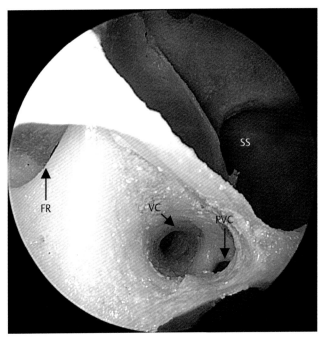

Fig. 16.24 Dry bone specimen image of the right sphenopalatine foramen (*SPF*). The vertical portion of the palatine bone (*VPB*) divides into two processes, the orbital process (*OP*), and the sphenoidal process (*SP*), and the SPF is located in between. *MT*, middle turbinate; *IT*, inferior turbinate.

Fig. 16.25 Close up image of a dry bone specimen following the widening of the right sphenopalatine foramen, and removal of the sphenoidal process of the palatine bone. The Vidian canal (*VC*) can be seen clearly with the palatovaginal canal (*PVC*) located more medially. *SS*, sphenoid sinus; *FR*, foramen rotundum.

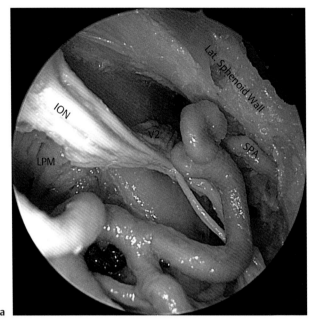

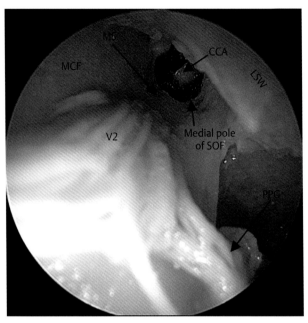

Fig. 16.26 (**a**) Endoscopic cadaveric image taken of the right pterygopalatine fossa. The maxillary division of the trigeminal nerve (*V2*) can be seen exiting the foramen rotundum before it divides into the infraorbital nerve (*ION*) and zygomatic nerve. *LPM,* lateral pterygoid muscle; *SPA,* sphenopalatine artery. (**b**) Closer image of V2 exiting the foramen rotundum, with the middle cranial fossa laterally, maxillary strut superiorly, and the supraorbital fissure posteriorly. Note how the maxillary strut (*MS*) is the strut of bone that separates the foramen rotundum and its contents (*V2*) from the supraorbital fissure. The supraorbital fissure (*SOF*) forms the anterior wall of the cavernous sinus, and as such the intracavernous carotid artery (*CCA*) can be seen in the distance. The medial pole of the SOF has been outlined. *LSW,* lateral sphenoid wall.

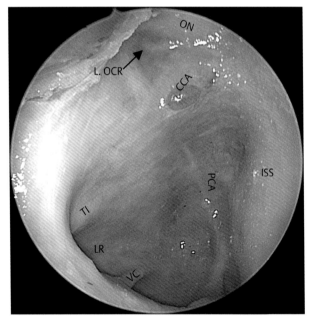

Fig. 16.27 Cadaveric dissection image taken of the right sphenoid sinus through a maximal sphenoidotomy. The Vidian canal (*VC*) and trigeminal impression (*TI*) for the maxillary division of the trigeminal nerve can be clearly seen. If the sphenoid sinus is well pneumatized then the lateral recess (*LR*) can be seen, a depression in the lateral sphenoid wall between the VC and the TI. The lateral opticocarotid recess (*L. OCR*) can be seen. This depression corresponds to pneumatization of the optic strut (the bony bridge that separates the optic canal from the superior orbital fissure). Further pneumatization into the optic strut may result in a pneumatized anterior clinoid process, which will place the optic nerve on a mesentery. *ISS,* intersinus septum; *ON,* optic nerve; *CCA,* anterior genu of the intracavernous carotid artery; *PCA,* paraclival carotid artery.

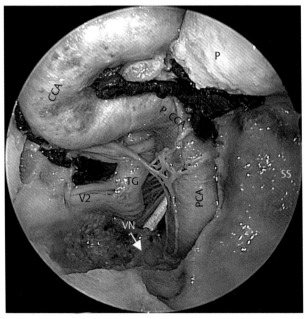

Fig. 16.28 Cadaveric dissection image of the lateral sphenoid wall following bone removal. *P,* pituitary gland; *CCA,* intracavernous carotid artery; *V2,* maxillary division of the trigeminal nerve; *TG,* trigeminal ganglion; *VN,* Vidian nerve; *PCA,* paraclival carotid artery; *P. CCA,* posterior genu of the intracavernous carotid artery; *SS,* sphenoid sinus.

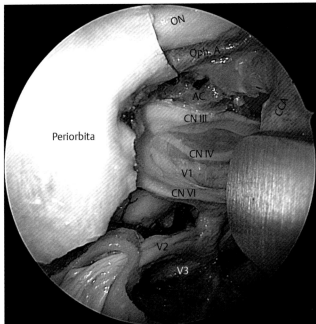

Fig. 16.29 Cadaveric dissection image of the right lateral wall of the sphenoid sinus. The bone has been removed and the anterior genu of the intracavernous carotid artery (*CCA*) retracted medially. This allows clear visualization of the nerves within the dural layers of the lateral wall of the cavernous sinus. The abducens nerve (*CN VI*) can be visualized medially, running within the cavernous sinus. Note the periorbita of the orbital apex. The bone of the anterior clinoid (*AC*) process has been left in place, positioned within the lateral opticocarotid recess. *ON*, optic nerve; *Oph. A*, ophthalmic artery; *CN III*, occulomotor nerve; *CN IV*, trochlear nerve; *V1*, ophthalmic division of the trigeminal nerve; *V2*, maxillary division of the trigeminal nerve; *V3*, mandibular division of the trigeminal nerve.

Fig. 16.30 Cadaveric dissection of the right lateral sphenoid wall following removal of the lateral sphenoid wall. Dissection has continued anteriorly to the pterygopalatine fossa inferiorly and the orbital apex superiorly. In this image, the periorbita has been retracted superiorly. Note the remnant of the maxillary strut (*MS*), the strut of bone that separates the foramen rotundum from the superior orbital fissure/orbital apex. The Vidian nerve (*VN*) can be seen moving into the posterior aspect of the pterygopalatine fossa and enters the pterygopalatine ganglion (*PPG*). The relationship between the foramen rotundum (*FR*) and the temporal lobe (*TL*) can be seen clearly. *V2*, maxillary division of the trigeminal nerve; *PN*, pharyngeal nerve; *PCA*, paraclival carotid artery; *CCA*, intracavernous carotid artery; *SS*, sphenoid sinus; *TG*, trigeminal ganglion.

be seen in **Fig. 16.29** leaving the lateral wall of the cavernous sinus to enter the orbital apex periorbita. In **Fig. 16.30** the space between the lateral wall of the sphenoid and the medial wall of the temporal fossa has been dissected, with the dura of the temporal fossa excised to reveal the medial side of the temporal lobe. In this image, the periorbita of the orbital apex has been retracted with a Freer dissector. Analysis of the maxillary nerve can clearly show the path in which tumors in this region may take. Heading posteriorly, they may enter the cavernous sinus and invade the intracavernous structures such as the intracavernous carotid artery. Moving medially, they will expand into the lateral wall of the sphenoid sinus. If a tumor pushed laterally then it would enter the middle cranial fossa.

Endoscopic Anatomy of the Region of the Middle Cranial Fossa

To access the region of the middle cranial fossa and foramen ovale, further removal of the lateral wall of the sphenoid is necessary (**Fig. 16.30**). To achieve this, both the Vidian nerve in the floor of the sphenoid sinus and the maxillary nerve in the lateral wall of the sphenoid are exposed and the bone around these nerves removed with a diamond bur (**Fig. 16.30**).

The Vidian canal leads directly to the second genu of the paraclival internal carotid artery as it turns vertically and runs up the lateral wall of the sphenoid toward the pituitary fossa. **Figure 16.30** shows the relationship between the Vidian canal and the maxillary nerve as the bone is removed between these structures. This bone removal exposes the space between the middle cranial fossa plate and the lateral wall of the sphenoid both below and above the maxillary nerve. As the bone removal continues posteriorly, the foramen ovale and the mandibular branch of the trigeminal nerve are seen, which are lateral and anterior to the carotid artery (see **Fig. 16.32**). The Vidian nerve is medial and marks the position of the carotid at the junction of the floor and posterior wall of the sphenoid. Directly above the foramen ovale in the lateral wall is the cavernous sinus (CS) and above the cavernous sinus is the orbital apex (OA). The space above the maxillary nerve is just below the orbital apex and a space is formed between the lateral wall of the sphenoid and the bone of the middle cranial fossa. Tumors expanding into this space can cause compression of the orbital apex. The relationship of the orbital apex, lateral wall of sphenoid, and medial wall of the middle cranial fossa is demonstrated in **Figs. 16.31** and **16.32**.

The final dissection of the lateral wall of the sphenoid exposes the cavernous sinus anterior to the paraclival carotid artery and the posterior genu of the intracavernous

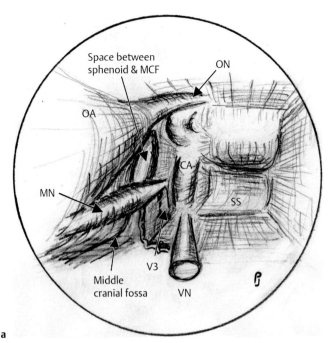

a

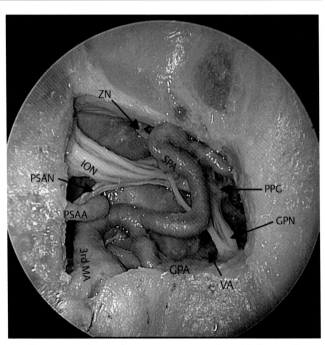

b

Fig. 16.31 (**a**) Illustrates the important relationships between the right maxillary nerve and the supraorbital fissure and the pterygopalatine fossa as viewed from anterior. (**b**) The maxillary nerve exits the foramen rotundum and crosses the roof of the pterygopalatine fossa and occupies the gap created by the supraorbital fissure. This relationship is important as it helps one to understand how tumors spread from one fossa to another and, on occasion, into the orbital apex. *OA*, orbital apex; *VN*, Vidian nerve; *PPG*, pterygopalatine ganglion; *GPC*, greater palatine canal; *GPA*, greater palatine artery; *GPN*, greater palatine nerve; *SPA*, sphenopalatine artery; *ION*, infraorbital nerve; *ZN*, zygomatic nerve; *PSAA*, posterior superior alveolar artery; *PSAN*, posterior superior alveolar nerve; *3rd MA*, third division of maxillary artery.

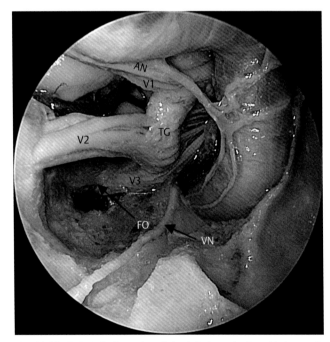

Fig. 16.32 Cadaveric dissection of the right lateral sphenoid sinus wall. Bone has been removed at the lateral recess (between the Vidian nerve and the maxillary division of the trigeminal nerve). This allows identification of foramen ovale (*FO*), with the mandibular division (*V3*) moving through this canal almost immediately after leaving the semilunar shaped trigeminal ganglion (*TG*). Note that the dura between V1 and V2, and V2 and V3 has been removed. *VN*, Vidian canal; *V2*, maxillary division of trigeminal nerve; *V1*, ophthalmic division of trigeminal nerve; *AN*, abducens nerve.

carotid artery. If the remaining bone of the lateral wall of the sphenoid is removed, the cavernous sinus and mandibular branch of the trigeminal nerve (V3) will be exposed above the foramen ovale (**Fig. 16.32**). Further bone removal laterally will remove the bone overlying the medial middle temporal fossa and expose the underlying dura. Although dura covers the cavernous sinus as it is approached from the sphenoid sinus, this covering is very thin and tenuous with multiple small veins joining or leaving the cavernous sinus so that such a dissection can be quite bloody and the bleeding difficult to control. The relationship of the Vidian nerve (VN), carotid artery (CA), cavernous sinus (CS), V2, V3, foramen ovale, and middle cranial fossa (MCF) can be appreciated in **Figs. 16.28**, **16.29**, **16.30**, and **16.32**.

Endoscopic Anatomy of the Infratemporal Fossa

Once the bone overlying the posterior wall of the maxillary sinus has been removed, the pterygopalatine fossa and infratemporal fossa are seen (**Fig. 16.33**). The infraorbital nerve (MN) can be seen at the junction of the infratemporal fossa and orbit. These fossae are covered by periosteum and the contents are exposed by removing the periosteum. Both fossae contain fat, blood vessels, and nerves. The fat and blood vessels usually lie anteromedial to the neural structures. Once the fat has been removed, the underlying maxillary artery and muscles of the infratemporal fossa can be seen. The superior and inferior heads of the lateral pterygoid muscle (LP) can be seen originating directly behind the

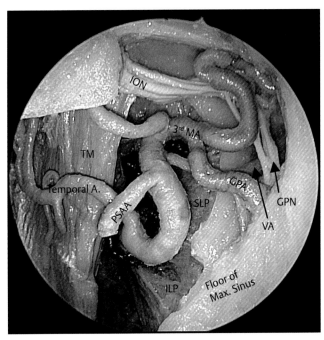

Fig. 16.33 Cadaveric dissection image following the removal of the lateral wall, floor, and posterior wall of the right maxillary sinus. This image reveals the temporalis muscle (*TM*) located just deep to the lateral wall of the maxillary sinus. The superior (*SLP*) and inferior (*ILP*) heads of the lateral pterygoid muscle can be seen where they attach and cover the superficial surface of the lateral pterygoid plates. *GPN*, greater palatine nerve; *VA*, Vidian artery; *GPA*, greater palatine artery; *SPA*, sphenopalatine artery; *ION*, infraorbital nerve; *PSAA*, posterior superior alveolar artery; *3rd MA*, third division of the maxillary artery.

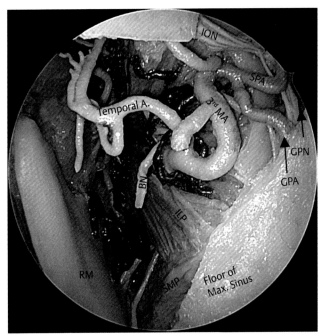

Fig. 16.34 Cadaveric dissection of the right infratemporal fossa following removal of the temporalis muscle revealing the ramus of the mandible (*RM*). With an angled endoscope, the superficial head of the medial pterygoid muscle (*SMP*) can also be visualized. Note that the medial pterygoid muscle has both a superficial head and a deep head. The superficial head lies just superficial to the inferior head of the lateral pterygoid muscle (*ILP*). The maxillary artery enters the infratemporal fossa between the superior and inferior head of the lateral pterygoid muscles. *GPN*, greater palatine nerve; *GPA*, greater palatine artery; *SPA*, sphenopalatine artery; *ION*, infraorbital nerve; *3rd MA*, third division of the maxillary artery.

greater palatine canal with the maxillary artery entering the infratemporal fossa between the two heads of the lateral pterygoid muscle. As one moves farther laterally, the temporalis muscle (TM) comes into view. Removing the temporalis muscle reveals the ramus of the mandible (**Fig. 16.34**). With the use of an angled endoscope looking inferiorly, the superficial head of the medial pterygoid muscle can be appreciated.

◆ Tumors Involving the Maxillary Sinus, Pterygopalatine Fossa, and Infratemporal Fossa

Antrochoanal Polyp

Antrochoanal polyps commonly form from the posterior wall of the maxillary sinus. These tumors need to have the site of origin resected to prevent recurrence. The first step is to perform a large middle meatal antrostomy and to expose the site of origin of the tumor. If the entire site can be easily accessed through the middle meatal antrostomy then the tumor and the site of origin are resected with a margin of normal mucosa around the attachment. If the site of origin

is not easily accessible through a middle meatal antrostomy, a canine fossa trephination should be performed and the microdebrider or Freer elevator placed through the trephine site and the origin of the polyp resected with the margin of normal tissue.

Inverting Papilloma

The other most common benign tumor involving the maxillary sinus is inverting papilloma (IP). Small IP tumors of the maxillary sinus that do not arise from the anterior wall of the maxillary sinus can be resected by creating a large middle meatal antrostomy and a canine fossa trephine (described in Chapter 5). The endoscope can be placed into the maxillary antrostomy while the dissecting instrument is placed through the canine fossa puncture. This can be reversed with the endoscope being placed through the canine fossa puncture and instrument through the maxillary antrostomy. Using this technique, almost the entire maxillary sinus can be accessed. The only area where access may not be adequate is the anterior face of the maxillary sinus. Tumors located on the anterior face may require a prelacrimal approach or endoscopic medial maxillectomy for adequate access and complete resection. All other small or localized tumors can be resected using this two-site approach.

Large or Anterior Wall Maxillary Sinus Tumors

If a tumor cannot be accessed with the canine fossa trephination or it originates from a large area or from the anterior wall of the maxillary sinus, either a prelacrimal approach (as described earlier) or an endoscopic medial maxillectomy should be performed. If additional access is required when doing a medial maxillectomy, the frontal process of the maxilla can be drilled away. This can be combined with a transseptal access to improve the angulation to the anterior wall as described earlier in this chapter. All walls of the maxillary sinus should be able to be accessed and the tumor and underlying mucosa should be removed. In **Fig. 16.35** the patient has a large inverting papilloma extending laterally beyond the limits of the maxillary sinus.

This inverting papilloma was based on the inferior turbinate. Resection of the medial maxilla removed a large part of the tumor origin. In addition, the tumor took origin from the adjacent floor and posterior wall of the maxillary sinus. This could be easily accessed after endoscopic medial maxillectomy. The bone in the region of origin of the tumor was able to be drilled with a diamond bur to ensure no tumor had infiltrated into bony crevices seen in the region of new bone formation classically associated with the tumor origin.

The following patient presented with an inverting papilloma that took origin around a region of new bone formation on the lateral and anterior wall of the maxillary sinus. This anterior and lateral area was able to be accessed (after an endoscopic medial maxillectomy) with a 70-degree diamond bur and the origin of the tumor completely cleared with drilling of the underlying bone (**Fig. 16.36**). It is common for inverting papilloma to originate from a region of new bone formation and therefore it is important to drill away this new bone as mucosa may invaginate into the bony crevices associated with new bone and failure to remove this may result in tumor recurrence.[8]

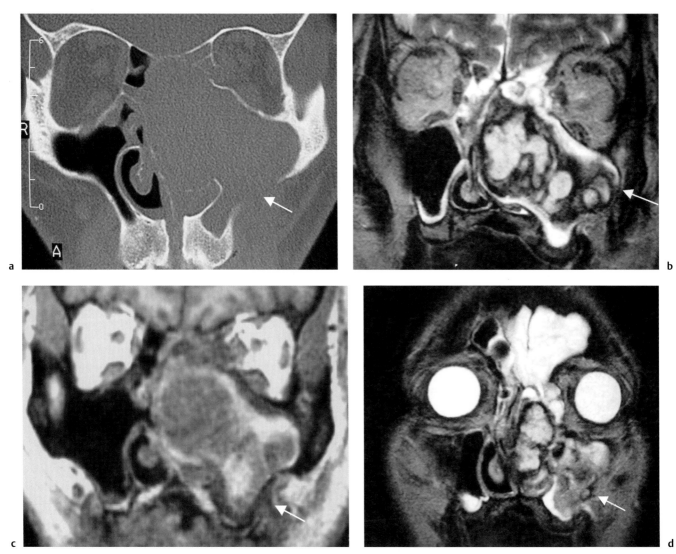

Fig. 16.35 A large inverting papilloma eroding the lateral wall of the maxillary sinus (*white arrow*). The CT (**a**), MRI (**b**), T1 protocol (**c**), and T2 protocol (**d**) show the tumor's extent. (**d**) MRI (T2 protocol) shows an obstructed frontal sinus with mucus lighting up in the frontal sinus.

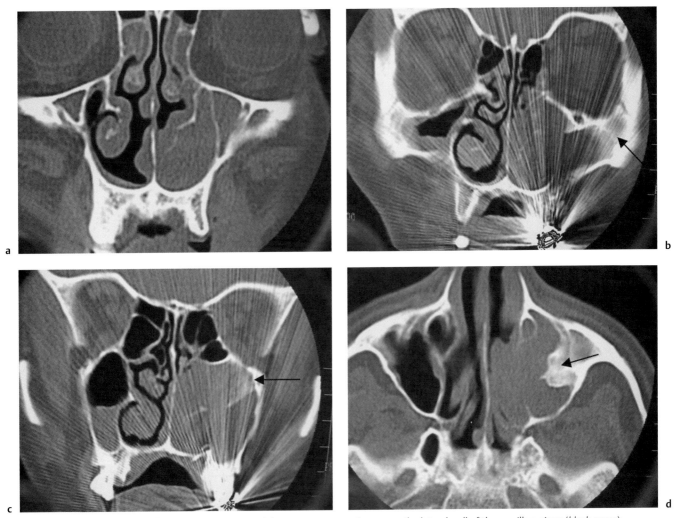

Fig. 16.36 (a–d) Inverting papilloma originating around the neo-osteogenesis seen on the lateral wall of the maxillary sinus (*black arrow*).

◆ Results of the Endoscopic Resection of Inverted Papillomas

Patients with inverting papilloma were classified according to the classification of Krouse[4] presented in **Table 16.1**.

The published series of patients who have undergone endoscopic resection of inverting papillomas, including those patients with large and extensive lesions who have had an endoscopic medial maxillectomy as part of the tumor resection, is presented in **Table 16.2**. As can be seen from these results and from recent publications by Krouse[9] and a review article by Melroy and Senior,[10] the results obtained by endoscopic removal of inverting papillomas are better than those achieved in the past using an open approach. The recurrence rates of inverting papilloma with open procedures averages at 18%, whereas those performed endoscopically average 12%.[10]

Juvenile Nasopharyngeal Angiofibroma

There is currently widespread acceptance that juvenile nasopharyngeal angiofibroma (JNAs) occupying the nasal cavity alone or with extension into the pterygopalatine fossa or adjacent sinuses can be managed endoscopically.[6,10] The first step is to embolize the tumor within 24 hours of the surgery to reduce its vascularity. If the embolization is done prior to 24 hours, significant collateral blood supply may open and the tumor may regain a degree of its vascularity. The second step is to perform a large middle meatal

Table 16.1 Staging system for inverted papilloma as proposed by Krouse[4]

Stage	Extent of Tumor
I	Tumor confined to nasal cavity; no malignancy
II	Tumor involving the ostiomeatal complex, and ethmoids and/or medial wall of maxillary sinus; no malignancy
III	Tumor involving the inferior, superior, lateral, or anterior wall of maxillary sinus, sphenoid, and/or frontal sinus; no malignancy
IV	All extranasal/extrasinus tumors; all tumors associated with malignancy

Table 16.2 Presentation, origin, stage, procedure, and outcome for endoscopic removal of inverting papilloma, including patients who underwent medial maxillectomy for removal of the inverting papilloma[5]

Case	Age and Sex	Symptoms	Origin	Stage	Endoscopic Procedure	Current Status and Follow-up
1.[a]	51M	Left nasal obstruction, rhinorrhea	Left maxillary antrum, lamina papyracea, sphenoid sinus	IV	Medial maxillectomy, canine fossa puncture, ethmoidectomy, sphenoidotomy, and clearance of the frontal recess	Had recurrence of tumor after 4 months in left infratemporal fossa; surgically cleared and now disease free after 3 years
2.	54M	Left nasal obstruction, epistaxis	Left maxillary sinus and inferior turbinate	II	Medial maxillectomy, canine fossa puncture and DCR	Disease free
3.	71M	Right nasal obstruction, rhinorrhea	Right uncinate process	II	MMA	Disease free
4.	41M	Left nasal obstruction (previous lateral rhinotomy for IP)	Left lamina papyracea, frontal sinus	III	MMA, ethmoidectomy, sphenoidotomy, and endoscopic Lothrop procedure	Disease free
5.	74M	Left nasal obstruction	Left nasal septum	I	Middle meatal antrostomy, ethmoidectomy	Disease free
6.	72M	Asymptomatic	Left middle turbinate	I	Resection of middle turbinate, ethmoidectomy, sphenoidotomy	Disease free
7.	46M	Left nasal obstruction	Left maxillary sinus	II	MMA, ethmoidectomy, and sphenoidotomy	Disease free
8.	53M	Right frontal sinusitis (previous lateral rhinotomy for IP)	Right maxillary sinus floor	III	Medial maxillectomy and canine fossa puncture	Disease free
9.	60F	Right nasal obstruction, rhinorrhea	Right maxillary sinus floor	III	MMA and canine fossa puncture	Disease free
10.	78F	Right epistaxis and nasal obstruction	Right maxillary sinus floor	III	Medial maxillectomy, ethmoidectomy, DCR, and canine fossa puncture	Disease free
11.	53M	Left nasal obstruction (previous Caldwell Luc)	Left maxillary sinus floor	III	MMA, ethmoidectomy, and frontal recess clearance	Disease free
12.	44M	Right nasal obstruction	Left middle meatus	I	MMA, ethmoidectomy, middle turbinectomy	Disease free
13.	67M	Left nasal obstruction	Sphenoid and posterior ethmoids	III	MMA, ethmoidectomy, superior turbinectomy, and extended sphenoidotomy	Disease free
14.	58F	Right nasal obstruction and blood-stained discharge	Posterior septum	I	Sphenoethmoidectomy, septal and middle, and superior turbinate resection	Disease free
15.	71M	Right nasal obstruction	Right middle meatus and medial wall maxillary sinus	II	Ethmoidectomy, frontal recess clearance, middle turbinectomy, medial maxillectomy, and canine fossa puncture	Disease free
16.	50F	Left nasal obstruction, epistaxis and discharge	Left superior rim of maxillary sinus ostium	II	Anterior ethmoidectomy, MMA, and canine fossa puncture	Disease free
17.	56M	Right nasal obstruction	Middle meatus on posterior rim of maxillary ostium	II	Ethmoidectomy and MMA	Disease free

[a]Recurrence found associated with squamous cell carcinoma deposits.

Abbreviations: DCR, dacryocystorhinostomy; IP, inverting papilloma; MMA, middle meatal antrostomy.

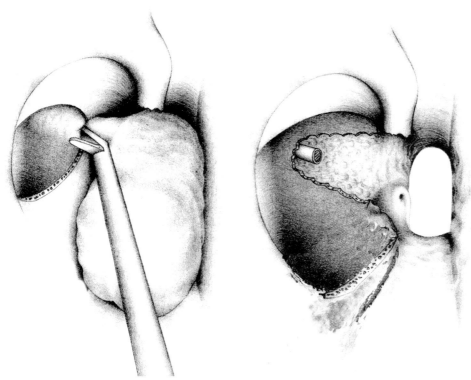

a

b

Fig. 16.37 (**a**) The nasal component of the tumor has been mobilized and the large middle meatal antrostomy performed. A 45-degree through-biting Blakesley is used to remove the posterior wall of the maxillary sinus.

(**b**) The tumor has been removed and the pterygopalatine fossa exposed. The maxillary artery is seen in the tumor bed.

antrostomy with removal of the posterior fontanelle and a sphenoethmoidectomy to provide access over the top of the tumor into the sphenoid sinus. Thereafter the intranasal component of the tumor is mobilized with a malleable suction Freer* (Integra). Often it is stuck to the septum and posterior bony choana but there is always a surgical plane directly on the tumor surface. If there is sufficient room in the nose, the tumor does not need to be debulked but if the nasal component is very large this may need to be resected before any extension of the tumor is dealt with. For tumors with a large intranasal and nasopharyngeal component, it is important to mobilize the nasopharyngeal component at this stage as well. The nasopharyngeal component is always stuck to the nasopharyngeal wall and mobilization is performed using the coblation wand. Once mobilization is complete, the tumor is divided at its entry into the sphenopalatine foramen using the coblation wand. The concomitant tissue removal and hemostasis achieved with the coblation wand reduces bleeding from the cut surface of the tumor. The nasal and nasopharyngeal components are then delivered via the nasopharynx through the mouth. Next, the extension of tumor into the pterygopalatine fossa needs to be exposed. The posterior wall of the maxillary sinus is removed, starting at the pterygopalatine foramen and moving laterally until the tumor in the pterygopalatine fossa and the attached maxillary artery is exposed (**Fig. 16.37**). Large tumor extensions into the pterygopalatine fossa need to be dealt with as described in the following section.

◆ Large Juvenile Nasopharyngeal Angiofibromas[11]

The most common benign tumor involving the pterygopalatine fossa (and infratemporal fossa) is the JNA. These tumors normally originate in the region of the opening of the Vidian canal and expand into the pterygopalatine fossa. Large tumors that extend into the infratemporal fossa will usually have a large intranasal component that may extend into nearby sinuses, especially the sphenoid sinus. Other benign tumors seen in this region are rare but may include inverting papillomas extending from the nasal cavity or tumors originating from the nerve sheath (schwannomas), cartilage, or muscle. The reason why there has been debate about the most appropriate method for removing these tumors is the significant vascularity that is associated with these tumors. Massive bleeding can occur during tumor resection and if the surgeon is not prepared or unable to manage such hemorrhage, complications can result. There are two significant steps that are now possible to allow these large JNAs to be tackled endoscopically. The first step is to preoperatively embolize the tumor thereby significantly reducing the vascularity and improving visualization during resection[6,11] (**Fig. 16.38**).

The second step is the two-surgeon approach that allows the second surgeon to place a high-volume suction in the operative field when bleeding is problematic and alternatively to place traction on the tumor facilitating the dissection.[6,11]

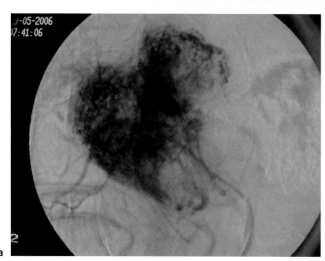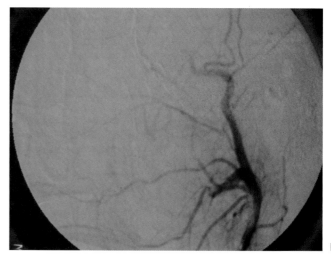

Fig. 16.38 (**a**) The significant vascular blush of the tumor can be seen, and in (**b**) this blush has been removed by embolization of the maxillary artery feeding the tumor.

Before surgery is performed, a large JNA needs careful assessment to decide if it is endoscopically resectable. Large JNAs tend to expand into potential spaces and to follow pathways of least resistance. In the pterygopalatine fossa and infratemporal fossa, a number of areas need to be critically evaluated before the surgeon decides if the tumor is endoscopically resectable.[11] In the pterygopalatine fossa the supraorbital fissure needs to be closely evaluated. There is a potential space between the lateral wall of the sphenoid and the middle cranial fossa, as seen in the previous anatomical review of this region. The tumor can infiltrate around the infraorbital nerve and enter the potential space above the nerve and expand this space. Further growth will cause the tumor to push posteriorly toward the cavernous sinus and the anterior genu of the cavernous carotid artery. Such a case is illustrated in **Fig. 16.39** where the tumor abuts the cavernous sinus and carotid and compresses the orbital apex within this potential space by expanding the supraorbital fissure.

In this case (**Fig. 16.39**) the maxillary nerve would be completely surrounded by tumor and it would be unlikely that the tumor could be separated from the nerve and indeed the nerve needed to be sacrificed during the dissection. In most cases where the tumor does not expand through the supraorbital fissure, the nerve is pushed upward by the tumor and can usually be dissected free from the tumor. The nerve should be identified proximally in the maxillary sinus early in the dissection and followed posteriorly. The nerve can often be separated from the tumor by peeling the nerve off the top of the tumor. Staying on the surface of the tumor, the tumor is pushed inferiorly and the nerve gently separated from the tumor. From the posterior wall of the maxillary sinus to the foramen rotundum the nerve hangs in a crescentic manner. As long as this anatomy is kept in mind as the nerve is followed posteriorly over the top of the tumor, the nerve can be kept intact. If the nerve transgresses through the tumor, it may need to be sacrificed. The suction dissection instruments are used to separate the nerve from the tumor. Fibrous tissue that will not dissect away is divided with endoscopic soft

tissue scissors from the Wormald Skull Base set* (Integra). These scissors come in 3- and 5-mm blade lengths with left-curved, right-curved, up-turned, and straight blades in both sizes.

The other region that is often involved in the spread of JNAs is the Vidian canal.[11] The tumor grows in this region in close proximity to the mouth of the Vidian canal. This funnel-shaped opening allows the tumor to grow down the canal and expand the canal. This region, and particularly the Vidian canal, should always be assessed on both CT and MRI. It is vitally important to understand the anatomy and relationships of the Vidian canal and to be able to assess tumor spread in this region. As was demonstrated earlier in this chapter, the Vidian canal runs in the floor of the sphenoid in an anteroposterior direction toward the carotid artery as it moves from its lacerum segment into its cavernous segment. Tumor may expand this canal and erode the floor of the sphenoid and, in some cases (**Fig. 16.40**), abut the carotid artery. It is our belief that failure to fully evaluate the Vidian canal at the time of removal of the JNA is one of the biggest causes of tumor recurrence. Small pieces of tumor lying within the canal can easily be missed and may grow progressively over time after tumor removal.

◆ Endoscopic Two-Surgeon Technique for Tumors of the Pterygopalatine Fossa and Infratemporal Fossa[6,11]

Although excellent access is provided by an endoscopic medial maxillectomy, the key to successful endoscopic removal of large JNAs is having two surgeons operating at the same time.[6,11] This is achieved by providing access to the tumor bed for the second surgeon through the septum. At the beginning of the procedure a Freer (hemitransfixion) incision is made on the opposite side to that of the tumor. Using standard septoplasty techniques, the mucosa

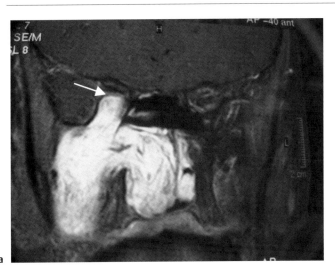
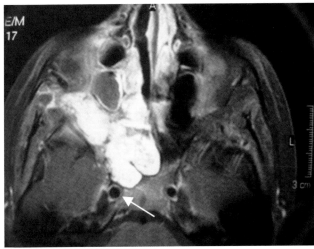

a

b

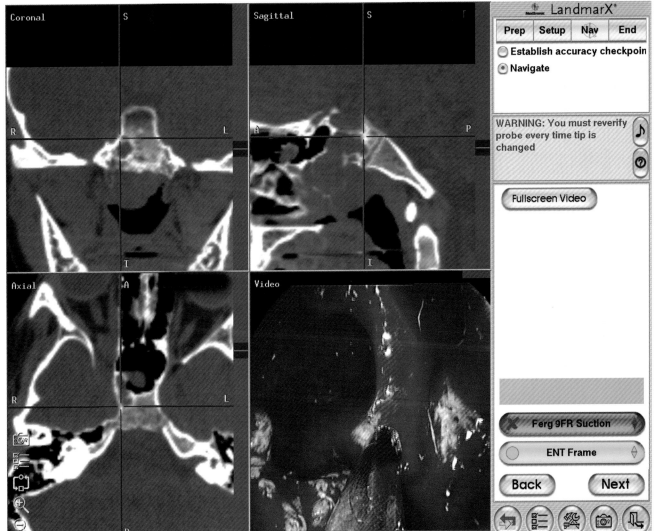

c

Fig. 16.39 (a) The tumor extends around the infraorbital nerve into the space between the lateral wall of the sphenoid sinus and the temporal lobe and significantly compresses the orbital apex (*white arrow*). (b) The tumor can be seen extending posteriorly into this space and abutting the cavernous sinus and carotid artery (*white arrow*). (c) In the intraoperative image guidance picture, the suction probe is placed in this space between the lateral wall of the sphenoid and temporal lobe after tumor resection as can be seen by the *crosshairs* on the adjacent CT scans.

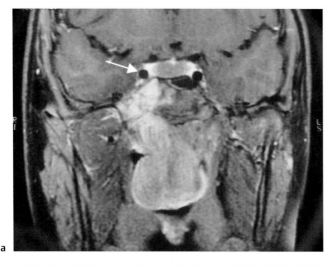

a

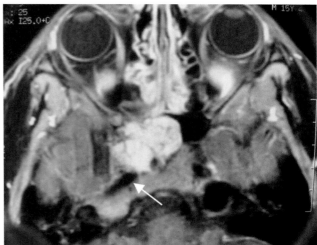

b

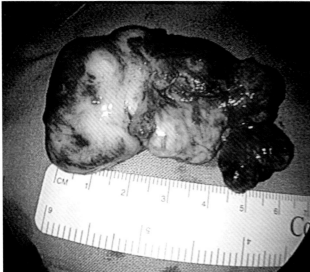

c

Fig. 16.40 (**a**) The tumor fills the nasopharynx, and expands the Vidian canal posteriorly until it abuts the internal carotid artery (*white arrow*). (**b**) This abutment of the carotid artery (*white arrow*) is seen in the axial MRI. (**c**) After endoscopic removal of the tumor, it is placed on a ruler for evaluation of its size.

is elevated off the cartilage of the septum. The cartilage of the septum is preserved but most of the posterior bony septum is resected. At the point where access is required, a horizontal incision is made in the opposite septal mucosa to allow instruments placed through the opposite nostril and into the Freer incision to cross the septum and access the tumor region on the opposite side of the nose (**Fig. 16.41**). An alternative is to perform a posterior septectomy to allow the second surgeon access to the contralateral side through this posterior septectomy.

During removal of the tumor, the second surgeon can provide significant traction on the tumor. This traction is vital to help the primary surgeon keep the dissection progressing around the posterior region of the tumor. This rotation of the tumor will also allow the feeding vessel (usually the maxillary artery) to be identified and clipped or cauterized before it is divided. If significant bleeding occurs, then a large volume suction can be placed in the field and allow the skull base angled vascular clamps (Integra) to be placed on the bleeding vessels and the vessel to be either clipped or cauterized with the suction bipolar forceps.

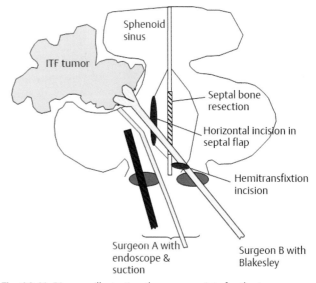

Fig. 16.41 Diagram illustrating the access points for the two-surgeon technique.

Once the tumor is removed, the tumor bed can be closely inspected to ensure no tumor remnant remains, especially in the region of the Vidian canal. If remnants are seen, they are carefully removed. Once hemostasis is achieved with the suction bipolar forceps, the preserved mucosa from the posterior wall of the maxillary sinus is replaced. Surgicel (Ethicon; Somerville, NJ) or Gelfoam powder (Pfizer; Kalamazoo, MI) can be placed in the cavity if required and the horizontal incision in the septal mucosa is sutured. This stitch is continued anteriorly as a through and through plication suture of the septum until it is brought out at the base of the Freer incision and used as a continuous suture to close this incision.

The final step is to ensure that the lacrimal sac is adequately exposed to prevent postoperative stenosis and epiphora. Without intraoperative management of lacrimal sac, the incidence of postoperative epiphora has been described to be as high as 30%.[7]

◆ Results of Endoscopic Removal of Juvenile Nasopharyngeal Angiofibromas

In a series of 18 consecutive patients with angiofibroma managed endoscopically, 12 patients had extensive disease requiring endoscopic medial maxillectomy.[6,11] The classification of Radkowski et al[12] was used to classify the patients and the distribution of the patients in each category is presented in **Table 16.3**. Only patients classified as either IIC or IIIA required endoscopic medial maxillectomy for an entirely endoscopic removal of their tumor.

All patients described in this series have had regular postoperative MRI scans. In two patients, there was residual tissue enhancement with contrast in the region of the Vidian canal. Both of these patients have had repeated MRI scans over a number of years without any enlargement of this enhancing area and are monitored monthly for any change. Whether this enhancement reflects disease recurrence or increased tissue vascularity is unclear but revision

surgery will only be offered if this tissue shows growth on repeated MRI scans. The rest of the patients are currently disease free with an average follow-up time of 6 years. The patient numbers have increased from the recently published series[6,11] to include all patients operated upon over the last 10 years.

Schwannoma Involving the Pterygopalatine and Infratemporal Fossae

Medial maxillectomy also provides access to other tumors that may involve the pterygopalatine and infratemporal fossa. In **Fig. 16.42** a schwannoma of the maxillary nerve involves the entire pterygopalatine fossa and extends significantly into the infratemporal fossa. Medial maxillectomy allows access to the entire posterior wall of the maxillary sinus and after its removal to the tumor.

Fig. 16.43 illustrates the tumor seen in **Fig. 16.42** after endoscopic medial maxillectomy and tumor removal. It was confirmed histologically to be a schwannoma.

Malignant Tumors Involving the Nasal Cavity, Sinuses, and Pterygopalatine and Infratemporal Fossae

Currently the role of endoscopic resection for the management of malignant tumors involving the pterygopalatine fossa and infratemporal fossa is unclear.[13,14] Recently, there have been some studies published utilizing endoscopic resection for malignant tumors of the nasal cavity and sinuses but the authors have stressed that long-term follow-up is not available for these patients and that radical resection with open approaches remains the gold standard.[13,14] In our practice patients are offered standard external approaches and radical resection if the tumor involves the orbit or does not have a well-defined margin. This is especially true for squamous carcinoma. If the tumor margin is well defined on radiology then endoscopic tumor removal with postoperative radiotherapy with or without chemotherapy is offered. Most malignancies in the nose and sinuses have a pushing front and do not infiltrate through the orbital periosteum or dura. These tumors are usually soft and there is usually a surgical plane between the tumor and the natural boundaries of the nose and sinuses. In some instances where there is localized infiltration of the tumor into the dura or orbital periosteum, this can be endoscopically resected and, in the case of the dura, repaired.

The principle of malignant tumor removal is to first debulk the tumor to create space in the nose in which to operate. This is easily done with a Blakesley forceps (to allow tumor to be sent for histology) and a microdebrider blade. No attempt is made to remove tumor from surrounding structures. Once there is space to operate then a surgical plane is established between the tumor and the lamina papyracea or, if absent, the orbital periosteum. In the region of the skull base this plane is established between the

Table 16.3 Radkowski et al[12] classification of juvenile angiofibromas

Stage	Description	n = 18
IA	Limited to nose and nasopharyngeal area	1
IB	Extension into one or more sinus	0
IIA	Minimal extension into pterygopalatine fossa	2
IIB	Occupation of the pterygopalatine fossa without orbital erosion	5
IIC	Infratemporal fossa extension without cheek or pterygoid plate involvement	4
IIIA	Erosion of the skull base (middle cranial fossa or pterygoids)	6
IIIB	Erosion of skull base with intracranial extension with or without cavernous sinus involvement	0

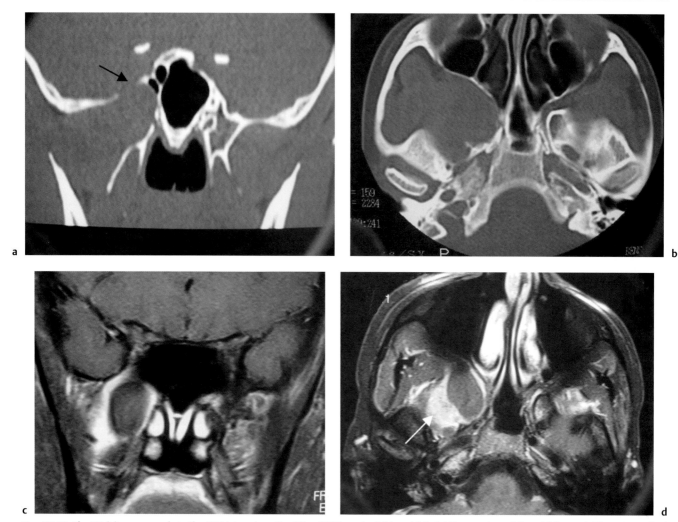

Fig. 16.42 The CT (**a**) corresponds to the MRI (**c**) as does the CT and MRI marked (**b**) and (**d**). (**a**) The erosion of the middle cranial fossa is marked with a *black arrow*. (**d**). The extension of the tumor into the infratemporal fossa is marked with a *white arrow*.

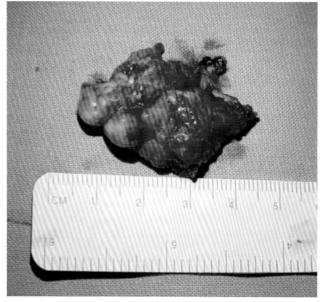

Fig. 16.43 Resected schwannoma from patient shown in **Fig. 16.42**.

skull base and, if absent, the dura. To start the dissection, the junction of the tumor and lateral nasal wall is found anteriorly and a malleable suction Freer is used to elevate the mucosa anterior to the tumor, establishing the plane between mucosa and bone. This allows the surgical plane to be established around the margins of the tumor. If this plane is followed either onto the exposed orbital periosteum or dura, tumor can be dissected off the periosteum or dura without its disruption. In this way, it is usually possible to remove all macroscopic tumors that do not invade these structures and allows preservation of the underlying periosteum and dura. If, however, the tumor invades the periosteum or dura then the dura/periosteum is resected. In the following case example the patient presented with a sinonasal undifferentiated carcinoma (SNUC) (**Fig. 16.44**). The surgical plan was to attempt endoscopic tumor removal but if necessary to combine endoscopic resection with a craniotomy. At the time of surgery, complete macroscopic resection was achieved endoscopically and we

felt that there would be no additional benefit in performing a craniotomy. The patient underwent postoperative radiotherapy and to date is still disease free (5+ years of follow-up).

In the following case example a patient presented with a chondrosarcoma with significant proptosis, diplopia, and nasal obstruction (**Fig. 16.45**). He was elderly (85 years) and in poor general health and the Combined Oncology Head and Neck Clinic felt that he would not be suitable for craniofacial resection and so he was offered endoscopic resection and radiotherapy. The tumor was debulked and after space was created, a good surgical plane was able to be established anterior to the tumor origin. The tumor was then able to be dissected off the dura and the orbital periosteum. There was no invasion into the dura or orbital periosteum. An endoscopic medial maxillectomy was performed to improve lateral access. Complete macroscopic tumor removal was achieved and the patient was offered postoperative radiotherapy.

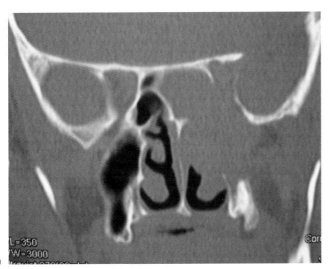

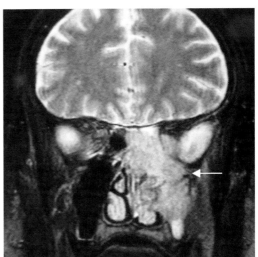

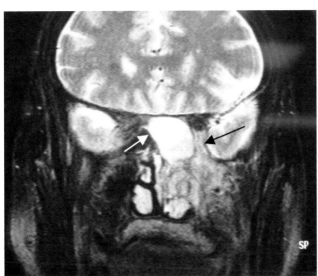

Fig. 16.44 (a) CT scan shows erosion of the lateral wall of the sphenoid, erosion of the upper pterygoid plates, and widening of the supraorbital fissure. (b) MRI scan shows extension of the tumor into the infratemporal fossa (*white arrow*) and (c) extension of tumor through the supraorbital fissure into the potential space between the lateral wall of the sphenoid and the temporal lobe (*black arrow*). The sphenoid is filled with mucus (*white arrow*).

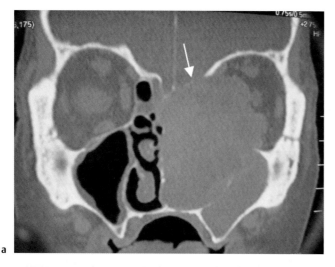

a

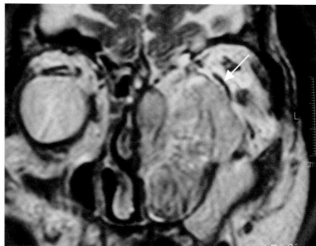

b

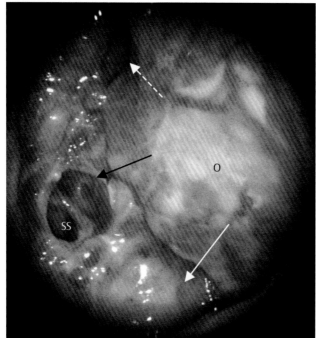

c

Fig. 16.45 (**a**) CT scan shows the skull base has been eroded (*white arrow*) and there is significant compression of the orbit. (**b**) MRI scan shows the compression rather than invasion of the orbit is illustrated by the medial rectus (*white arrow*) being pushed up against the optic nerve. (**c**) The postoperative picture clearly shows the sphenoid sinus (*SS*) and orbit (*O*) can be clearly seen with the posterior ethmoid artery (*black arrow*), maxillary sinus (*white arrow*), and frontal ostium visible (*broken white arrow*).

◆ Postoperative Care

Broad-spectrum antibiotics are continued for 10 days after surgery. Douching of the nose with saline is started immediately postoperatively. Crusting will usually continue until mucosal healing has taken place. If the patient requires radiotherapy then this may worsen during and immediately after radiotherapy. In most patients crusting is not problematic in the long term although some patients (who have had radiotherapy) can continue to have significant crusting if mucociliary drainage is not reestablished after some months. Topical douches with an ampule (2 mL of 1 mg/mL) of budesonide diluted in 240 mL of saline is used to wash the nasal cavity and sinuses once daily. This is highly effective and, if successful, can be used for months or even years to keep the patient symptom free.

◆ Conclusion

Knowledge of the anatomy of the pterygopalatine and infratemporal fossae, supraorbital fissure, and adjacent parasphenoid region including the Vidian canal is essential if tumors in these areas are to be endoscopically addressed. This chapter presents a detailed overview of this anatomy and the various endoscopic surgical techniques used to address this region.

References

1. Hyams VJ. Papillomas of the nasal cavity and paranasal sinuses. A clinicopathological study of 315 cases. Ann Otol Rhinol Laryngol 1971; 80(2):192–206
2. Keleş N, Değer K. Endonasal endoscopic surgical treatment of paranasal sinus inverted papilloma—first experiences. Rhinology 2001;39(3): 156–159
3. Sukenik MA, Casiano R. Endoscopic medial maxillectomy for inverted papillomas of the paranasal sinuses: value of the intraoperative endoscopic examination. Laryngoscope 2000;110(1):39–42
4. Krouse JH. Development of a staging system for inverted papilloma. Laryngoscope 2000;110(6):965–968
5. Wormald PJ, Ooi E, van Hasselt CA, Nair S. Endoscopic removal of sinonasal inverted papilloma including endoscopic medial maxillectomy. Laryngoscope 2003;113(5):867–873
6. Wormald PJ, Van Hasselt A. Endoscopic removal of juvenile angiofibromas. Otolaryngol Head Neck Surg 2003;129(6):684–691
7. Vrabec DP. The inverted Schneiderian papilloma: a 25-year study. Laryngoscope 1994;104(5 Pt 1):582–605
8. Chiu AG, Jackman AH, Antunes MB, Feldman MD, Palmer JN. Radiographic and histologic analysis of the bone underlying inverted papillomas. Laryngoscope 2006;116(9):1617–1620
9. Krouse JH. Endoscopic treatment of inverted papilloma: safety and efficacy. Am J Otolaryngol 2001;22(2):87–99
10. Melroy CT, Senior BA. Benign sinonasal neoplasms: a focus on inverting papilloma. Otolaryngol Clin North Am 2006;39(3):601–617, x
11. Douglas R, Wormald PJ. Endoscopic surgery for juvenile nasopharyngeal angiofibroma: where are the limits? Curr Opin Otolaryngol Head Neck Surg 2006;14(1):1–5
12. Radkowski D, McGill T, Healy GB, Ohlms L, Jones DT. Angiofibroma. Changes in staging and treatment. Arch Otolaryngol Head Neck Surg 1996;122(2):122–129
13. Batra PS, Citardi MJ. Endoscopic management of sinonasal malignancy. Otolaryngol Clin North Am 2006;39(3):619–637, x–xi
14. Stamm AC, Pignatari SS, Vellutini E. Transnasal endoscopic surgical approaches to the clivus. Otolaryngol Clin North Am 2006;39(3):639–656, xi

17 Endoscopic Resection of the Eustachian Tube and Postnasal Space

◆ Introduction

The most common tumor of the postnasal space is nasopharyngeal carcinoma. Fortunately, these tumors are radiosensitive and there is seldom a need for surgical excision. In rare cases, nasopharyngeal carcinoma that has recurred despite repeated radiotherapy may need surgical excision. In these cases, recurrent tumor is best managed by external procedures such as the maxillary swing technique, transmaxillary approach, facial translocation, transcervico-mandibulo-palatal, infratemporal fossa, and lateral infratemporal middle fossa.[1–7] These recurrent carcinomas are usually only suitable for endoscopic excision if the tumor has not extensively infiltrated the surrounding structures.[8,9] When a patient has previously undergone radiotherapy there is usually significant fibrosis that will often obliterate surgical planes making surgical dissection very difficult. If the tumor significantly infiltrates the surrounding tissue, it is removed by traditional techniques with appropriate vascular control. However, there are a small number of rare benign and malignant tumors that occur in the postnasal space and eustachian tube that are nonresponsive to radiotherapy and are best treated by primary surgical excision. Examples of these are the minor salivary gland tumors (benign and malignant), malignant melanomas, and juvenile angiofibromas. These tumors usually have an identifiable plane and a pushing front that will allow identification of the surgical plane and can be excised endoscopically even if there is limited extension into the parapharyngeal space. Endoscopic resection is appealing as it allows a complete resection of the tumor with minimal morbidity in contrast to the external approaches that have significant associated morbidity. To perform endoscopic resections in this region, a detailed knowledge of the anatomy is necessary.

◆ Anatomy

The key anatomical landmark is the medial pterygoid plate. The relationship of the medial pterygoid plate, medial pterygoid muscle, tensor palatini, levator palatini, and eustachian tube needs to be understood. If the postnasal space is viewed endoscopically the medial pterygoid plate, eustachian tube, and fossa of Rosenmüller can be clearly seen (**Fig. 17.1**).

In order to access the eustachian tube (ET), the medial pterygoid plate needs to be removed and the underlying medial pterygoid muscle exposed (**Figs. 17.2** and **17.3**). Note how the tensor palatine muscle forms a natural surgical plane as it attaches to the anterior aspect of the ET (**Fig. 17.4**). Inferiorly, the ET lies on the levator palatini muscle as it moves laterally to its attachment to the skull base (**Fig. 17.4**). The lateral pterygoid muscle attaches to the lateral aspect of the lateral pterygoid plate and is usually not seen in the dissection unless there is significant infratemporal fossa extension of the tumor. Just anterior to where the ET attaches to the skull base, the mandibular branch (V3) of the trigeminal nerve is seen (**Fig. 17.5**). Directly posterior to V3, in the apex of the fossa of Rosenmüller, the internal carotid artery can be seen (**Figs. 17.2** and **17.5**).

◆ Surgical Approach

The nose is prepared in the standard fashion. A pterygopalatine fossa block is placed through the mouth and greater palatine canal into the pterygopalatine fossa. The first step for this surgery is to remove the posterior half of the inferior turbinate. A large middle meatal antrostomy is done with exposure of the posterior wall of the maxillary sinus (**Fig. 17.6**). The middle meatal antrostomy is taken down to the floor of the nose and the mucosa over the medial pterygoid plate is elevated (**Fig. 17.7**).

In order to access this region a two-surgeon approach is advocated. The use of both nostrils allows greater angulation and, if significant bleeding occurs, clearance of blood, so that surgery can continue. The first step is to raise a Hadad pedicled septal flap on the contralateral side (see Chapter 20) to the tumor. The posterior aspect of the tumor side of the

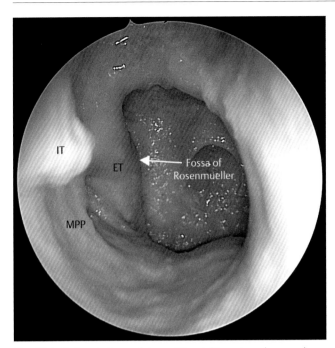

Fig. 17.1 Cadaveric image taken of the right postnasal space showing the posterior attachment of the inferior turbinate (*IT*) to the vertical portion of the palatine bone. The right medial pterygoid plate (*MPP*) can be seen as a mucosal prominence directly anterior to the eustachian tube (*ET*). The fossa of Rosenmüller can be seen behind the ET.

septum is mobilized by making superior and inferior horizontal incisions then, by joining them with a posterior vertical incision, creating an anterior pedicled flap. This flap is now rotated anteriorly and fixed with a 30 Vicryl (Ethicon; Somerville, NJ) plication suture. Additionally, to help the passage of instruments in and out of the nose during the two-surgeon approach, a 5–6 × 1.5 cm piece of thin silastic can be placed across the columella and the limbs pushed down each nostril and sutured with silk plication suture placed in the same manner as the septal suture. This results in the removal of the posterior half of the septum and gives great access to both sides of the postnasal space for the two-surgeon approach. This access allows the ET and tumor to be placed on traction when dissection is being performed in the lateral regions of the postnasal space that increases the safety by pulling the ET and tumor medially lessening the risk to the carotid artery (**Fig. 17.8**).

The next step is to remove the bone of the medial pterygoid plate using a Stylus skull base curved diamond bur (Medtronic ENT) (**Fig. 17.3**). As the bone is removed, the descending palatine artery is exposed. This needs to be cauterized using the suction bipolar then divided. This gives the surgeon access to the medial pterygoid muscle and the lateral pterygoid plate. The medial pterygoid muscle is surrounded by a dense venous plexus and sharp dissection of this muscle can result in significant venous bleeding. We prefer to use the coblation wand to remove this muscle as this can be done without significant bleeding.

There is a natural surgical plane anterior to the ET. This is formed by the cartilaginous anterior aspect of the ET and

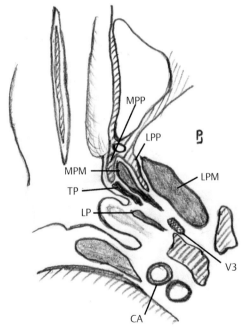

a

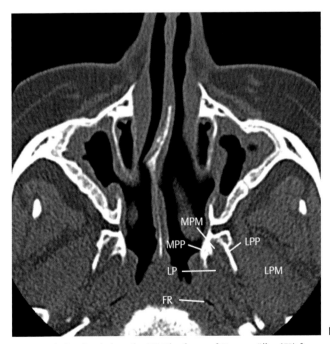

b

Fig. 17.2 In diagram (**a**) and axial CT scan (**b**), the medial pterygoid plate (*MPP*) and lateral pterygoid plate (*LPP*) are identified. The medial pterygoid muscle (*MPM*) is seen between these two plates. The lateral pterygoid muscle (*LPM*) is seen lateral to the LPP. The levator palatini (*LP*) attaches to the medial aspect of the eustachian tube, whereas the

tensor palatine lies below the ET. The fossa of Rosenmüller (*FR*) forms most of the posterior boundary of the ET. Note the relationship of the mandibular nerve (*V3*) and the carotid artery (*CA*) to the apex of the fossa of Rosenmüller and V3.

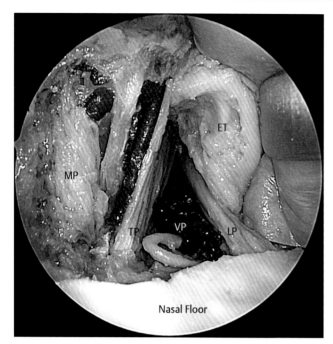

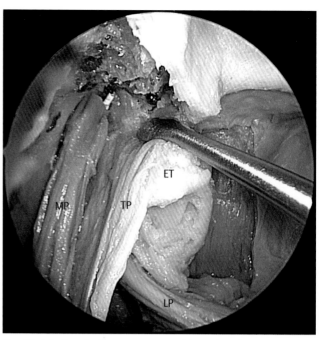

Fig. 17.3 Cadaveric dissection image taken with a 70-degree endoscope of the right eustachian tube (*ET*). A mucosal flap has been elevated revealing the cartilaginous ET. The right medial pterygoid plate has been drilled away, revealing the deep head of the medial pterygoid muscle (*MP*), along with the tensor palatini (*TP*) and levator palatini (*LP*) muscles. The fibrofatty tissue located between the TP and LP has been removed to reveal a vascular plexus (*VP*).

Fig. 17.4 Cadaveric dissection image of the right side demonstrating tensor palatini (*TP*) attaching to the anterior aspect of the cartilaginous eustachian tube (*ET*). *LP*, levator palatini; *MP*, medial pterygoid muscle.

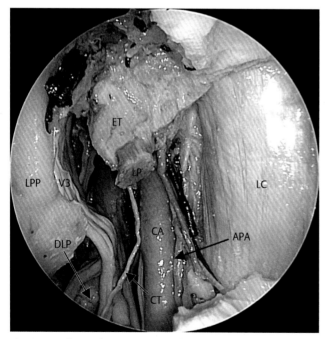

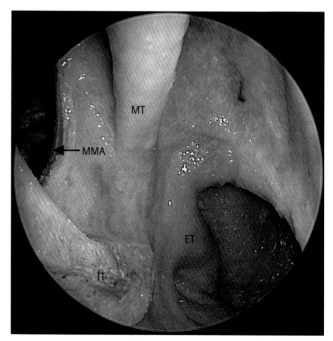

Fig. 17.5 Cadaveric dissection image taken with a 30-degree endoscope following resection of the majority of the cartilaginous eustachian tube (*ET*), and only a remnant stump can be seen, which attaches to the skull base. Directly anterior to this remnant is the mandibular branch of the trigeminal nerve (*V3*). Directly posterior is the carotid artery (*CA*), seen directly posterior to the attachment of the levator palatini muscle (*LP*). This muscle is a good landmark to the point that the artery enters the carotid canal. *LPP*, lateral pterygoid plate; *DLP*, deep lobe of the parotid gland; *CT*, chorda tympani; *APA*, ascending pharyngeal artery; *LC*, longus capitis.

Fig. 17.6 Cadaveric dissection image taken of the right nasal cavity. A large middle meatal antrostomy has been performed. The posterior attachment of the middle turbinate (*MT*) and inferior turbinate (*IT*) to the lateral nasal wall is clearly visualized. The inferior turbinate has been excised.

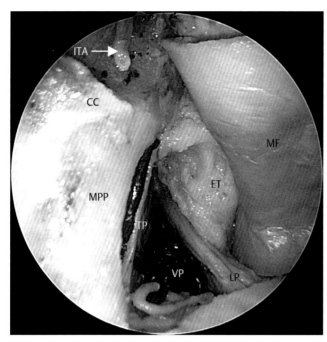

Fig. 17.7 Cadaveric dissection image shows the mucosal flap (*MF*) over the medial pterygoid plate (*MPP*) has been elevated and the cartilaginous eustachian tube (*ET*) and levator palatini (*LP*) muscle has been exposed. The conchal crest (posterior attachment of the inferior turbinate to the palatine bone) can be clearly seen. The fibrofatty tissue between the tensor palatini muscle (*TP*) and levator palatini muscles (*LP*) has been excised to reveal a rich vascular plexus (*VP*). The inferior turbinate (*ITA*) branch from the sphenopalatine artery can be visualized.

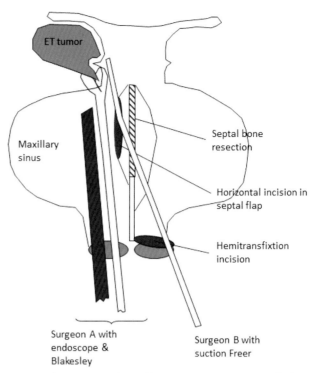

Fig. 17.8 The resection of septal bone is more posterior as is the horizontal incision in the elevated septal mucosal flap. The two-surgeon technique allows greater flexibility in instrument placement and better angulation to the region of the tumor.

the attached fibrous aponeurosis of the tensor palatini. If the aponeurosis is followed inferiorly the tensor palatini muscle fibers can be seen (**Fig. 17.9**). The surgical removal of the medial pterygoid plate and partial removal of the medial pterygoid muscle with establishment of the anterior surgical plane can be also appreciated (**Fig. 17.10**).

The next step is to release the ET inferiorly and posteriorly (**Fig. 17.11**). These horizontal and posterior incisions are made with the coblation wand to minimize bleeding. The horizontal incision cuts through the tensor and levator palatini muscles and further dissection enters the parapharyngeal space. The dissection is continued laterally directly

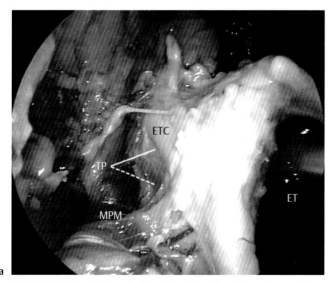

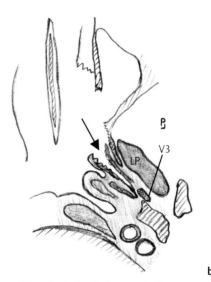

Fig. 17.9 (**a**) The right eustachian tube (*ET*) orifice defines the medial extent of the dissection. The medial pterygoid muscle (*MPM*) is being swept laterally with the dissector exposing the anterior cartilage of the ET (*ETC*). Attached to this cartilage is the tensor palatini (*TP*) fibrous aponeurosis

(*solid white line*) with its muscle fibers seen below (*broken white line*). (**b**) The resection of the inferior turbinate, posterior medial maxilla, medial pterygoid plate, and medial pterygoid muscle can be appreciated. The *solid black arrow* indicates the surgical plane anterior to the ET but medial to V3.

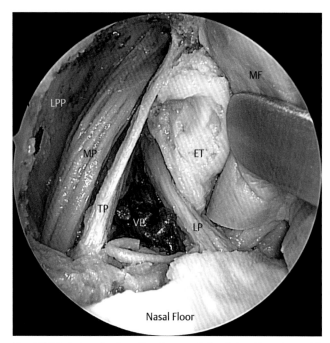

Fig. 17.10 Cadaveric dissection image of the right side, taken with a 30-degree endoscope. The medial pterygoid plate has been drilled away revealing the lateral pterygoid plate (*LPP*) once some fibers of the deep head of the medial pterygoid muscle (*MP*) have been resected. *TP*, tensor palatini; *VP*, vascular plexus; *LP*, levator palatini; *ET*, eustachian tube; *MF*, mucosal flap.

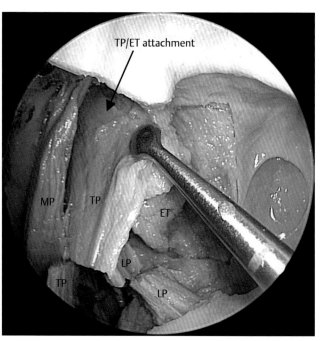

Fig. 17.11 Cadaveric dissection demonstrating the inferior horizontal incision taken through the tensor palatini (*TP*) and levator palatini (*LP*) muscles. The attachment of the TP muscle to the anterior cartilaginous eustachian tube (*ET*) can be clearly seen with a surgical plane directly anterior to this. The ET has been retracted medially and posteriorly. *MP*, deep head of the medial pterygoid muscle.

under the ET thereby mobilizing the ET from the parapharyngeal space. If the fossa of Rosenmüller is to be included in the resection, the posterior incision is made onto the longus capitis muscle. The surgical plane is anterior to the fascia of this muscle. If the plane is deep to these muscles the carotid artery and jugular vein are at increased risk in the most lateral extent of the fossa (**Fig. 17.5**).

The ET complex is relatively immobile until the fibrous attachment of the ET to the skull base is cut. As this tissue is tough, these incisions need to be done with sharp instruments such as the angled scissors from the Skull Base Set* (Integra). It is not advisable to use a scalpel to perform this step as the internal carotid artery is at risk during this maneuver. It is better to use the natural curve of the scissors angled medially (away from the carotid). In addition, the second surgeon should place the ET under traction thereby allowing each cut made with the scissors to be more effective and less likely to damage the internal carotid.

Once the ET has been removed, the surrounding anatomical structures can be clearly identified (**Fig. 17.12**). Further dissection in **Fig. 17.13** demonstrates the lateral pterygoid plate, mandibular branch of the trigeminal nerve, ascending pharyngeal artery, a portion of the deep lobe of the parotid gland, the cervical carotid artery entering the petrous temporal bone, and also the longus capitis muscle. Above and lateral to the attachment of the ET to the skull base is the mandibular branch (V3) of the trigeminal nerve. The internal carotid artery is usually posterior and in some patients more lateral than V3.

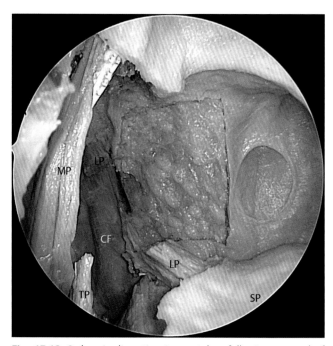

Fig. 17.12 Cadaveric dissection image taken following removal of the cartilaginous eustachian tube. The carotid fascia (*CF*) can be seen overlying the carotid artery just behind the stump of the levator palatini (*LP*) muscle. This muscle is a good landmark for entry of the carotid artery into the carotid canal, which is directly posterior to the attachment of the levator palatini muscle to the skull base. *TP*, tensor palatini muscle; *MP*, deep head of the medial pterygoid muscle; *SP*, soft palate.

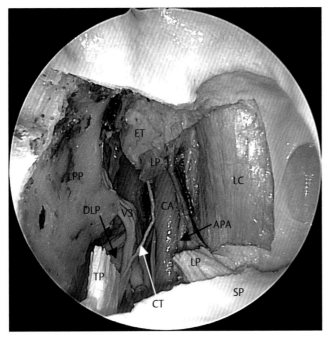

Fig. 17.13 Cadaveric dissection image taken with a 30-degree endoscope, with the removal of the carotid fascia and deep lobe of the medial pterygoid muscle on the right side. This reveals the lateral pterygoid plate (*LPP*) and the mandibular branch of the trigeminal nerve (*V3*) just anterior to the attachment of the eustachian tube (*ET*) to the skull base. *LC*, longus capitis muscle; *LP*, levator palatini muscle; *TP*, tensor palatini muscle; *SP*, soft palate; *CA*, carotid artery; *APA*, ascending pharyngeal artery; *CT*, chorda tympani; *DLP*, deep lobe of parotid gland.

◆ Postoperative Care

Hemostasis is achieved with the suction bipolar forceps. The pedicled septal flap is rotated into place to cover the dissection bed and edges are secured with Surgicel (Ethicon). The area is covered using a fibrin glue sealant. No packing

is placed. Broad-spectrum antibiotics are given for 10 days. In order to decrease postoperative crusting, the patient performs regular nasal douches using the squeeze bottle nasal wash method. Nasal toilet is performed at 2 weeks postoperatively and as necessary thereafter. A repeat MRI scan is performed to ensure that there is no tumor recurrence at 6 and 12 months and yearly thereafter.

◆ Case Examples

We have had three patients in recent years in whom we have performed this surgery. The first patient had a malignant melanoma of the mucosa within the ET and the second patient had a low-grade mucoepidermoid carcinoma originating within the ET lumen and protruding through the wall of the ET into the parapharyngeal space. A component of this tumor prolapsed into the nasopharynx and caused nasal obstruction. The third patient had a recurrent juvenile angiofibroma lateral and inferior to the ET.

The patient with the mucoepidermoid carcinoma presented with nasal obstruction and the following MRI demonstrated a postnasal space mass (**Fig. 17.14**). The patient was taken to theatre and the tumor prolapsing out of the ET orifice was removed and sent for histology and the diagnosis confirmed.

The surgeon who performed the biopsy confirmed tumor remained within the ET orifice and the patient was sent to the tumor board where it was decided that endoscopic excision was the best option for the patient. Computer-aided surgery (CAS) is an important part of the surgical plan. In these cases, both CT and MRI should be loaded and a "merge" performed. This tool allows the surgeon to move between CT and MRI and to adjust the image to have any percentage blend of CT and MRI. In this case, the tumor could not be visualized on CT scanning but could be visualized on MRI scanning. Merge allowed the blend between CT and MRI to

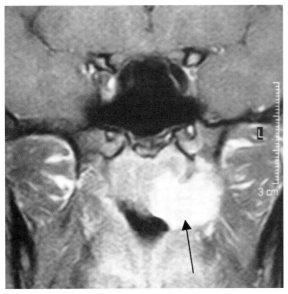
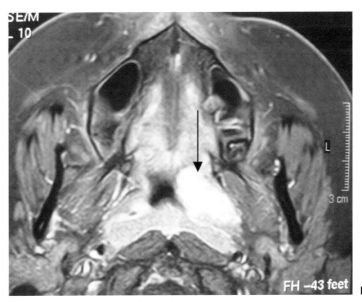

Fig. 17.14 The tumor is indicated by a *black arrow* in the coronal T1 MRI scan (**a**) and in the axial scan (**b**).

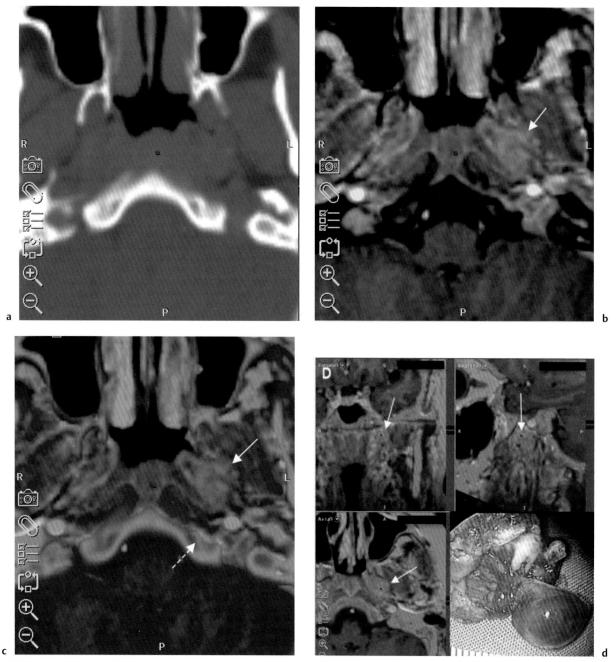

Fig. 17.15 In axial CT scan (**a**), the tumor is not clearly seen but the bony landmarks are visible. In MRI scan (**b**), the tumor is clearly seen (*white arrow*) but the bony landmarks are absent. In the merged (CT and MRI) scan (**c**) both the bony landmarks (*broken white arrow*) and tumor (*white arrow*) are clearly seen. (**d**) The intraoperative image guidance merged scan with the tumor (*white arrow*) and bony landmarks seen in all three planes. In addition, the resected eustachian tube and tumor can be seen.

be adjusted so that the bony landmarks (pterygoid plates) and the tumor were clearly visible (**Fig. 17.15**). In addition, if contrast is used, the internal carotid arteries can also be clearly seen.

This tumor, the melanoma, and angiofibroma were removed using the technique described. Biopsies of tissue remaining in the surgical bed after excision revealed no residual tumor. No additional treatment modalities were given to these patients and they have remained free of locoregional recurrence of disease. The melanoma patient has, however, developed distant metastasis.

◆ Key Points

If endoscopic surgery is to be contemplated in this area it is vitally important that the surgeon is familiar with the endoscopic anatomy of this region. The surgeon needs to create a mental three-dimensional (3D) image of the anatomy and be able to place the dissection at all times within the 3D picture. The new CAS guidance systems help significantly and the ability to merge the CT and MRI scan allows both bony and soft tissues to be accurately identified. Using the two-surgeon approach also adds significantly to the safety of the procedure as the second surgeon can keep the surgical field clear of blood and provide traction on the tumor at vital stages of the dissection. The biggest risk of this surgery is injury to the internal carotid artery and both the anesthetist and surgeon should have a surgical plan ready to put into action should this complication occur.

References

1. Fee WE Jr, Gilmer PA, Goffinet DR. Surgical management of recurrent nasopharyngeal carcinoma after radiation failure at the primary site. Laryngoscope 1988;98(11):1220–1226
2. Hsu MM, Ko JY, Sheen TS, Chang YL. Salvage surgery for recurrent nasopharyngeal carcinoma. Arch Otolaryngol Head Neck Surg 1997;123(3):305–309
3. Wei WI, Lam KH, Sham JS. New approach to the nasopharynx: the maxillary swing approach. Head Neck 1991;13(3):200–207
4. Hao SP, Tsang NM, Chang CN. Salvage surgery for recurrent nasopharyngeal carcinoma. Arch Otolaryngol Head Neck Surg 2002;128(1): 63–67
5. Morton RP, Liavaag PG, McLean M, Freeman JL. Transcervico-mandibulo-palatal approach for surgical salvage of recurrent nasopharyngeal cancer. Head Neck 1996;18(4):352–358
6. Fisch U. The infratemporal fossa approach for nasopharyngeal tumors. Laryngoscope 1983;93(1):36–44
7. Schramm VL Jr, Imola MJ. Management of nasopharyngeal salivary gland malignancy. Laryngoscope 2001;111(9):1533–1544
8. Yoshizaki T, Wakisaka N, Murono S, Shimizu Y, Furukawa M. Endoscopic nasopharyngectomy for patients with recurrent nasopharyngeal carcinoma at the primary site. Laryngoscope 2005;115(8): 1517–1519
9. Roh JL, Park CI. Transseptal laser resection of recurrent carcinoma confined to the nasopharynx. Laryngoscope 2006;116(5):839–841

18 Anatomy of the Sphenoid and Adjacent Structures of Importance during Skull Base Surgery

◆ Anatomy of the Sphenoid

When the sphenoid sinus is opened and entered with an endoscope, the surgeon should be able to identify if the sinus is the dominant sinus. The intersinus septum usually attaches to the lateral wall of the sphenoid in the region of the carotid artery. If the anterior face of the pituitary fossa is visible then the surgeon is in the dominant sinus (**Fig. 18.1**). If the sinus is small and if the septum implants on the lateral wall, the pituitary fossa should not be seen and the surgeon should be in the nondominant sinus. This should be correlated to the CT scan images. Once the intersinus septum is removed (usually with a through-biting Blakesley or diamond bur—twisting should be avoided to avoid possible damage to the carotid artery by fracturing bone), the normal structures should be identifiable. The pituitary fossa is seen in the midline with the anterior genu of the cavernous carotid seen on either side. As the carotids are followed superiorly, the optic nerves are seen at the junction of the side wall and roof. There is often a depression between the optic nerve and carotid in a well-pneumatized sphenoid which represents a pneumatization of the optic strut and is termed the opticocarotid recess (OCR) (**Fig. 18.2**). Between the medial aspect of the optic nerve at the point where it leaves the sphenoid and the anterosuperior medial region of the carotid is a slight thickening of bone termed the medial OCR and corresponds to pneumatization into the medial clinoid process. On the lateral wall, the V2 branch of the trigeminal nerve can be seen as well as the Vidian nerve in the floor of the sinus. Posterior in the midline below the pituitary fossa the clivus is visible. Depending on the sphenoid pneumatization, this bone may be either thick or quite thin. On either side of the clivus is the vertical paraclival portions of the carotid (**Fig. 18.2**). These are important landmarks for any surgical approach to the clivus.

Above the pituitary fossa is the tuberculum sella—this is a thickened area of bone that forms the junction between the anterior face of the pituitary fossa and the roof of the sphenoid (termed the planum sphenoidale).

◆ Anatomy of the Pituitary Fossa

Bone is removed from cavernous sinus to cavernous sinus, onto the floor of the fossa and up to the tuberculum sella. Care must be taken as the tuberculum sella is approached as there is a fold of dura that comes down with the tuberculum sella and if this is grabbed with the Kerrison punch, a cerebrospinal fluid (CSF) leak will result. Once the bone over the pituitary fossa has been removed, the underlying periosteum is exposed. Between the periosteum and the dura is a potential space. This space is occupied by venous channels that connect the cavernous sinuses in the upper and lower regions of the pituitary (**Fig. 18.3**). In most macroadenomas, these venous channels are obliterated by the pressure from the enlarging tumor. However, in microadenomas and tuberculum sella meningiomas, these venous plexuses remain and can bleed significantly when opened. Bipolar cautery may seal the channels but often the most effective way is to use the Aquamantas system from Medtronic ENT. This system uses radiofrequency energy and saline to seal venous channels. If this fails then Gelfoam powder (Pfizer; Kalamazoo, MI) mixed into a paste by adding saline (or Floseal [Baxter; Deerfield, IL] or Surgiflo [Ethicon; Somerville, NJ]) can be used. This is injected directly into the open venous channels and pressure is applied with a neurosurgical pattie.

◆ Lateral Wall of the Pituitary Fossa

The lateral wall of the pituitary fossa is formed by the cavernous sinus and the cavernous portion of the carotid artery. It is important for the surgeon to have a clear understanding of the carotid artery in the lateral wall of the pituitary fossa. The cavernous carotid has three parts: the horizontal, anterior genu, and clinoid. The horizontal starts at the posterior genu and is frequently seen in the lateral wall of the sella during pituitary surgery. The anterior genu is usually only in the lateral wall of the sphenoid and is infrequently seen

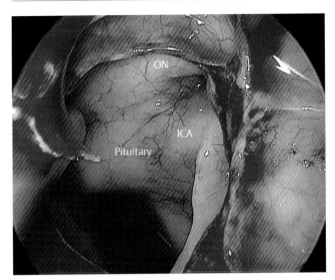

Fig. 18.1 The suction rests on the pituitary sella with a clear view of the carotid artery (*ICA*) and the optic nerve (*ON*) indicating that the surgeon is in the dominant sphenoid sinus.

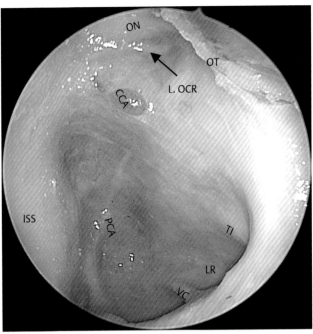

Fig. 18.2 Cadaveric dissection image taken of the left sphenoid sinus through a maximal sphenoidotomy. The Vidian canal (*VC*) and trigeminal impression (*TI*) of the maxillary division of the trigeminal nerve can be clearly seen. If the sphenoid sinus is well pneumatized, then the lateral recess (*LR*) can be seen, a depression in the lateral sphenoid wall between the VC and the TI. The lateral opticocarotid recess (*L. OCR*) can be seen. This depression corresponds to pneumatization of the optic strut (the bony bridge that separates the optic canal from the superior orbital fissure). Further pneumatization into the optic strut may result in a pneumatized anterior clinoid process which will place the optic nerve on a mesentery. The optic tubercle (*OT*) is the bone located at the junction of the orbital apex and the sphenoid sinus. *ISS*, intersinus septum; *ON*, optic nerve; *CCA*, anterior genu of the intracavernous carotid artery; *PCA*, paraclival carotid artery.

in the sella unless the tumor has pushed significantly anteriorly. The carotid may then reenter the lateral wall of the sella and tumor may push in between the horizontal portion and the upper part of the genu before the carotid leaves the cavernous sinus. As it leaves the cavernous sinus the carotid oculomotor membrane thickens to form the lower fibrous ring around the carotid. Above this ring is the clinoid section of the carotid which is short. The upper fibrous ring is

formed by the continuation of the thickened falciform ligament (**Fig. 18.4**). Tumor is routinely removed from the lateral wall with suction and standard pituitary curettes, so knowing where to expect the carotid is important for the surgeon so that care is taken not to apply any pressure over the carotid. Tumor may also need to be followed into the cavernous sinus so this anatomical understanding is crucial for the surgeon to understand where tumor may be followed. **Fig. 18.5** shows the normal course of the carotid in the lateral wall and the areas where extra care needs to be taken.

◆ Anatomy of the Cavernous Sinus

It is important to understand the anatomy of the cavernous sinus in patients in whom tumor extends into this area. If the surgeon enters the cavernous sinus from the pituitary fossa, this is usually following a tumor extension through the dura above the horizontal portion of the cavernous carotid and posterior to the anterior genu (**Fig. 18.5**). If tumor is chased lateral to the carotid, the lateral wall of the cavernous sinus may be exposed. The third nerve can be seen running horizontally in the lateral wall. As the cavernous carotid forms

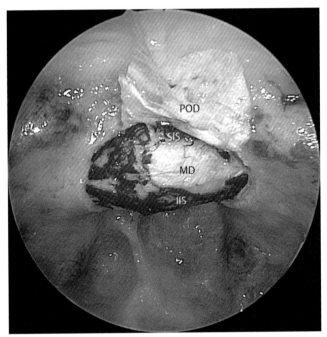

Fig. 18.3 Cadaveric dissection illustrating the exposure of the sella. In this dissection, just the periosteal layer of dura (*POD*) has been reflected, exposing the superior (*SIS*) and inferior intercavernous dural sinus (*IIS*). These sinuses run between the periosteal layer of dura and the meningeal layer of dura (*MD*).

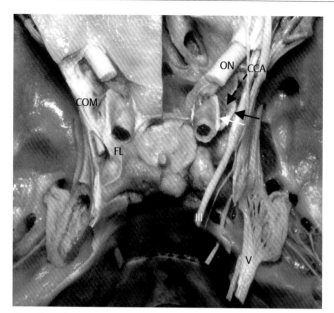

Fig. 18.4 This image is split with the left side illustrating the two fibrous rings (*black* and *white arrows*) encircling the clival carotid. On the right side, the carotid oculomotor membrane (*COM*) (*black arrow*) left side is still intact whereas the falciform ligament (*FL*) (*white arrow*) left side has been partially trimmed away from the carotid. Note how the carotid oculomotor membrane covers the oculomotor nerve (*III*). *ON*, optic nerve; *CCA*, clinoid carotid artery; *COM*, carotid oculomotor membrane; *FL*, falciform ligament; *V*, fifth nerve.

the anterior genu and becomes the clinoid carotid, the tumor may envelop this as well. It is usually not possible to chase tumor in the region of the clinoid carotid as the lower fibrous ring formed by the carotid oculomotor membrane is tough and will prevent further exploration (**Fig. 18.5**). If tumor grows anterior and lateral to the anterior genu of the cavernous carotid, the cavernous sinus may be entered via a separate incision through the dura lateral to the anterior genu. Great care should be taken with this incision and the surgeon should confirm the position of the carotid with image guidance as well as an intranasal Doppler. Gentle suction clearance of tumor in this region will often reveal the third nerve lateral and superiorly in the cavernous sinus (**Figs. 18.6 and 18.7**). If inferior dissection is performed around the anterior genu, the sixth nerve may be seen hugging its anterolateral border and traversing the cavernous sinus from medial to lateral (**Fig. 18.7**). Sympathetic branches from the carotid are often picked up by the sixth nerve as it passes the carotid. Inferiorly in the lateral wall of the cavernous sinus, the Gasserian ganglion and its branches V1, V2, and V3 can be seen (**Fig. 18.7**). Note the cavernous sinus is always above V2 which does leave an anatomical pathway under V2 into the middle cranial fossa (**Fig. 18.7**).

◆ Anatomy of the Vidian Nerve

Clinically, the Vidian nerve is always followed from the pterygopalatine fossa posteriorly into the floor of the sphenoid. It can often be seen in a well-pneumatized sphenoid as it forms an inferior ridge in the floor of the sphenoid (**Fig. 18.2**).

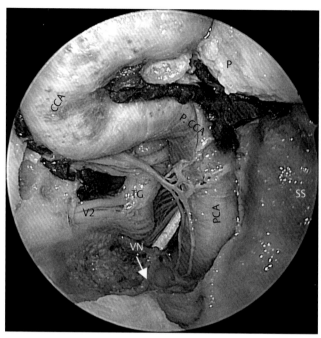

Fig. 18.5 Cadaveric dissection image of the lateral sphenoid wall following bone removal. *P*, pituitary gland; *CCA*, intracavernous carotid artery; *V2*, maxillary division of the trigeminal nerve; *TG*, trigeminal ganglion; *VN*, Vidian nerve; *PCA*, paraclival carotid artery; *P. CCA*, posterior genu of the intracavernous carotid artery; *SS*, sphenoid sinus.

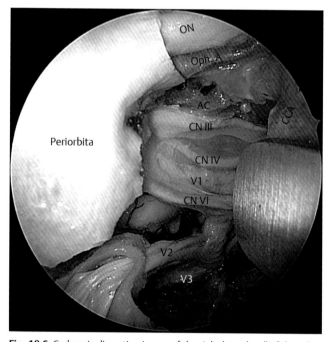

Fig. 18.6 Cadaveric dissection image of the right lateral wall of the sphenoid sinus. The bone has been removed and the anterior genu of the intracavernous carotid artery (*CCA*) retracted medially. This allows clear visualization of the nerves within the dural layers of the lateral wall of the cavernous sinus. The abducens nerve (*CN VI*) can be visualized medially, running within the cavernous sinus. Note the periorbita of the orbital apex. The bone of the anterior clinoid (*AC*) process has been left in place, positioned within the lateral opticocarotid recess. *ON*, optic nerve; *Oph. A*, ophthalmic artery; *CN III*, oculomotor nerve; *CN IV*, trochlear nerve; *V1*, ophthalmic division of the trigeminal nerve; *V2*, maxillary division of the trigeminal nerve; *V3*, mandibular division of the trigeminal nerve.

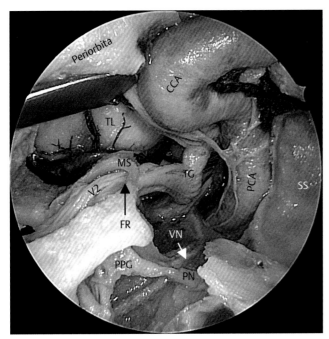

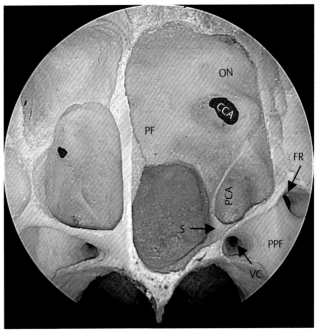

Fig. 18.7 Cadaveric dissection of the right lateral sphenoid wall following removal of the lateral sphenoid wall. Dissection has continued anteriorly to the pterygopalatine fossa inferiorly and the orbital apex superiorly. In this image, the periorbita has been retracted superiorly. Note the remnant of the maxillary strut (*MS*), the strut of bone that separates the foramen rotundum from the superior orbital fissure/orbital apex. The Vidian nerve (*VN*) can be seen moving into the posterior aspect of the pterygopalatine fossa and enters the pterygopalatine ganglion (*PPG*). The relationship between the foramen rotundum (*FR*) and the temporal lobe (*TL*) can be seen clearly. *V2*, maxillary division of the trigeminal nerve; *PN*, pharyngeal nerve; *PCA*, paraclival carotid artery; *CCA*, intracavernous carotid artery; *SS*, sphenoid sinus; *TG*, trigeminal ganglion.

Fig. 18.8 This dry bone image of the sphenoid sinus within the body of the sphenoid. It clearly demonstrates how the Vidian canal (*VC*) communicates with the pterygopalatine fossa (*PPF*) anteriorly, and the foramen lacerum posteriorly. The Vidian canal runs in the floor of the sphenoid sinus, and frequently has a sphenoid sinus septation (*S*) attaching to the roof of the canal. The foramen lacerum is the location of the supralacerum genu of the carotid artery, where the horizontal petrous carotid artery turns upward to become the paraclival carotid artery (*PCA*). The Vidian canal and nerve is a vital landmark in surgical dissection in this area. *PF*, pituitary fossa; *FR*, foramen rotundum; *CCA*, anterior genu of the cavernous carotid artery.

It forms an important lateral boundary when surgeons remove the floor of the sphenoid in preparation for approaching the clivus (**Fig. 18.8**). If the Vidian nerve is followed posteriorly it initially approaches the supralacerum genu of the carotid artery at its medial aspect but then moves laterally and over the top of the petrous portion of the carotid (**Fig. 18.7**). If the Vidian nerve is been followed to the petroclival genu, this anatomical relationship needs to be clearly understood otherwise the carotid may be inadvertently damaged during this dissection. In the petrous region of the carotid the deep petrosal nerve (sympathetic fibers) joins with the greater superficial petrosal nerve (parasympathetic fibers) to form the Vidian nerve.

◆ Anatomy of the Clivus

The clivus is flanked by the paraclival carotids and extends from the floor of the sphenoid up to the floor of the pituitary fossa. The thickness of the bone of the clivus varies depending upon the pneumatization of the sphenoid. The first step in transclival approaches to the posterior fossa is to accurately identify both paraclival carotids. This prevents inadvertent injury. With the paraclival carotids visible, the bone of the

clivus can be removed to expose the periosteum. Between the periosteum and the dura are a collection of venous lakes: the basilar plexus. These can bleed extensively and often require the dura to be opened, rolled, and bipolared to stem the bleeding. Again, the Aquamantas from Medtronic ENT is useful for stopping bleeding from these venous lakes. Additionally, Gelfoam paste or Surgiflo is used with neuropatties in an attempt to fill these venous lakes and stem the bleeding. One of the most important structures encountered in this region is the sixth nerve. The sixth nerve leaves the pons just lateral to the vertebrobasilar junction and moves laterally, traversing the post fossa (termed the cisternal segment) until it enters the dura (at Dorello's point) and runs between the dura and the clival periosteum in the space between the layers called Dorello's canal (**Figs. 18.9** and **18.10**). Dorello's point can usually be found just behind the carotid about midway between the sphenoid floor and pituitary fossa. A good landmark is the dorsal meningeal artery found just medial to the entry of the nerve into Dorello's canal. Other landmarks include the distance from the posterior clinoid, which averages 20 mm and usually 10 mm from the midline. Dorello's canal runs just below the gulfar venous plexus. This venous plexus is formed between dura and periosteum and is made up of the inferior petrosal venous sinus, the posterior part of the cavernous sinus, and the basilar venous plexus. These all

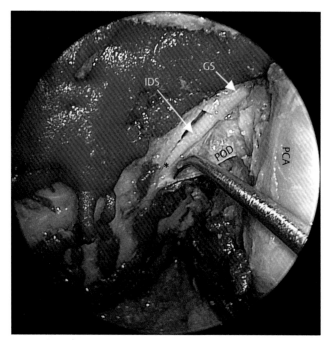

Fig. 18.9 Cadaveric dissection of the left middle clivus (taken with a 30-degree endoscope) demonstrating the different segments of the abducens nerve. The abducens nerve moves through the posterior cranial fossa (cisternal segment) before perforating through the meningeal layer of dura (marked by *asterisk*). Then the nerve enters a channel between the meningeal layer of dura and the periosteal layer of dura (*POD*). This segment is called the interdural segment (*IDS*). In this dissection, a leaf of periosteal dural (*POD*) has been incised and reflexed to clearly visualize the abducens nerve running within. The nerve then enters the confluence of dural sinus, made up of the superior and inferior petrosal sinuses, the basilar plexus, and the cavernous sinus. Here it is called the gulfar segment (*GS*). *PCA*, paraclival carotid artery.

join in this region and the nerve runs in the floor of this so-called gulfar segment. Another landmark in this area is the sphenopetrosal ligament (Gruber's) that is formed from the posterior clinoid process and lateral aspect of the dorsum sella to the petrous apex. After the nerve enters the back of the cavernous sinus below the horizontal portion of the cavernous carotid, it travels forward and hugs the inferior aspect of the anterior genu of the carotid before traversing the cavernous sinus on the lateral wall of the cavernous sinus. From here it enters the superior orbital fissure and into the orbit.

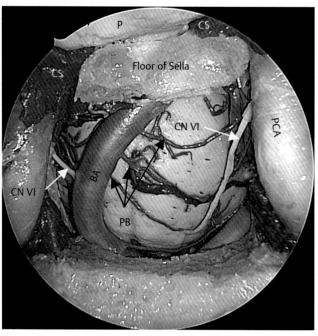

Fig. 18.10 Cadaveric dissection following removal of the middle one-third of the clivus and dura. The very tortuous basilar artery (*BA*) can be seen. Its pontine branches (*PB*) can be clearly seen. *CN VI*, abducens nerve; *CS*, cavernous sinus; *P*, pituitary gland; *PCA*, paraclival carotid artery.

Anatomy of V2

The maxillary branch of the trigeminal nerve leaves the cavernous sinus from the Gasserian ganglion and precedes horizontally toward the foramen rotundum and the pterygopalatine fossa. In a well-pneumatized sphenoid, a well-defined ridge is formed in the lateral wall called the trigeminal impression (**Fig. 18.2**). The sphenoid may also pneumatize under the nerve thinning the bone between the sphenoid and the middle cranial fossa. This pneumatization may also develop into the upper root of the pterygoid plates. This thin plate between the middle cranial fossa and a laterally pneumatized sphenoid is a common site for prolapse of dura and the development of a spontaneous CSF leaks.

19 Endoscopic Resection of Clival and Posterior Cranial Fossa Tumors

◆ Introduction

Tumors of the clivus and posterior cranial fossa are very difficult to access via traditional neurosurgical approaches. In the past, skull base teams would approach the petroclival region either by a lateral or anterior route. The lateral route was via an extended middle cranial fossa approach,[1] whereas the anterior route could be transmaxillary, transoral, or transcervical.[2,3] All of these approaches involve significant resection of normal structures with inevitable associated morbidity.[1-4] Even after such a resection, the final surgical access was usually limited. The operating microscope did not allow a view around the corner and if the tumor extended beyond the exposed area, resection under direct vision was not possible.

The advantage of the endoscopic transsphenoidal approach is that it allows access to the entire clivus down to the atlas of the cervical spine. It also allows early identification of the vital vascular structures with clear visualization of both carotid arteries and the cavernous sinuses and associated neurological structures.[4] The most common tumor presenting in the clival region is a chordoma. Although complete resection of the tumor and the surrounding bone is optimal, this is often not possible due to the location and surrounding vital structures.[2,5] It is accepted that as complete a resection as is possible should be performed.[5] In most cases clival chordomas are slow growing and if surgery can be combined with radiotherapy (especially proton beam radiotherapy), this gives the patient the best possible chance of prolonged survival.[2,5] Because curative surgery is often not possible, the morbidity associated with tumor debulking should be as limited as possible. These factors make an endoscopic approach to these tumors attractive as it provides the best possible chance of complete surgical removal with the least surgical morbidity.[4,5] In order to remove the clival tumor and any associated intracranial extension, a clear understanding of the anatomy of this region is essential.

◆ Anatomy of the Clivus, Posterior Cranial Fossa, and Cavernous Sinus

The Clivus

The clivus extends from the dorsum sella to the foramen magnum (**Figs. 19.1** and **19.2**). The thickness of the clivus depends on the pneumatization of the sphenoid and can vary significantly. When this bone is thick, it may hold significant venous channels (**Fig. 19.3**). This makes removal of the bone a slow process as significant bleeding can occur as the cancellous bone is opened. This is generally quickly controlled by packing the area with Gelfoam (Pfizer; Kalamazoo, MI) paste made up from combining Gelfoam powder and saline into a paste. Further drilling will provoke more bleeding which requires repacking and this process can make bone removal tedious. However, there is no quick and easy solution to the control of the bleeding in this area. The lateral borders of the dissection of the clivus are the paraclival carotid arteries and these need to be exposed at the beginning of the dissection to avoid inadvertent damage (**Fig. 19.4**). The inferior limit of the dissection is usually the floor of the sphenoid but should access be required to the basiocciput, foramen magnum, or even lower to the first cervical vertebra, the entire sphenoid floor should be removed (**Fig. 19.4**).

Complete removal of the clivus exposes the dura of the posterior fossa. Bone behind the inferior portion of the paraclival carotid arteries can be removed so that the arteries stand proud of the lateral margins (**Fig. 19.5**). The limit to which this bone can be removed is determined by the 45-degree angle that the carotid arteries make as they run in their canals through the petrous temporal bone. This region where the petrous portion of the carotid artery turns vertically in the floor of the sphenoid is where bone should be removed to access the petrous apex. In some patients, a large cholesterol granuloma may thin down the bone separating

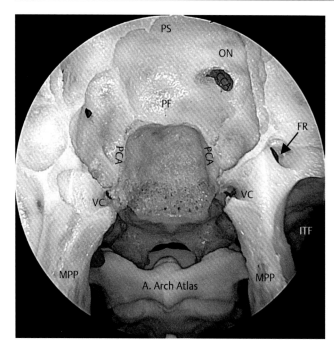

Fig. 19.1 Dry skull dissection with the floor of the sphenoid sinus drilled away revealing the middle and lower thirds of the clivus. The Vidian canals (VC) can be seen bilaterally at the level of the floor of the sphenoid sinus. PS, planum sphenoidale; PF, pituitary fossa; ON, optic nerve; CCA, anterior genu of the intracavernous carotid artery; FR, foramen rotundum; PCA, paraclival carotid artery; MPP, medial pterygoid plate; FR, foramen rotundum; A. Arch Atlas, anterior arch of atlas; ITF, infratemporal fossa.

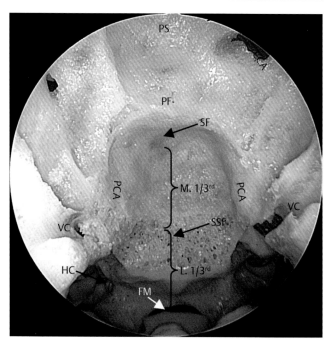

Fig. 19.2 Dry bone specimen demonstrating the middle and lower thirds of the clivus. The middle third (M. 1/3rd) begins at the sella floor (SF) and extends to the floor of the sphenoid sinus (SSF), and the lower third (L. 1/3rd) extends from the floor of the sphenoid sinus to the foramen magnum (FM). The upper third corresponds to the dorsum sella, and visualization is obstructed by the pituitary gland. A pituitary transposition allows visualization of the upper third of the clivus. VC, Vidian canal; HC, hypoglossal canal; PCA, paraclival carotid artery; PF, pituitary fossa; PS, planum sphenoidale; CCA, anterior genu of the intracavernous carotid artery.

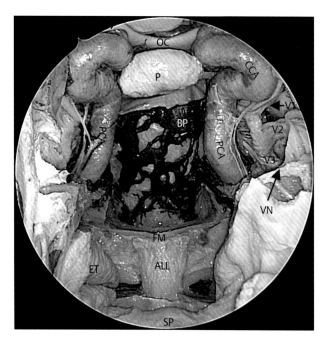

Fig. 19.3 Cadaveric dissection demonstrating the large venous channels within the clivus that constitute the basilar plexus (BP) that can cause significant bleeding during surgery. OC, optic chiasm; P, pituitary gland; CCA, anterior genu of the intracavernous carotid artery; PCA, paraclival carotid artery; VN, Vidian nerve; FM, foramen magnum; ET, eustachian tube; ALL, anterior longitudinal ligament; SP, soft palate; V1, ophthalmic division of the trigeminal nerve; V2, maxillary division of the trigeminal nerve; V3, mandibular division of the trigeminal nerve.

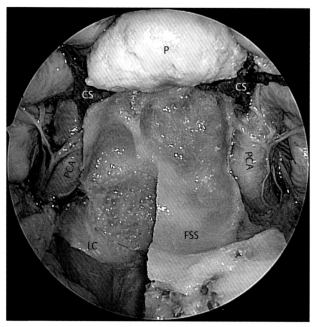

Fig. 19.4 Cadaveric dissection demonstrating the identification of the paraclival carotid arteries (PCA), the lateral borders of the dissection. If dissection is to continue to the lower clivus then the entire floor of the sphenoid sinus can be removed. The longus capitis muscle (LC) attaches firmly to the floor of the sphenoid sinus (FSS). CS, cavernous sinus; P, pituitary gland.

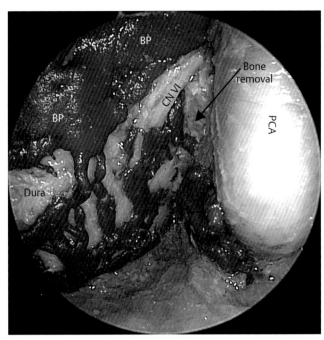

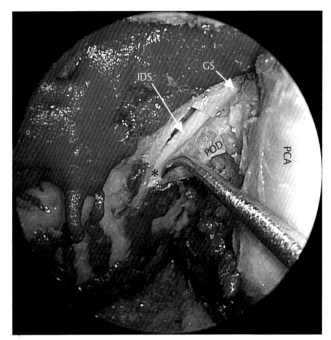

Fig. 19.5 Cadaveric dissection image taken with a 30-degree endoscope. Bone has been removed behind the paraclival carotid artery (*PCA*) so that the arteries stand proud of the lateral margins. *BP*, basilar plexus; *PCA*, paraclival carotid arteries; *CN VI*, abducens nerve; *, gulfar segment of the abducens nerve.

Fig. 19.6 Cadaveric dissection of the left middle clivus (taken with a 30-degree endoscope) demonstrating the different segments of the abducens nerve. The abducens nerve moves through the posterior cranial fossa (cisternal segment) before perforating through the meningeal layer of dura (marked by *asterisk*). Then the nerve enters a channel between the meningeal layer of dura and the periosteal layer of dura (*POD*). This segment is called the interdural segment (*IDS*). In this dissection, a leaf of periosteal dural (*POD*) has been incised and reflexed to clearly visualize the abducens nerve running within. The nerve then enters the confluence of dural sinus, made up of the superior and inferior petrosal sinuses, the basilar plexus, and the cavernous sinus. Here it is called the gulfar segment (*GS*). *PCA*, paraclival carotid artery.

the granuloma from the sphenoid, allowing the granuloma to be drained through the sphenoid.

Posterior Cranial Fossa

The dura has two layers: a periosteal layer and a meningeal layer. The extensive and rich venous plexus—the basilar plexus—runs between the periosteal and meningeal layers of the dura. Exposure of the clival periosteum can result in significant bleeding. In a patient with a recurrent meningioma previously removed through external approach, bleeding of 3 L was encountered. One of the ways to seal off these venous sinuses is to open the dura and bipolar the two layers together; alternatively, the Aqamantas from Medtronic ENT has proved very useful for these venous lakes. In this patient, a combination of bipolar and Floseal (Baxter; Springfield, IL) failed to control the bleeding and it was felt that the patient had lost too much blood to proceed. Surgery was stopped and muscle patches placed over the venous lakes and surgery rescheduled for 2 weeks later. At this operation, there was minimal bleeding and the tumor was successfully addressed. Before the dura is opened, the surgeon needs to have a clear understanding of where the sixth nerve is likely to be. As seen in Chapter 18, the sixth nerve enters Dorello's canal (canal formed by the periosteal and dural layers about midway up the middle third of the clivus just below the posterior meningeal artery) and then progresses to the gulfar region behind the carotid artery (**Figs. 19.5** and **19.6**). The gulfar region is formed by the junction of the inferior and superior petrosal sinus, basilar plexus, and posterior region of the

cavernous sinus. All of these sinuses are between the periosteal and meningeal layers of dura. A general landmark for this region is the junction of the floor of the pituitary with the vertical paraclival section of the carotid. Once the dura of the posterior cranial fossa has been opened, the contents of the posterior cranial fossa can be seen (**Figs. 19.7** and **19.8**). The first and most notable structure seen is the basilar artery which is usually covered with arachnoid (**Fig. 19.8**). **Figs. 19.9**, **19.10**, **19.11**, **19.12**, **19.13**, and **19.14** demonstrate the structures that are easily visualized. In most patients, the segments of the brainstem that can be easily visualized are the upper part of the medulla, the pons, and the lower edge of the midbrain. The vessels that are seen are the basilar artery, the posterior cerebral arteries, the superior cerebellar, and the anterior inferior cerebellar artery. Depending on the state of the brain, a variable number of the cranial nerves can be seen. Dehydration of the brain by the administration of mannitol may enlarge the space around the brainstem and allow easier visualization of the nerves.

Pituitary Translocation for Access to the Upper Third of the Clivus

Tumors extending behind the pituitary gland are usually unresectable unless the upper third of the clivus is removed.

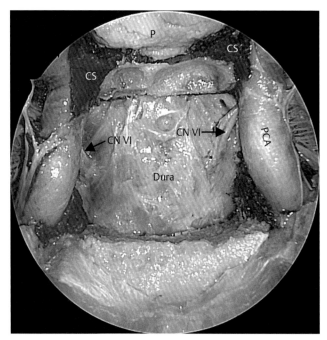

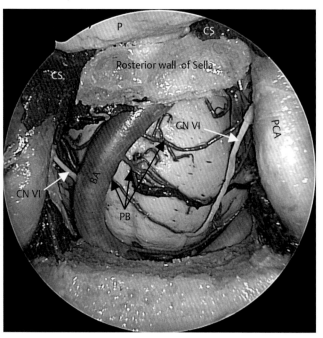

Fig. 19.7 Cadaveric dissection of the middle third of the clivus with removal of the basilar plexus and exposing the dura. The abducens nerves (*CN VI*) can be seen bilaterally as they perforate the meningeal dura and become the interdural segments of cranial nerve six. *CS*, cavernous sinus; *PCA*, paraclival carotid arteries; *P*, pituitary gland.

Fig. 19.8 Cadaveric dissection following removal of the middle third of the clivus and dura. The basilar artery (*BA*) can be seen very tortuous. Its pontine branches (*PB*) can be clearly seen. *CN VI*, abducens nerve; *CS*, cavernous sinus; *P*, pituitary gland; *PCA*, paraclival carotid artery.

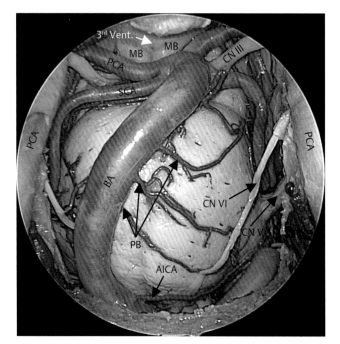

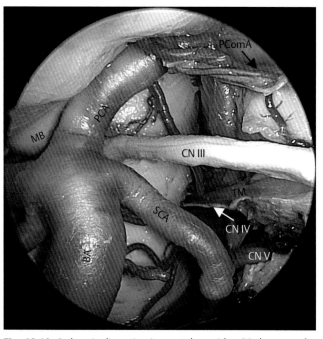

Fig. 19.9 Cadaveric dissection with removal of the upper third and middle third of the clivus with visualization of the posterior cerebral arteries (*PCA*), superior cerebellar arteries (*SCA*), and the oculomotor nerve in between (*CN III*). *3rd Vent*, third ventricle; *MB*, mammillary bodies; *PCA*, posterior cerebral arteries; *SCA*, superior cerebellar arteries; *CN III*, oculomotor nerve; *PCA*, paraclival arteries; *BA*, basilar artery; *PB*, pontine branches; *CN VI*, abducens nerve, *CN V*, trigeminal nerve; *AICA*, anterior inferior cerebellar artery.

Fig. 19.10 Cadaveric dissection image taken with a 30-degree endoscope following removal of the superior third of the clivus, visualizing the small trochlear nerve seen running along the tentorial membrane edge. *BA*, basilar artery; *PCA*, posterior cerebral artery; *SCA*, superior cerebellar artery; *CN III*, oculomotor nerve; *CN IV*, trochlear nerve; *CN V*, trigeminal nerve; *TM*, tentorial membrane; *PComA*, posterior communicating artery; *MB*, mammillary body.

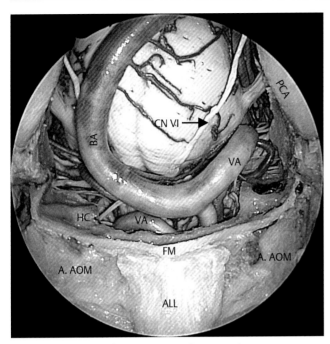

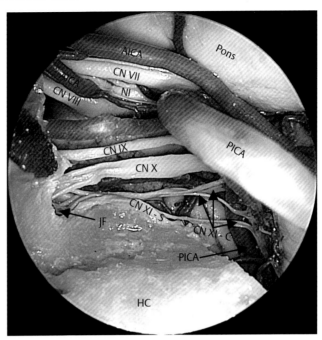

Fig. 19.11 Cadaveric dissection image demonstrating structures seen following dissection of the lower third of the clivus. Note how the basilar arteries and vertebral arteries can be extremely tortuous in their course. *ALL*, anterior longitudinal ligament; *A. AOM*, anterior atlanto-occipital membrane; *FM*, foramen magnum; *HC*, hypoglossal canal; *VA*, vertebral arteries; *BA*, basilar artery; *CN VI*, abducens nerve; *PCA*, paraclival carotid artery.

Fig. 19.12 Cadaveric dissection with image taken just above the skeletonized hypoglossal canal (*HC*) at the cerebellopontine angle. The anterior inferior cerebellar artery (*AICA*) can be seen intimately associated with the vestibulocochlear nerve (*CN VIII*), facial nerve (*CN VII*), and the nervus intermedius (*NI*). The posterior inferior cerebellar artery (*PICA*) can be seen running between the vagus (*CN X*) and spinal and cranial portions of the accessory nerves (*CN XI – S, CN XI – C*).

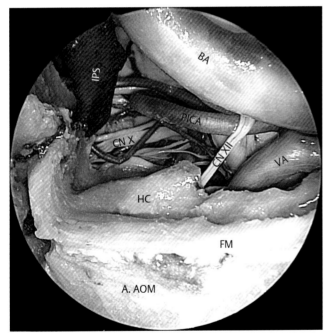

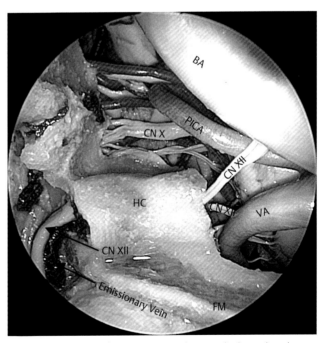

Fig. 19.13 Cadaveric dissection image taken following dissection of the right lower third of the clivus. As the posterior inferior cerebellar artery (*PICA*) courses from the vertebral artery (*VA*) it frequently runs through the rootlets that make up the hypoglossal nerve (*CN XII*). It may tent these rootlets as it courses to the cerebellomedullary fissure to run intimately with the cranial nerves eleven to nine. *CN X*, vagus nerve; *HC*, hypoglossal canal; *IPS*, inferior petrosal sinus; *BA*, basilar artery; *FM*, foramen magnum; *A. AOM*, anterior atlanto-occipital membrane.

Fig. 19.14 Cadaveric dissection image showing the hypoglossal nerve exiting the hypoglossal foramen with its corresponding vein that communicates the internal jugular vein with the basilar plexus. *HC*, hypoglossal canal; *CN XII*, hypoglossal nerve and rootlets; *FM*, foramen magnum; *VA*, vertebral artery; *PICA*, posterior inferior cerebellar artery; *BA*, basilar artery; *CN X*, vagus nerve.

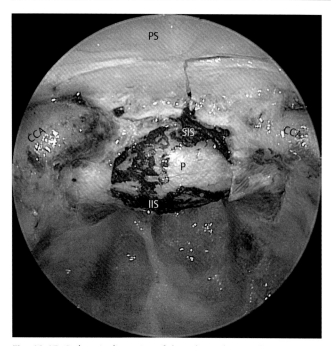

Fig. 19.15 Cadaveric dissection of the sphenoid sinus, demonstrating the removal of bone over the anterior genu of the intracavernous carotid arteries, sella, tuberculum sella, and the posterior half of the planum sphenoidale (*PS*). *CCA*, anterior genu of the intracavernous carotid artery; *IIS*, inferior intercavernous sinus; *SIS*, superior intercavernous sinus; *P*, pituitary gland.

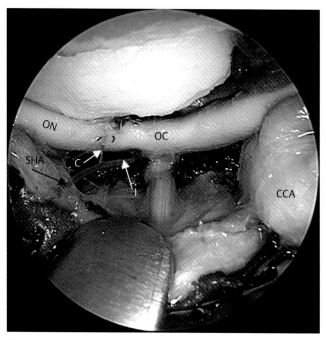

Fig. 19.16 Cadaveric dissection allowing visualization into the subchiasmatic cistern. The superior hypophyseal artery (*SHA*) can be seen giving off its chiasmatic (*C*) and infundibular (*I*) branches. *ON*, optic nerve; *OC*, optic chiasm; *CCA*, cavernous carotid artery.

To do this, the pituitary gland must either be translocated anteriorly, partially resected, or, in patients with hypopituitarism with a nonfunctional gland, removed. Before the gland can be translocated, space needs to be created for the gland to be positioned in the planum sphenoidale. The first step is to remove all the bone over the pituitary fossa onto the carotid arteries. Then, remove the bone overlying the tuberculum sella and over the posterior half of the planum sphenoidale (**Fig. 19.15**). This bone is removed from optic nerve to optic nerve and wider on the planum sphenoidale. The dura is incised and the subchiasmatic cistern inspected (**Fig. 19.16**) The diaphragm of the pituitary should be visualized and divided with skull base scissor up to the pituitary stalk (**Fig. 19.17**). Next, to translocate the gland, the periosteum and dura layers over the anterior aspect of the gland need to be separately identified and the plane between these layers clearly established. As the gland is mobilized, the dentate ligaments that hold the pituitary gland in place are identified and divided (**Fig. 19.18**). The inferior hypophysial artery will need to be divided to allow mobilization of the gland (**Figs. 19.19** and **19.20**). Dissection needs to proceed carefully otherwise the thin layer covering the cavernous sinus can be easily penetrated resulting in substantial venous bleeding. This can be controlled by Gelfoam paste and pressure with a neuropattie, but this should be avoided if possible. Once the gland is fully mobile it can be translocated into the region of the planum sphenoidale (**Figs. 19.20, 19.21,** and **19.22**). The upper third of the clivus is now visible and can be removed (**Fig. 19.23**). An inverted Y-shaped osteotomy is made with the stem in the midline. A 1- to 2-mm high-speed

Stylus diamond bur (Medtronic ENT) is used to perform these osteotomies (**Fig. 19.24**). Once the posterior clinoids are fully mobile, a combination of a blunt hook and dissector is used to gently peel the clinoids out of their periosteal layer. Remember that the posterior clinoid abuts both the intracranial

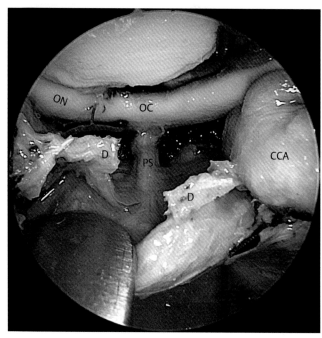

Fig. 19.17 Cadaveric dissection image demonstrating the incised diaphragma (*D*) to the pituitary stalk (*PS*). *ON*, optic nerve; *OC*, optic chiasm; *CCA*, cavernous carotid artery.

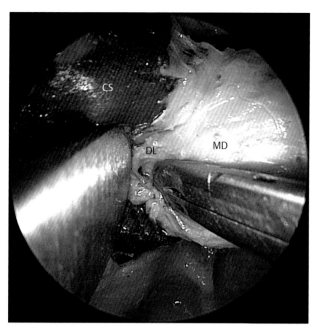

Fig. 19.18 Cadaveric dissection in the plane between the periosteal layer of dura and the meningeal layer of dura (*MD*) covering the right side of the pituitary gland. The pituitary dentate ligaments (*DL*) can be clearly visualized. *CS*, cavernous sinus.

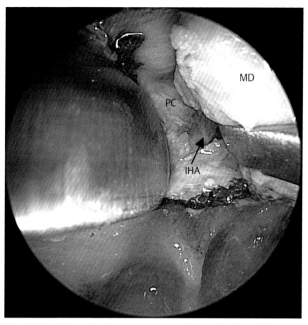

Fig. 19.19 Cadaveric dissection image of the right side of the pituitary gland. Dissection has occurred between the periosteal layer of dura and the meningeal layer of dura (*MD*) as far posteriorly as the dorsum sella. The inferior hypophyseal artery (*IHA*) is visualized as the base of the posterior clinoid (*PC*).

carotid artery and the posterior genu of the intracavernous carotid artery simultaneously, and is at risk during this maneuver (**Figs. 19.23** and **19.24**). Now the dura can be opened and the suprasellar anatomy fully visualized. An alternative is to resect a third of the pituitary gland and use this corridor

to remove the upper third of the clivus. During this procedure, the residual gland is compressed laterally to provide additional space. This does not give the access of the pituitary translocation but is technically easier and, in our patients, there remained pituitary function after this procedure.

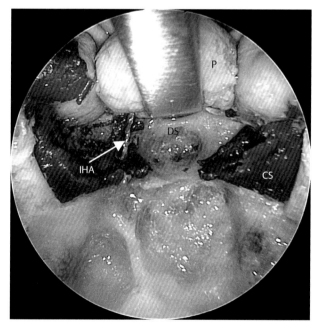

Fig. 19.20 Cadaveric dissection image of the pituitary gland tethered from its transposed position by the inferior hypophyseal artery (*IHA*). In this image, the meningeal and periosteal layers of dura have been removed. The IHA needs to be ligated and cut to allow complete transposition between the carotid arteries. The dorsum sella (*DS*) can be visualized. *P*, pituitary gland; *CS*, cavernous sinus.

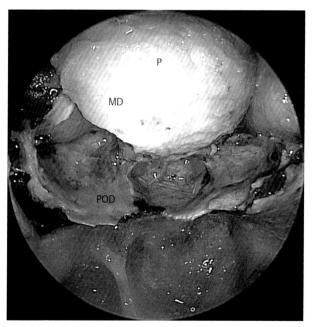

Fig. 19.21 Cadaveric dissection with preservation of the meningeal (*MD*) and periosteal layers (*POD*) of dura, and the pituitary gland (*P*) transposed between the carotid arteries.

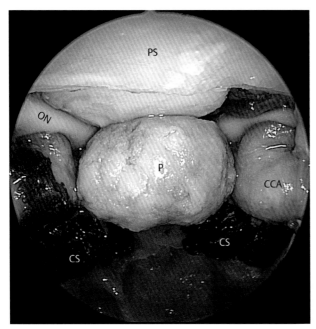

Fig. 19.22 Cadaveric dissection image with removal of the layers of dura. The pituitary gland (*P*) lies in its transposed position against the planum sphenoidale (*PS*), and between the cavernous carotid arteries (*CCA*). *ON*, optic nerve; *CS*, cavernous sinus.

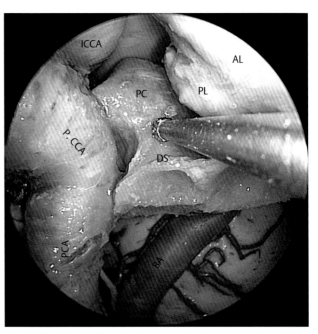

Fig. 19.23 Cadaveric dissection demonstrating the osteotomies at the base of the posterior clinoids (*PC*) for separation with the body of the dorsum sella (*DS*). *P. CCA*, posterior genu of the intracavernous carotid artery; *PCA*, paraclival carotid artery; *ICCA*, intracranial carotid artery; *BA*, basilar artery; *PL*, posterior lobe of the pituitary gland; *AL*, anterior lobe of the pituitary gland.

Once the dura of the upper third of the clivus is removed, the first structure encountered is Liliequist membrane. This is a condensation of arachnoid that attaches to the posterior clinoids and third nerves and has a semicircular aperture through which the basilar artery can pass (**Fig. 19.25**).

Once the pituitary has been translocated or removed, a better perspective of the cranial nerves in the posterior fossa can be achieved. In **Fig. 19.26** the telescope is turned laterally and the sixth cranial nerve can be seen just below the carotid artery and again in the cavernous sinus behind the carotid

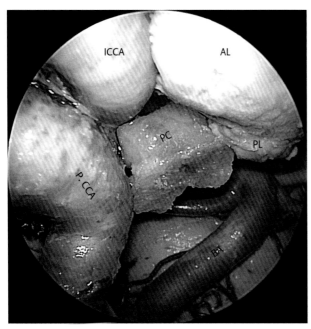

Fig. 19.24 Cadaveric dissection image demonstrating the close anatomical relationship of the posterior clinoid (*PC*) with both the intracranial carotid artery (*ICCA*) and the posterior genu of the intracavernous carotid artery (*P. CCA*). *AL*, anterior lobe of the pituitary gland; *PL*, posterior lobe of the pituitary gland; *BA*, basilar artery.

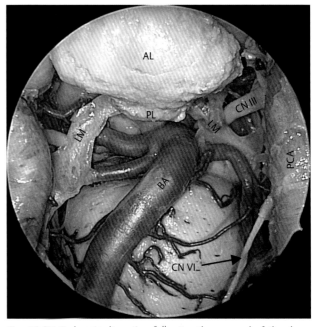

Fig. 19.25 Cadaveric dissection following the removal of the dorsum sella allowing visualization of Liliequist membrane (*LM*), a condensation of arachnoid membrane with a semicircular hole through which the basilar artery (*BA*) passes before dividing into its terminal branches. *AL*, anterior lobe of the pituitary gland; *PL*, posterior lobe of the pituitary gland; *CN III*, oculomotor nerve; *CN VI*, abducens nerve; *PCA*, paraclival carotid artery.

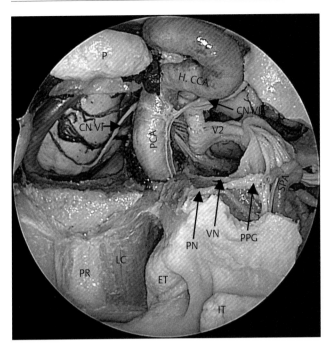

Fig. 19.26 Cadaveric dissection image taken with a 70-degree endoscope. The abducens nerve (*CN VI*) can be seen passing behind the paraclival carotid artery (*PCA*) to run parallel with the horizontal portion of the intracavernous carotid artery (*H. CCA*). Here the nerve is located between the carotid artery medially, and the ophthalmic division of the trigeminal nerve laterally. *P*, pituitary gland; *V2*, maxillary division of the trigeminal nerve; *PN*, pharyngeal nerve; *VN*, Vidian nerve; *PPG*, pterygopalatine ganglion; *SPA*, sphenopalatine artery; *ET*, eustachian tube; *IT*, inferior turbinate; *LC*, longus capitis; *PR*, pharyngeal raphe.

artery. The third cranial nerve can be seen exiting the brainstem between the posterior cerebral artery and the superior cerebellar artery (**Fig. 19.10**). The thin fourth cranial nerve can also be seen in the edge of the tentorium (**Fig. 19.10**).

If the 30-degree endoscope is advanced farther into the posterior cranial fossa, the rest of the cranial nerves can be seen (**Fig. 19.4**). The trigeminal nerve exits the lateral aspect of the pons with the thin fourth cranial nerve below it (**Fig. 19.10**). The fifth cranial nerve enters Meckel's cave before passing into the cavernous sinus. Below the fifth cranial nerve, the seventh, eighth, and the nervus intermedius can be seen exiting the brainstem and entering the internal auditory meatus (see **Figs. 19.12** and **19.28**). Although in this cadaver (**Fig. 19.27**) there seems to be space between the brainstem and the skull base, this is not always the case in patients and therefore caution should be exercised when contemplating removing tumors from the lateral regions of the posterior cranial fossa. To evaluate the seventh and eighth nerves, the lateral end of the pontomedullary sulcus is inspected and the facial and vestibulocochlear nerves can be seen emerging from the brainstem, with nervus intermedius located between these nerves, and intimately related to the anterior inferior cerebellar artery (AICA) vessels (**Figs. 19.12** and **19.27**). The nervus intermedius mostly arises as a single trunk between the vestibulocochlear and the facial nerve, but may arise from as many as four rootlets. In **Fig. 19.12** we can visualize three rootlets. In most cases, the AICA vessel passes just below the facial and vestibulocochlear nerves on its way around the brainstem, but it may also pass through or above

as seen in this example as it passes through the facial and vestibulocochlear nerves (**Fig. 19.12**). The AICA gives off a labyrinthine artery, subarcuate arteries, and the recurrent perforating branches to the brainstem. The facial nerve enjoys a consistent relationship to the junction of the glossopharyngeal/vagus/spinal accessory nerves within the medulla. The facial arises 2 to 3 mm above the most rostral rootlet.

Inferior to the seventh and eighth cranial nerves, the ninth and tenth cranial nerves can be seen entering the jugular foramen (**Fig. 19.12**). The AICA can in some patients (54%) loop a variable distance into the internal auditory meatus before giving off its labyrinthine branch (**Fig. 19.27**). The glossopharyngeal, the vagus, and the accessory nerves arise from rootlets lined along the postolivary sulcus (a shallow groove between the olive and the posterolateral surface of the medulla). The glossopharyngeal and vagus nerves arise at the level of the superior third of the olive, whereas the spinal accessory rootlets arise along the posterior margin of the inferior two-thirds of the olive and from the lower medulla and upper segments of the spinal cord. The glossopharyngeal nerve arises as a line of one or two rootlets from the upper medulla, just below the facial nerve. The posterior inferior cerebellar artery (PICA) arises from the vertebral artery at the level of the medulla and typically travels dorsally between the vagus and the accessory nerves, as seen in **Fig. 19.28**. It then continues to reach the surface of the inferior cerebellar peduncle, where it dips to supply the cerebellomedullary fissure and terminates by supplying the suboccipital surface of the cerebellum. The choroid plexus is located directly behind these nerves as it spills out of the foramen of Luschka, located at the lateral margin of the pontomedullary sulcus (**Fig. 19.29**). The flocculus is visible just behind the facial and

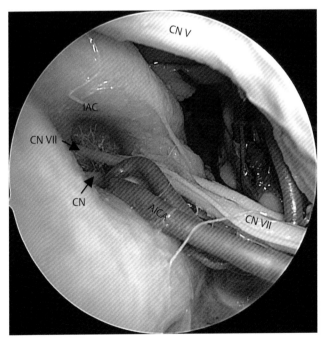

Fig. 19.27 Cadaveric dissection image taken with a 70-degree endoscope. The right internal auditory canal (*IAC*) can be clearly visualized with the meatal segment of the anterior inferior cerebellar artery (*AICA*) entering the meatus. This vessel then loops between the facial (*CN VII*) and vestibulocochlear nerves. *CN*, cochlear nerve; *CN V*, trigeminal nerve.

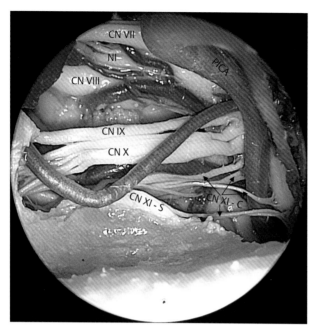

Fig. 19.28 Cadaveric dissection image demonstrating the posterior inferior cerebellar artery (*PICA*) running between the vagus (*CN X*) and the cranial accessory nerve rootlets (*CN XI-C*) at the position where the nerves exit the brainstem. *CN VII*, facial nerve; *CN VIII*, vestibulocochlear nerve; *NI*, nervus intermedius; *CN IX*, glossopharyngeal nerve; *CN XI-S*, spinal accessory nerve

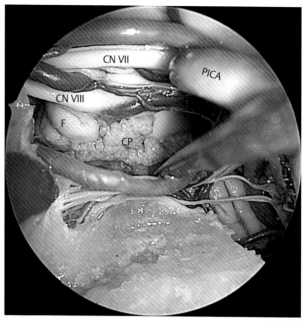

Fig. 19.29 Cadaveric dissection image on the right side with retraction inferiorly of the glossopharyngeal and vagus nerves to reveal the choroid plexus (*CP*) as it spills out of the foramen of Luschka. The flocculus (*F*) can also be visualized laterally, just behind the facial (*CN VII*) and vestibulocochlear nerves (*CN VIII*). *AICA*, anterior inferior cerebellar artery; *PICA*, posterior inferior cerebellar artery.

the vestibulocochlear nerves (**Fig. 19.29**). The hypoglossal nerve arises from a series of rootlets originating from the preolivary sulcus at the medulla, a groove between the olive and the medullary pyramid. The rootlets of the hypoglossal nerve may stretch over the posterior surface of the vertebral artery (**Fig. 19.14**). The PICA may transverse either around or between these rootlets before they enter the hypoglossal canal. The hypoglossal nerve then exits this canal often with a venous lake that joins the internal jugular vein (**Fig. 19.14**).

Cavernous Sinus

The cavernous sinus may be involved in clival tumors, particularly chordomas, and it is therefore important to understand the relationship of the cranial nerves within the cavernous sinus as discussed in Chapter 18. The most important relationship in clival tumors is the sixth nerve as it is the most vulnerable. Its cisternal segment is easily engulfed with intradural tumor extension and its cavernous segment is often involved in the gulfar regions and in Dorello's canal where it lies between layers of dura and periosteum (**Figs. 19.6**, **19.9**, and **19.26**).

The other cranial nerves that may be involved in tumor extension into the cavernous sinus are the third, fourth, and fifth cranial nerves. **Fig. 19.30** is a diagrammatic representation of the contents of the cavernous sinus adjacent to the pituitary gland, and **Fig. 19.31** shows these nerves as they run in the lateral wall of the cavernous sinus on their way to the orbital apex and superior orbital fissure (the cavernous carotid artery has been retracted medially).

The contents of the cavernous sinus are seldom seen during surgery as it is only possible to open the cavernous

sinus if tumor has infiltrated it and obliterated the venous sinusoids. However, in such cases, it is important to know the anatomy of the cavernous sinus so that these important structures are not damaged during resection of such tumors. In **Fig. 19.31** the carotid artery is swung medially to expose the contents of the cavernous sinus. Note how the third cranial nerve is a large nerve in the lateral roof of the sinus with the smaller, less easily visible fourth cranial nerve directly below it. The sixth cranial nerve is seen to enter the sinus lower down and from the posterior inferior aspect then to traverse from inferior to superior abutting the anterior genu of the carotid artery. If this nerve is moved medially, the V1

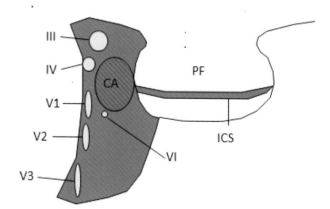

Fig. 19.30 This diagrammatic representation of the right cavernous sinus shows the carotid artery (*CA*) within the cavernous sinus. The sixth nerve is the most medial nerve, whereas the third, fourth, and fifth tend to run against the lateral wall of the cavernous sinus. The intercavernous venous sinus (*ICS*), which connects one sinus to the other, is demonstrated.

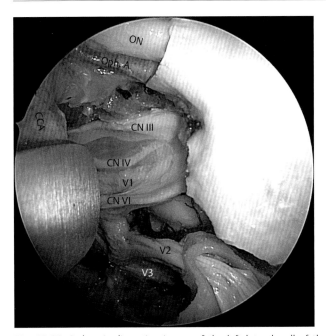

Fig. 19.31 Cadaveric dissection image of the left lateral wall of the sphenoid sinus. The bone has been removed and the anterior genu of the intracavernous carotid artery (*CCA*) retracted medially. This allows clear visualization of the nerves within the dural layers of the lateral wall of the cavernous sinus. The abducens nerve (*CN VI*) can be visualized medially, running within the cavernous sinus. *ON*, optic nerve; *Oph. A*, ophthalmic artery; *CN III*, oculomotor nerve; *CN IV*, trochlear nerve; *V1*, ophthalmic division of the trigeminal nerve; *V2*, maxillary division of the trigeminal nerve; *V3*, mandibular division of the trigeminal nerve.

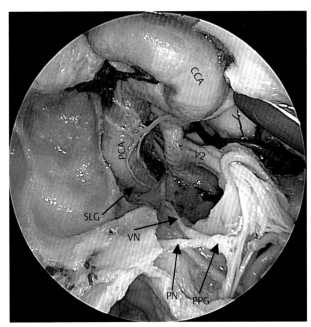

Fig. 19.32 Cadaveric dissection image of the lateral sphenoid wall on the left side demonstrating the Vidian nerve (*VN*) coursing laterally toward the supralacerum genu (*SLG*), located at the junction of the vertical paraclival carotid artery (*PCA*) with the horizontal petrous carotid artery. *PCA*, paraclival carotid artery; *CCA*, anterior genu of the intracavernous carotid artery; *V2*, maxillary division of the trigeminal nerve; *VN*, Vidian nerve; *PN*, pharyngeal nerve; *PPG*, pterygopalatine ganglion.

and V2 branches of the fifth cranial nerve can be seen. V3 is in the same surgical plane but lies more inferiorly.

◆ Surgical Technique for Clivus and Posterior Cranial Fossa Lesions

The first step is to raise a Hadad pedicled septal flap and place it in the maxillary sinus which had been widely opened. The opposite septum is mobilized, as in Chapter 20, to cover the donor site of the pedicled septal flap thereby removing the posterior half of-the septum and creating enough space for a two-surgeon approach. This anteriorly based flap is secured with a 3-0 Vicryl (Ethicon; Somerville, NJ) suture. Silastic may again be placed over the columella, as in Chapter 17, to facilitate bilateral passing of instruments. Next, the superior turbinate is removed and bilateral large sphenoidotomies are created. The floor of the sphenoid is resected with a curved high-speed diamond bur (Medtronic ENT). The lateral landmarks for this resection are the Vidian nerves. These are identified at the beginning of the resection and all bone between these nerves is removed. As the supralacerum genu of the carotid is approached, remember that the Vidian nerve is on the medial side of the genu but as it progresses onto the carotid it travels lateral and over the top of the carotid (**Fig. 19.32**). It is important to resect all of the floor as failure to do so will result in the anterior sill of the floor of the sphenoid driving the instruments upward toward the pituitary (**Fig. 19.33**).

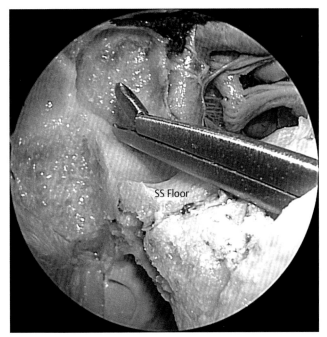

Fig. 19.33 Cadaveric dissection demonstrating that instrumentation without adequate removal of the floor of the sphenoid sinus results in a straight instrument being driven high into the middle third of the clivus beneath the pituitary fossa. Removal of the floor of the sphenoid sinus (*SS*) will allow access to the junction of the posterior sphenoid floor and adjacent clivus.

The next step is to identify the vertical paraclival carotid arteries thereby delineating the lateral limits of the mid third of the clival dissection (**Fig. 19.3**). Usually this is done with an angled high-speed diamond bur (Medtronic ENT), which allows the carotids to be exposed with a thin layer of bone protecting them. Image guidance and intraoperative Doppler plays an important role in correctly identifying the arteries so that the bone overlying the arteries can be thinned until transparent and the arteries clearly identified. If the drill inadvertently contacts the adventitia of the wall of the carotid it will usually not damage the wall as long as the artery is

immediately recognized. Prolonged contact between the bur and wall is dangerous and may lead to a lesion of the artery. If the tumor extends inferolateral to the carotid canals it can be followed as long as it is kept in mind that the petrous temporal portion of the carotid runs at about 45 degrees to the vertical portion of the carotids. In a patient with a chordoma such an extension can be removed with a curved diamond bur. In certain situations, the 40- or 70-degree diamond burs (Medtronic ENT) may be useful for very laterally based lesions (**Fig. 19.34**).

If the tumor breaches the clival dura and protrudes intracranially then this portion of the tumor may be separated

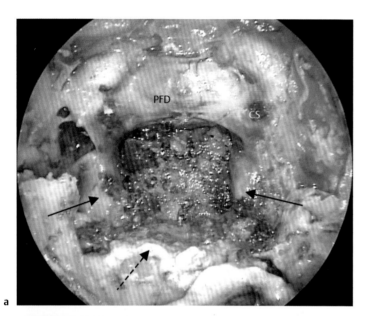
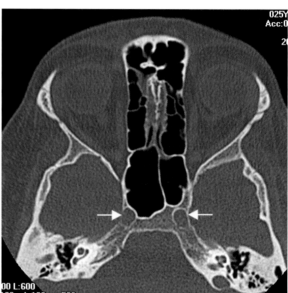
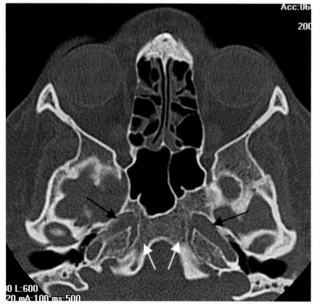
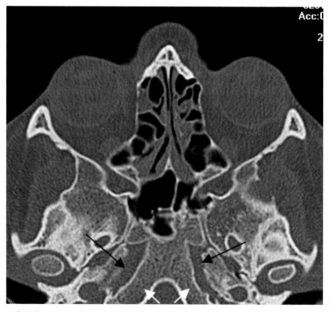

Fig. 19.34 (**a**) The vertical portions of the carotid arteries have been exposed (*solid black arrows*). Superiorly the dura overlying the pituitary fossa (*PFD*) has been exposed and the cavernous sinus (*CS*) on both sides can be clearly seen. Note the intercavernous venous sinus connecting the two sinuses. Inferiorly, the floor of the sphenoid has been drilled away until almost adjacent to the clival dura (*broken black arrow*).

(**b**) The vertical portions of the carotid arteries are seen (*white arrows*) with the clivus between the carotids. (**c,d**) Axial CTs in which the petrous portions of the carotid arteries and foramen lacerum are marked with *black arrows* and the posterolateral portions of the clivus behind the arteries marked with *white arrows*. Note how the petrous portion of the carotid runs at a 45-degree angle to the vertical portions of the arteries.

from the clival component by sharp dissection using the endoscopic skull base scissors* (Integra). The residual tumor protruding from the clivus into the posterior cranial fossa is now accessible without the surgeons having to work around the often bulky clival component. The dural opening should be visualized and can be further enlarged with the scissors to allow an endoscopic view of the intracranial tumor component. Clival chordomas are usually soft and amenable to debulking with gentle suction. Care must be taken to ensure that the tumor is not entangled with the sixth nerve or any of the vascular structures of the brainstem. Traction on a tumor wrapped around a brainstem perforator may cause catastrophic bleeding and hemorrhage into the brainstem and intraoperative death. In this situation, it is vitally important for the otolaryngologist and neurosurgeon to work closely as a team. The malleable skull base blunt hook and probe* (Integra Wormald Skull Base Set) are used to mobilize the tumor while gentle traction is applied and the tumor is gently delivered through the dural defect into the sphenoid. Angled endoscopes and malleable suctions* (Integra Wormald Skull Base Set) are used to visualize the intracranial cavity to ensure no residual tumor remains. If residual

tumor is seen, a suction regulator is placed in the suction line to reduce the amount of suction. The malleable skull base suction* (Integra) is then placed through the dural defect onto the residual tumor. The suction control port of this instrument is very wide so that if a vessel or nerve is inadvertently sucked into the end of the instrument, removal of the finger from the suction port will remove all suction at the tip and the vascular structure or nerve will be released uninjured.

◆ Case Examples and Results

This middle-aged woman presented with a large clival chordoma that protruded into the sphenoid sinus, abutting both internal carotid arteries and extending intracranially where it abutted the basilar artery (**Fig. 19.35**).

This patient was managed with a two-surgeon approach with bilateral large sphenoidotomies, removal of the posterior septum, and removal of the floor of the sphenoid. Once access had been achieved, both vertical portions of

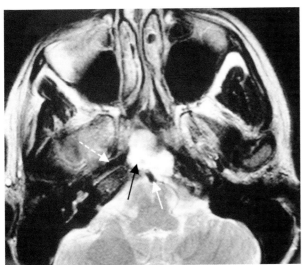

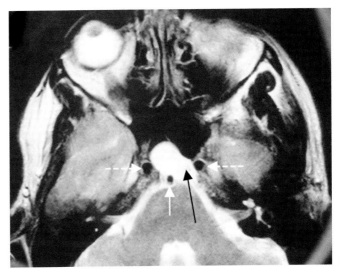

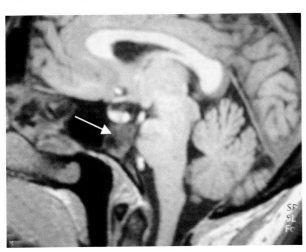

Fig. 19.35 (**a,b**) On the axial MRI, the chordoma (*black arrow*) can be seen between the carotid arteries (*broken white arrows*) and abutting the basilar artery (*solid white arrow*). (**c**) On the parasagittal MRI scan, the lesion can be seen in the clivus below the pituitary and abutting the pons.

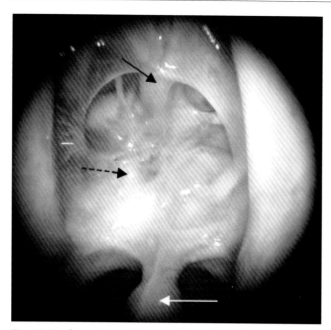

Fig. 19.36 This endoscopic image of the sphenoid indicates the residual septum (*white arrow*), intersinus septum of the sphenoid (*black arrow*), and the region of the reconstruction of the posterior fossa wall (*broken black arrow*).

the carotids were exposed with a rough diamond bur. The remaining bony clivus was removed with exposure of the clival dura with a central deficit through which the chordoma entered the posterior cranial fossa. Utilizing the two-surgeon approach the intracranial portion of the tumor was slowly mobilized under direct vision. A 30-degree endoscope was used to visualize the inferior intracranial extension of the tumor. The malleable blunt tip and curved probes were used to gently dissect the arachnoid from the tumor and the tumor was delivered into the sphenoid and removed. Reconstruction of the skull base was achieved initially with fat alone but the patient developed a cerebrospinal fluid (CSF) leak about 1 month after surgery and the repair was then augmented with fascia lata. This repair remains intact after 8 years' follow-up (**Fig. 19.36**). To date there is no evidence of a recurrent disease on MRI scanning.

The second case example is a middle-aged man who presented with partial sixth cranial nerve palsy. MRI scans showed a lesion extending from internal carotid to internal carotid and extending inferior and lateral to the vertical portions of the carotids. The intracranial extension indents the anterior surface of the pons and displaces the basilar artery laterally (**Fig. 19.37**).

The other area that should always be assessed is the possible inferior bony extension of these tumors. If the CT scans of this case are reviewed, the inferolateral extension behind the petrous temporal portions of the internal carotids can be seen (**Fig. 19.38**). There is significant bony erosion of this part of the clivus down toward the foramen magnum.

In this patient, more bony erosion is seen on the right side (*white arrow*) in the petrous apex.

This patient was approached with a two-surgeon standard pituitary exposure with wide sphenoidotomies, septal resection, and floor of sphenoid resection. Once the tumor was fully in view, the vertical paraclival portions of the internal carotid arteries were exposed from the base of the sphenoid to the floor of the pituitary fossa using a diamond bur. The dura of the entire floor of the pituitary was then exposed. This delineates the superior and lateral margins of the dissection. Next, the floor of the sphenoid was drilled away and the tumor followed laterally behind the vertical portions of the internal carotids and posteriorly until the posterior cranial fossa dura was exposed. Once dura was exposed inferiorly (at the base of the clivus), laterally (behind the carotids), and superiorly at the pituitary–clivus junction, the tumor was felt to be fully mobile. The tumor was placed under slight traction and a gush of CSF was seen as the intracranial component was displaced in the posterior fossa dural defect. Using the skull base endoscopic scissors* (Integra), the sphenoid/clival component of the tumor was divided from the intracranial extension at the level of the posterior fossa dura. Once the sphenoid component was removed, enough space was created so that the two surgeons could work comfortably on the remaining intracranial tumor. The dural defect was enlarged with the endoscopic skull base scissors and a view of the posterior cranial fossa obtained. Using the malleable right-angled hook and blunt tip probe (skull base instrument set, Integra), the intracranial component was gently mobilized and delivered through the dural defect. The endoscope was switched to a 30-degree endoscope and the posterior cranial fossa reexplored. Residual tumor was seen superiorly on the anterior face of the pons. A suction regulator was placed in the suction line, limiting the amount of suction, and the malleable frontal sinus suction was bent so it could be placed through the dural defect superiorly and the residual tumor indenting the pons was gently removed. Complete macroscopic tumor resection was achieved. The skull base defect was repaired with two layers of fascia lata. One layer was placed intracranially and the other on the dura from the sphenoid. Fibrin glue and a nasal pack were put in place. Unfortunately, the patient developed a CSF leak after the pack was removed. On reexploration, the dural repair was solid with a very thin stream of CSF seen coming from the junction between the pituitary dura and the repair. This region was opened and repaired with a bath-plug type fat plug and fibrin glue.

To date we have endoscopically removed 16 clival chordomas. Eight of the nine primary cases had radiotherapy with one patient having proton beam irradiation. Four of the seven revisions had undergone radiotherapy prior to presentation to us. In seven of the nine primary cases, complete macroscopic tumor resection was possible and, in this group, there has been no recurrence of tumor since resection with a mean follow-up of 4 years. In the partially resected patients, the residual tumor is growing very slowly and this is being monitored with sequential MRI scans. Further surgery will be offered if the tumor grows significantly or produces symptoms. In the seven revision cases, all had their primary surgery at

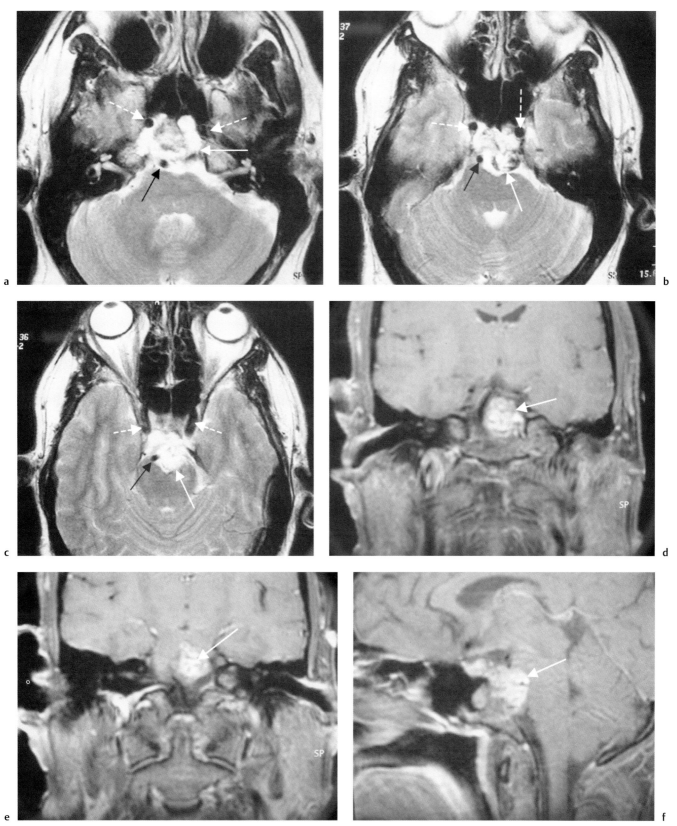

Fig. 19.37 (**a–c**) MRI T2-weighted axial scans in which the tumor (*white arrow*) is seen between the two vertical portions of the carotids (*broken white arrows*). It is also evident how the tumor indents the pons and displaces the basilar artery (*black arrow*) laterally. (**d,e**) In the coronal T1-weighted scans, the tumor can be seen indenting the pons (*white arrow*). This indentation can be fully appreciated on the parasagittal MRI T1-weighted scan (**f**). Note the significant posterior indentation of the tumor into the pons (*white arrow*).

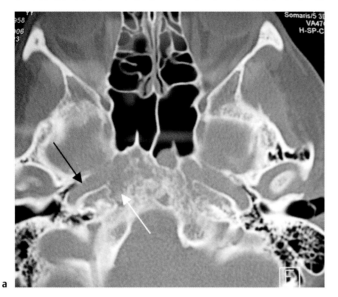

a

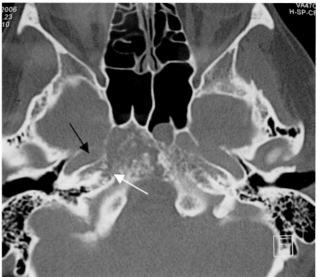

b

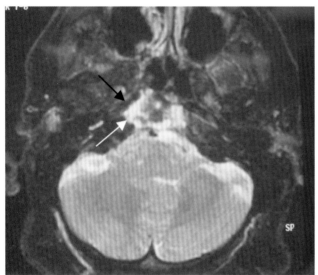

c

Fig. 19.38 (**a,b**) Axial CT scans and (**c**) T1-weighted MRI illustrate the horizontal portions of the internal carotid (*black arrow*) and the bony erosion immediately posterior to the carotid in the base of the clivus (*white arrow*).

other institutions. Five still have radiological residual disease with two patients deceased.

◆ Conclusion

Endoscopic resection of clival and posterior cranial fossa tumors presents a challenge to the skull base team. Successful management of these patients requires a detailed knowledge of the anatomy and a high level of endoscopic skill. The endoscopic skull base team, normally consisting of a rhinologist and neurosurgeon, needs to build their endoscopic expertise on less challenging cases such as with pituitary tumor resection and, once they have sufficient expertise, to then progress to clival and posterior cranial fossa tumors.

References

1. Brackmann DE, Arriaga MA. Surgery of the posterior cranial fossa. In: CW Cummings, ed. Otolaryngology Head and Neck Surgery. 4th ed. St Louis, MO: Mosby; 2005

2. Lanzino G, Dumont AS, Lopes MB, Laws ER Jr. Skull base chordomas: overview of disease, management options, and outcome. Neurosurg Focus 2001;10(3):E12

3. DeMonte F, Diaz E Jr, Callender D, Suk I. Transmandibular, circumglossal, retropharyngeal approach for chordomas of the clivus and upper cervical spine. Technical note. Neurosurg Focus 2001;10(3):E10

4. Solares CA, Fakhri S, Batra PS, Lee J, Lanza DC. Transnasal endoscopic resection of lesions of the clivus: a preliminary report. Laryngoscope 2005;115(11):1917–1922

5. Giorgio F, Vittorio S, Fabio C, Giovanni F, Diego M, Ernesto P. The endoscopic transnasal transphenoidal approach for the treatment of cranial base chordomas and chondrosarcomas. Op Neurosurg Suppl 2006;59(1):50–57

20 Endoscopic Resection of Anterior Cranial Fossa Tumors

◆ Introduction

Endoscopic techniques for transnasal resection of anterior cranial fossa tumors were developed for tumors involving the nasal cavity, sinuses, and the anterior cranial fossa. However, experience with these tumors has led to the refinement of these techniques to address tumors of the anterior cranial fossa that do not have a nasal or sinus component. Although most of this experience has been with meningiomas, these techniques can also be used to address malignant nasal tumors that are primary intracranial or that extend intracranially. The first step toward a wholly endoscopic resection of malignant sinonasal tumors was the experience gained with endoscopic management of the sinonasal component of the tumor during a standard craniofacial resection. We found that the endoscopic resection of the sinonasal component could be effectively dealt with endoscopically as it can be with external traditional approaches. In the case of large tumors involving both nasal cavities, the endoscopic approach was more effective as it dealt with both sides as opposed to most of the external approaches which limited access to one side of the nose. A significant number of these malignant tumors attach to the skull base and associated orbit. During craniofacial resection, the skull base involved with tumor is completely excised.[1-3] The associated orbital involvement would, in most circumstances, be removed as a separate excision. We found that endoscopically resecting the sinonasal component afforded better visualization of the tumor, allowing the nonattached tumor to be extensively debulked and the regions of tumor attachment to be accurately identified. This in turn allowed a complete resection of the sinonasal and, if present, the orbital component. As the experience with anterior skull base tumor resections developed, the indications including the size and involvement of both the skull base and intracranial cavity have progressed. The most suitable malignant tumors are adenocarcinoma and esthesioneuroblastoma, which in general have a pushing rather than infiltrative front and are thus more easily addressed endoscopically. Squamous carcinoma can be resected but only if localized with minimal orbital or brain involvement. In the past the gold standard for resection of these malignancies was a craniofacial resection.[1] However, there is now increasing evidence that the wholly endoscopic resection yields comparable results.[2-6] Recently published series have reported similar morbidity and mortality rates and very similar local recurrence rates.[2,3,5,6] In addition, there are significant benefits for the patients undergoing wholly endoscopic resection, as uninvolved structures are not removed and this approach avoids skin incisions with improved cosmetic results.[2-6] In addition, those patients who are medically or otherwise unsuitable for a standard craniofacial resection, or who choose not to undergo this procedure, can be offered the endoscopic approach as an alternative. Endoscopic resection of the anterior skull base requires a detailed knowledge of the anatomy of this region.

◆ The Anatomy of the Anterior Skull Base

The anterior skull base consists of the orbital plates of the frontal bone with the cribriform plates (part of the ethmoid bone) separating them. These plates attach to the planum sphenoidale (lesser wing of the sphenoid bone) posteriorly (**Fig. 20.1**). The cribriform plate gives rise to the crista galli onto which the falx cerebri attaches anteriorly.

If the anterior skull base is approached endoscopically from front to back, the frontal bone (posterior wall of the frontal sinus), foveae ethmoidalis, and intervening cribriform plates can be seen (**Figs. 20.2** and **20.3**). Posteriorly, the foveae ethmoidalis and cribriform plates attach to the planum sphenoidale (**Fig. 20.4**). The important vascular structures within the anterior skull base are the anterior and posterior ethmoid arteries. Note how there is a space or a cell between the frontal sinus ostium and the anterior ethmoidal artery (**Fig. 20.5**). This is always the case as the artery usually runs in the base of the second lamella which is the upward continuation of the anterior face of the bulla ethmoidalis.

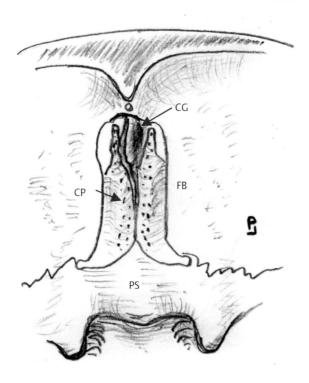

Fig. 20.1 This diagram illustrates the view of the anterior skull base from above (intracranial side). The crista galli (*CG*), cribriform plate (*CP*), orbital plate of the frontal bone (*FB*), and planum sphenoidale (*PS*) of the lesser wing of the sphenoid bone are visible.

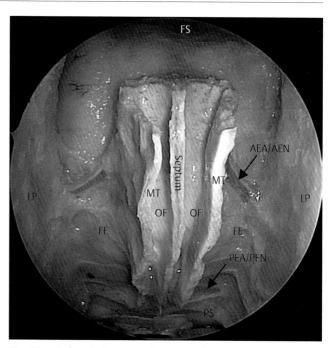

Fig. 20.2 Cadaveric dissection illustrating the anatomy of the anterior skull base following partial resection of both middle turbinates (*MT*) and nasal septum. The communal frontal sinus (*FS*) ostium can be seen anteriorly with both fovea ethmoidalis (*FE*) exposed. The lateral margins are the lamina papyracea (*LP*) and posteriorly the planum sphenoidale (*PS*) can be seen. *OF*, olfactory fossa; *AEA*, anterior ethmoidal artery; *PEA*, posterior ethmoidal artery; *AEN*, anterior ethmoidal nerve; *PEN*, posterior ethmoidal nerve.

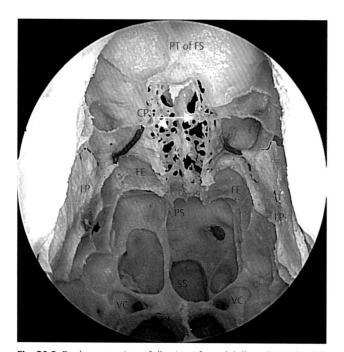

Fig. 20.3 Dry bone specimen following a frontal drillout shows the delicate cribriform plate (*CP*) and fovea ethmoidalis (*FE*). The nasal septum and middle turbinates have been completely resected. The sphenoid sinus (*SS*) can be seen posteriorly with the roof forming the planum sphenoidale (*PS*). The lamina papyracea (*LP*) is still intact. *VC*, Vidian canal; *PT of FS*, posterior table of frontal sinus.

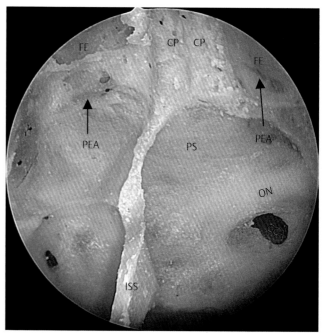

Fig. 20.4 Dry bone dissection image taken with a 30-degree endoscopic demonstrating the fovea ethmoidalis (*FE*) and cribriform plate (*CP*) junction with the planum sphenoidale (*PS*). This is marked approximately by the posterior ethmoidal artery (*PEA*). *ISS*, intersinus septum of sphenoid sinus; *ON*, optic nerve; *CCA*, anterior genu of the intracavernous carotid artery.

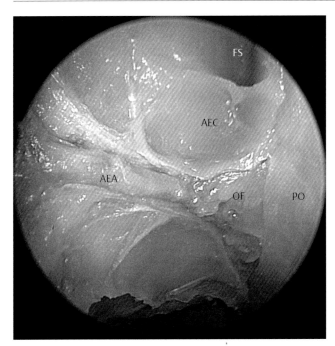

Fig. 20.5 Cadaveric dissection image of the left ethmoid cavity revealing the anterior ethmoidal artery (*AEA*) located one anterior ethmoidal cell (*AEC*) posterior to the frontal sinus (*FS*). *OF*, orbital fat; *PO*, periorbita.

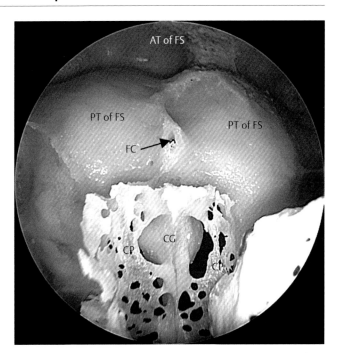

Fig. 20.6 Dry bone specimen following a frontal drillout procedure. This specimen clearly shows the close relationship between the frontal sinuses and the cribriform plate (*CP*), and hence the advantage of the drillout procedure for anteriorly based lesions. *AT of FS*, anterior table of frontal sinus; *PT of FS*, posterior table of frontal sinus; *FC*, foramen caecum; *CP*, cribriform plate; *CG*, crista galli.

One of the first decisions that needs to be made is whether the entire skull base needs to be resected. This is determined by the relationship between the anterior end of the tumor and the anterior ethmoidal artery (AEa). If the tumor approaches but does not come farther forward than the anterior ethmoidal artery, then the posterior skull base can be resected without the need to perform a frontal drillout procedure (grade 6 EFFS or modified Lothrop). Once the tumor encroaches past the anterior ethmoidal artery, a frontal drillout is necessary to be able to achieve the correct angle onto the tumor and be able to delineate the anterior arachnoid/tumor interface. This is necessary so that once the inside of the tumor has been debulked, the tumor arachnoid plane can be identified and the tumor wall collapsed into the tumor cavity allowing progressive resection of the tumor.

Resection of the skull base is only possible once the entire skull base has been exposed. This requires, as a first step, bilateral sphenoethmoidectomies with exposure of the skull base within the sphenoids, anterior and posterior ethmoids, and visualization of the frontal ostia. If the entire anterior skull base is to be resected, the frontal sinuses need to be drilled out with a grade 6 EFFS (Draf 3) procedure. The relationship between the cribriform plate and the frontal sinuses is clearly illustrated in this osteology model and illustrates the importance of performing a frontal drillout procedure for more anteriorly based tumors (**Fig. 20.6**). The other important structures that need to be identified are the anterior ethmoidal artery and the posterior ethmoidal artery. Note how the anterior ethmoidal artery has the anterior ethmoidal nerve running adjacent to it and how the lamina papyracea tents into the skull base as the anterior ethmoidal canal is formed (**Figs. 20.5 and 20.7**). This tenting

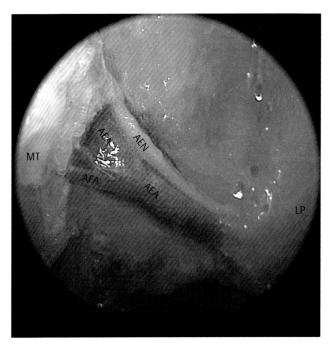

Fig. 20.7 Cadaveric dissection image demonstrating the left anterior ethmoidal artery (*AEA*) and nerve (*AEN*) running across the skull base toward the middle turbinate (*MT*) attachment. Here it can be seen dividing into several branches including the anterior falcine artery (*AFA*) to supply the falx cerebri. *LP*, lamina papyracea.

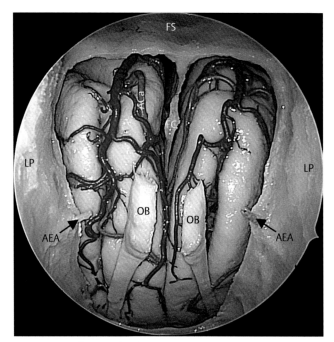

Fig. 20.8 Cadaveric dissection image: the skull base has been removed affording a view of the inferior aspect of both anterior cerebral lobes. The olfactory bulbs (*OB*), branches of the anterior cerebral artery (*ACa*), and cut inferior aspect of the falx cerebri (*FC*) can be seen. *FS*, frontal sinus; *AEA*, anterior ethmoidal artery; *LP*, lamina papyracea.

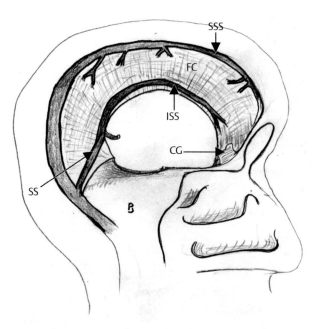

Fig. 20.9 The anterior attachment of the falx cerebri (*FC*) to crista galli (*CG*) is seen. Note the superior sagittal sinus (*SSS*) running in the superior aspect of the falx cerebri with in the inferior sagittal sinus (*ISS*) in the lower margin of the falx cerebri. The inferior sagittal sinus becomes the straight sinus (*SS*) after the it joins with the great cerebral vein.

of the lamina papyracea is important to understand when exposing and cauterizing the anterior ethmoidal artery. Our preferred technique is to expose the artery with a diamond bur then to use the suction bipolar to cauterize the artery. However, if the bur is too big or if the exposure is done over the lateral area on the triangular fat invagination, division of the artery with the bur may result in retraction of the artery into the orbit and orbital hematoma formation. This has happened in one case in which an anterior skull base tumor was being removed and required an immediate orbital decompression to relieve the pressure on the eye. The tumor resection continued uneventfully once this had been done. The posterior ethmoidal artery should be addressed in the same manner with exposure with a diamond bur and bipolar cautery. Once this has been done any residual septum is detached from the anterior skull base.

Once the skull base has been dropped down and removed, the anterior cranial fossa can be viewed (**Fig. 20.8**). The two olfactory bulbs and olfactory tracts are seen on the undersurface of the anterior cerebral hemispheres. The major vascular structures are the anterior cerebral arteries and branches from these arteries. The venous drainage of the anterior cranial fossa is via the superior and inferior sagittal sinuses. The superior sagittal sinus runs in the upper border of the falx cerebri, whereas the inferior sagittal sinus runs in the lower border of the falx cerebri (**Fig. 20.9**). Large anterior skull base tumors may have large veins draining into the inferior sagittal sinus which, if disrupted, can bleed significantly.

◆ Vascular Anatomy of the Anterior Cranial Fossa

Tumors that arise in the tuberculum sella region, planum sphenoidale, or posterior olfactory fossa can involve the anterior part of the circle of Willis and anterior cranial fossa vessels as they push posteriorly and superiorly (**Fig. 20.10**). **Fig. 20.11** gives an overview of the how the carotids enter the skull base and then form the anterior portion of the circle of Willis and go on to supply the anterior cranial fossa. The most common tumor in this region is the tuberculum sella meningioma but others include craniopharyngiomas and anterior/superior extension of pituitary tumors. When the tumor fills the subchiasmatic cistern, the superior hypophyseal vessels are also at risk and damage to these vessels can lead to ischemic damage of the optic nerves and chiasm with blindness. When the A1-AComm-A2 complex is surrounded by tumor, understanding the anatomy of this complex is vital for safe surgery to be performed in this region (**Fig. 20.10**). A detailed description of the anterior cerebral arteries is given in **Fig. 20.12**. A1 (first part of the anterior cerebral artery) is formed when the internal carotid divides into the middle and anterior cerebral arteries. It enters the lamina terminalis cistern and at this point is banded to the lateral aspect of the optic nerves by thick arachnoid bands.[7] The medial lenticulostriate arteries arise from the posterior and superior surface of the first half of A1 and supply the medial septum pellucidum, medial part of the anterior commissure and pallidum, pillars of the fornix, paraolfactory area, anterior limb of the internal capsule, anteroinferior part of the striatum,

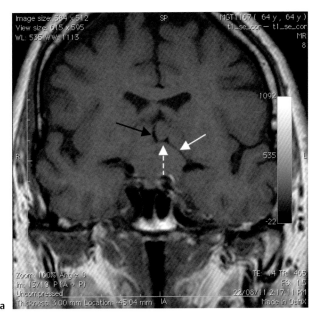
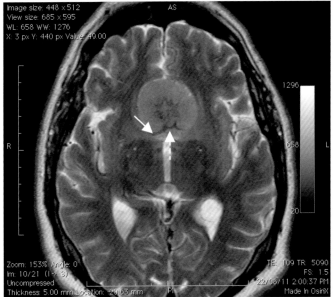

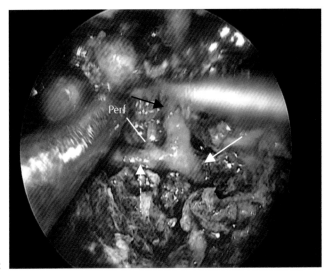
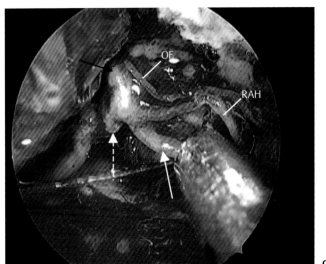

Fig. 20.10 (**a,b**) MRI scans show the A1 (*solid white arrow*) can be seen leaving the middle cerebral artery juncture toward the Acomm (*dashed white arrow*) with the A2s (*black arrow*) progressing superiorly. These vessels are all within the substance of the tumor. The clinical dissection of this tumor is seen in (**c**) and (**d**) with tumor encompassing the perforators (*Perf*) coming off the Acomm. Once all tumor had been removed, the vascular complex with A1–Acomm, A2, and the important branch of A1 (the recurrent artery of Hubner [*RAH*]) and the A2 branch (orbitofrontal [*OF*] artery) are clearly visible.

and anterior hypothalamus. Vessels arising from the second half of A1 are smaller and join the arterial plexus of the optic nerve, chiasm, and optic tract.[7,8] Once identified, the A1 vessel can be followed to the AComm and the recurrent artery of Heubner (**Figs. 20.10** and **20.12**). The recurrent artery of Heubner (RAH) is present bilaterally in 85% of patients, unilaterally in 11%, and absent in 4%.[8] It immediately courses posteriorly toward the trunk of A1 before entering the subarachnoid space and penetrating the brain at the junction of the medial and lateral olfactory stria. It is an important vessel to preserve as it supplies the head of the caudate and the anteroinferior internal capsule, anterior hypothalamus, and olfactory region. The other vitally important vessels in this region are the posterior perforating vessels from the AComm.

These branches can number from one to six and arise from the superior and posterior surface of AComm and course posteriorly to supply the infundibulum of the pituitary, optic nerve and chiasm, lamina terminalis, anterior perforating substance, corpus callosum, anterior commissure, limbic system, and associated regions of cortex. Deficits associated with injury to these arteries include serious and incapacitating memory deficits, personality changes, and electrolyte imbalances. Occlusion of A1 region can result in paraplegia of the lower extremities with sparing of the upper limbs, incontinence, abulic or motor aphasia, and frontal lobe symptoms.

The A2 has three main branches (**Figs. 20.10** and **20.12**). The RAH originates from the AComm–A2 junction or from the first few millimeters of A2 in 90% of patients (in the other

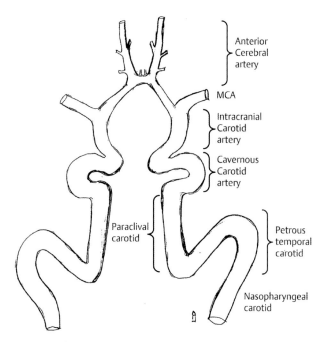

Fig. 20.11 The carotid bends laterally in the nasopharynx before entering the petrous temporal bone. It then swings anteriorly before becoming the paraclival carotid in the floor of the sphenoid and progresses vertically into the cavernous sinus and then enters the anterior cranial fossa giving off the middle cerebral artery (*MCA*) to become the anterior cerebral artery.

10% from the upper A1).[7,8] The other two branches are the orbitofrontal and frontopolar branches. The orbitofrontal usually originates from the first 5 mm of A2 at the junction of the lamina terminalis and callosal cisterns and has a downward and forward course, crossing the olfactory tract to the gyrus rectus. The frontopolar branch originates after the

orbitofrontal branch and travels anteriorly more medially across the subfrontal sulcus.

◆ Surgical Technique

The surgical removal of anterior skull base tumors requires a team consisting of an endoscopic sinus surgeon and a neurosurgeon. It is vitally important that both members of this skull base team have endoscopic skills. These are best learned doing pituitary tumor resections together as a team. Here the neurosurgeon learns how to manage the endoscope and how to work from the video monitor in two dimensions rather than with the microscope in three dimensions. The sinus surgeon learns how to manipulate intracranial tumors and surrounding neural and vascular structures. These hours spent on pituitary tumor resection build confidence within the skull base team, enabling benign or malignant nasal tumors with intracranial extension to be tackled.

The first steps for access are complete sphenoethmoidectomy with exposure of the entire skull base. If the tumor is relatively posteriorly sited with a relatively small intracranial extension, skull base resection can be performed without a frontal drillout procedure. In such cases the intracranial extension of tumor must be small and the resection of this extension should be possible without it being necessary to resect across the midline. Surgically, the skull base defect should be clearly delineated and then enlarged to expose uninvolved dura on all sides of the defect. The dura is then excised with a combination of endoscopic skull base scissors* (Integra) or scalpel with a normal margin of dura and the tumor extension and dura delivered into the nose.

However, if a complete resection of the anterior skull base is required, then the next step is to perform an endoscopic frontal drillout (EFSS grade 6) procedure allowing the

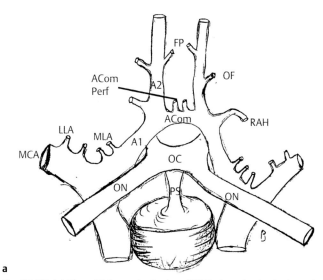

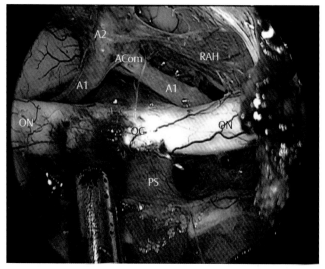

Fig. 20.12 (**a**) The middle cerebral artery (*MCA*) gives rise to the lateral lenticulostriate arteries (*LLA*) at the bifurcation complex. The medial lenticulostriate arteries (*MLA*) arise from the proximal section of A1. At the juncture of A1-Acomm-A2 the recurrent artery of Hubner (*RAH*) is given off. Acomm completes the anterior portion of the circle of Willis and has a number of perforating vessels (*ACom Perf*) that head posteriorly. In the first 5 mm of A2 the orbitofrontal (*OF*) artery is given off with the frontopolar (*FP*) artery staying more medially. (**b**) A clinical picture after removal of a tuberculum sella meningioma with a well-defined display of the anterior cerebral arteries.

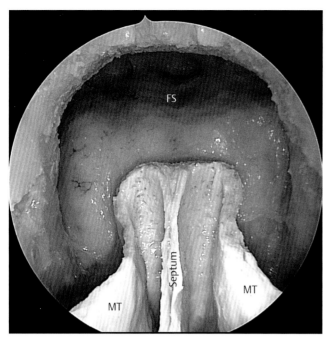

Fig. 20.13 Cadaveric dissection demonstrating the completion of a frontal drillout, with a maximized anterior/posterior dimension and complete removal of the intersinus septum. *MT*, middle turbinate; *FS*, frontal sinus.

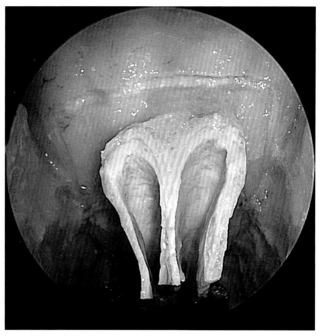

Fig. 20.14 Cadaveric dissection with osteotomies created using a diamond drill.

anterior aspect of the skull base to be delineated (**Fig. 20.13**). The nasal septum is separated from the skull base allowing visualization of the entire skull base from the frontal sinuses anteriorly to the anterior face of the pituitary fossa (**Fig. 20.2**). Both laminae papyracea should be on view forming the lateral limits of the resection. Before the skull base can be resected, the anterior and posterior ethmoidal arteries need to be identified and ligated or cauterized and divided. The technique of removing lamina papyracea to find the anterior artery as it enters the canal is not preferred as it risks rupture of the artery and with fat prolapse makes identification of the artery very difficult. An easier and safer technique is to run the diamond bur over the region of the anterior ethmoidal artery, removing the bone until the artery is exposed in its canal but not divided. The bone is removed over the artery with a malleable curette until the artery is fully exposed. The artery is then cauterized and divided. This is done bilaterally before the posterior ethmoidal arteries are also identified using the diamond drill on the skull base. The arteries usually enter the skull base at the junction of the posterior ethmoids and sphenoid and the drill is run over this region of the skull base until the artery is clearly identified, cauterized, and cut on both sides (**Fig. 20.4**).

The next step is to perform an endoscopic frontal drillout (EFFS grade 6) procedure as set out in Chapter 9. A septal window is performed and the frontal sinus opened bilaterally and communicated by removal of the intersinus septum (**Fig. 20.13**).

The final preparation step is to disconnect the nasal septum from the skull base. A straight through-cutting Blakesley is used to cut the nasal septum at its insertion to the skull

base. This isolates the skull base and allows the osteotomies to be made at the junction of the fovea ethmoidalis and lamina papyracea so that the skull base can be dropped into the nasal cavity (**Fig. 20.14**). A skull base diamond bur 3-mm (30,000 rpm) or Stylus high speed 3-mm diamond bur (Medtronic ENT) is used to create the osteotomies along the lines shown in **Fig. 20.14**. The dura is exposed but can be largely preserved. If necessary a 2- to 3-mm 40-degree forward-biting Kerrison punch can also be used to remove any residual bone to maximize the bony osteotomies to improve access for tumors with lateral extension. However, the osteotomies in the planum need to respect the optic nerve canals as their lateral landmarks. Next, the dura needs to be incised with a scalpel. The only residual attachment holding the skull base is the attachment of the falx cerebri to the crista galli (**Figs. 20.15** and **20.16**).

The falx cerebri often has vessels running in it and should be bipolar cauterized before being cut. This is done incrementally with the suction bipolar forceps (Integra) before each cut so maximal visualization is maintained during this process. The falx can extend posteriorly for some distance (often more than 1 cm) so care needs to be taken not to damage the vessels lying on each side of the falx. A curved endoscopic skull base scissors* (Integra) angled inferiorly is used to cut the falx cerebri and the skull base can then be dropped into the nasal cavity and removed (**Figs. 20.16** and **20.17**). To perform this maneuver, one surgeon puts downward pressure on the mobile skull base, putting any remaining attachments under stretch, allowing the second surgeon to either dissect free or cut any small residual attachments under visualization with magnification. If the posterior osteotomy is not 100% complete, this attachment can be gently fractured through the osteotomy lines

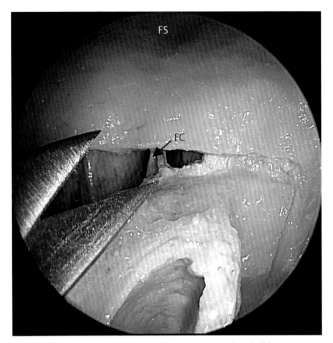

Fig. 20.15 Cadaveric dissection demonstrating the skull base scissor cutting the attachment of the falx cerebri (*FC*) to the crista galli.

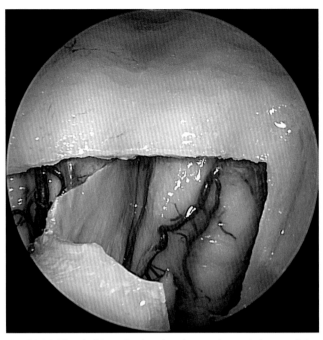

Fig. 20.16 The skull base is placed under traction and the remaining posterior falx cerebri still holds the skull base. This needs to be cut before the skull base can be dropped into the nose.

but the dura will need to be cut under direct vision. In most cases, limited extension of tumor through the skull base will be removed en bloc with the osteotomies placed through normal surrounding bone, similar to the technique for a craniofacial resection performed through a craniotomy.[9] Removal of the entire skull base in this fashion

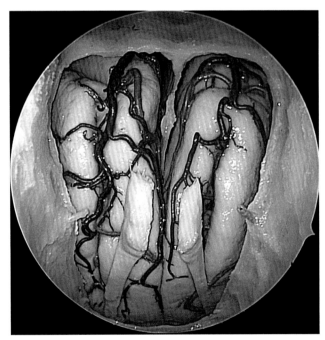

Fig. 20.17 The anterior skull base has been removed and both anterior cerebral gyri and olfactory bulbs are visible.

exposes the anterior cranial fossa and tumor that remains can now be dissected free. Such a dissection is again very delicate, requiring great endoscopic skill from both surgeons. The arachnoid plane needs to be developed and the tumor dissected from the arachnoid. Particularly for meningiomas that extend posteriorly onto the optic chiasm and superiorly and engulf the A1 (anterior cerebral artery prior to anterior communicating artery), AComm (anterior communicating artery), and A2 (anterior vertebral artery after AComm) complex, dissection of these vessels from the tumor is critical (**Fig. 20.10**). When the A1–A2 complex is engulfed in tumor, there are two routes to identifying the vessels and dissecting them free from the tumor. Once the bulk of the main tumor has been removed either with a Cusa Excel Ultrasonic aspirator (Integra Radionics; Burlington, MA) or Sonopet Ultrasonic aspirator (Stryker; Kalamazoo, MI), the arachnid plane is identified and the tumor wall delivered into the created cavity. This can be done superiorly looking for the frontopolar branch of A2 or for A2 itself or from below delivering the tumor superiorly into the cavity and identifying A1 (**Figs. 20.10** and **20.12**). With either technique once the vessels have been identified, the vessel is dissected free from the surrounding tumor by using a blunt hook (Integra endoscopic skull base set) and staying on the vessel wall and gently clearing tumor from the vessel wall. Alternatively, if it is felt that this cannot be safely done either due to the consistency of the tumor, position of the tumor, or endoscopic skill levels of the surgeons, then residual tumor should be left and the vessels not endangered.

Vessels that can be preserved are carefully dissected free from the tumor but vessels supplying the tumor are cauterized with bipolar forceps and divided.

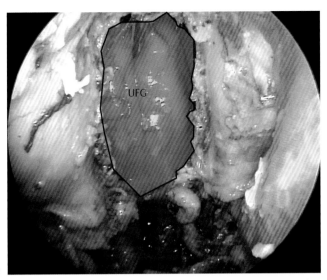
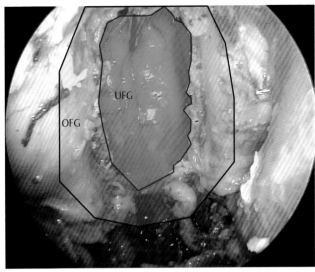

Fig. 20.18 In dissection (**a**) the fascia lata graft is placed as an underlay (*UFG*) on the inside of the cranial cavity and the edges smoothed out. In dissection (**b**) the second fascia lata graft is placed on the nasal surface of the defect as on overlay graft (*OFG*) again smoothing out the edges to ensure that the graft fits snugly around the entire defect.

◆ Skull Base Closure

If the dura or a large vessel, such as the intrasphenoid carotid artery, is exposed then coverage of this area is considered important for safe postoperative healing. In most cases this is done with a vascularized pedicled flap or, if this is not available, a free mucosal graft from the nose or fascia lata graft. An exposed carotid artery should not be left unprotected after surgery. All skull base cases have routine preparation of the thigh for the harvesting of fascia lata during the procedure and pituitary tumor cases have either the thigh or abdomen prepared for graft harvesting. In the past when large intra-arachnoid skull base access was needed for tumor resection, the defect was closed in layers utilizing fat then an underlay and overlay fascia lata or the acellular dermal graft AlloDerm (Life Cell; Branchburg, NJ) with a free mucosal graft over the top. In regions where intracranial high flow cerebrospinal fluid (CSF) cisterns have been opened, fat is placed intracranially and used to support the first underlay fascia lata graft or dural substitute graft. The underlay graft needs to extend 5–10 mm past the defect edges circumferentially (**Fig. 20.18**). In the anterior cranial fossa, especially when a frontal drillout procedure has been performed and the defect reaches the posterior wall of the frontal sinus, the underlay graft tends to slip posteriorly and all our leaks have come from the anterior edge of the defect. We now tend to secure this underlay graft anteriorly by placing two 1-mm holes through the skull base and either passing tails of the graft through these holes and "riveting" the graft or by placing a suture through the underlay graft and passing it through the holes and tying the two sutures together thereby fixing the graft anteriorly (**Fig. 20.19**).[10,11] It is important to ensure that the graft extends beyond the defect edges in all directions. This is best achieved with the malleable skull base probe (Integra) as it does not have a ball on the tip and will not drag an adjusted graft back out with it once the graft is properly positioned. The graft must not have any folds and must be smoothly adherent to the inner surface of the skull base. A thin ring of fat is placed at the defect edges on the underlay graft as a gasket to increase the seal of this layer. The second layer of fascia lata is placed as an overlay on the skull base, again ensuring that there are no folds and that it lies

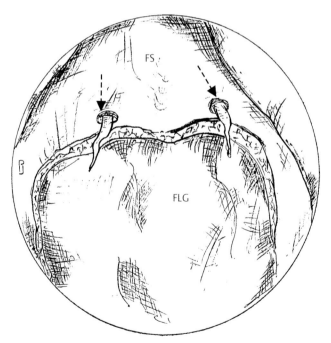

Fig. 20.19 In this patient, two small 1-mm holes (*broken arrows*) have been made through the anterior table anterior to the defect. Tails (*broken arrow*) of the underlay fascia lata graft (*FLG*) are pulled through these holes so that the anterior graft is "riveted" into the skull base. This prevents the graft from slipping posteriorly. In our experience this was the most common place for postoperative CSF leak. *FS*, frontal sinus.

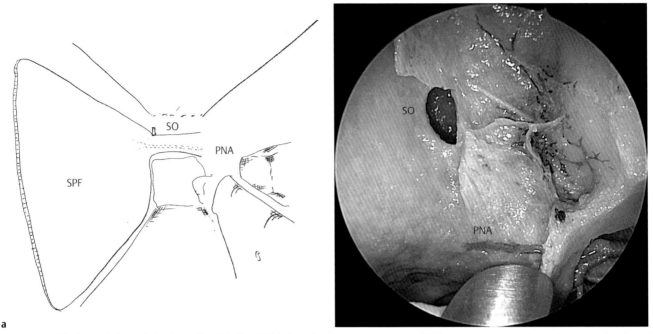

Fig. 20.20 (**a**) The Hadad vascularized septal pedicle flap (*SPF*) is based on the postnasal artery (*PNA*) and encompasses the entire mucosal surface of the septum. In the cadaver dissection (**b**) the PNA is clearly seen coming through the sphenopalatine foramen. *SO*, sphenoid ostium.

closely approximated to the skull base (**Fig. 20.18**). If a free mucosal graft is available this is placed over the second layer but is not essential. The edges of the overlay graft need to extend beyond the edges of the defect by about 10 mm in all directions and be placed onto bone denuded of mucosa. The edges of the graft are fixed with oxidized cellulose (Surgicel [Ethicon; Somerville, NJ]) and fibrin glue is applied to this layer followed by sheets of Gelfoam (Pfizer; Kalamazoo, MI). The Gelfoam ensures that the nasal pack does not stick to the grafts. The nasal cavity is packed with ribbon gauze soaked in the antiseptic BIPP (bismuth iodoform paraffin paste) or with an inflated intranasal balloon. We do not use the balloon as it is important to do an immediate postoperative CT if the balloon is used to ensure that the reconstruction has not been pushed intracranially by the balloon. This is not necessary with the BIPP pack as it is placed under direct vision and the packing force at all times controlled by the surgeon. This technique had a high postoperative CSF leak rate of around 15–30%.[10,11]

A recent important innovation by Hadad et al[12] where the vascularized pedicled septal flap was described has substantially altered the way that interarachnoid skull base defects are closed today (**Figs. 20.20** and **20.21**). This flap is based on the branch of the sphenopalatine artery—the postnasal artery (**Fig. 20.22**). This branch leaves the sphenopalatine foramen in its posterior superior aspect and travels along the anterior face of the sphenoid below the natural ostium of the sphenoid before reaching the posterior region of the septum. Here it divides into two main branches which, through the anastomosis with the anterior and posterior ethmoidal artery branches, supply the majority of the septum. The incisions for raising the flap are usually preformed after the sinuses have been fully opened and the middle turbinate resected.

Be aware that the posterior middle turbinate resection should not compromise the vascular pedicle of the flap. Performing the sinus surgery before raising the flap gives extra space and makes the procedure much simpler. It also allows the second surgeon to put parts of the flap under tension so that using a scissor is easier. My preference is to use a scalpel blade to make the incision for the flap although others use a Bovie unipolar needle that works just as well. The superior incision starts at the lower edge of the natural sphenoid ostium and proceeds toward the skull bases then comes anteriorly until just behind the mucocutaneous junction. It turns vertically onto the floor of the nose and then proceeds posteriorly to the posterior choana where it is taken along the inferior edge of the choana to the lateral nasal wall (**Fig. 20.21**). A suction Freer is used to raise the flap in the same way that a septoplasty is performed. Where the incisions have not gone through all the layers, the second surgeon places the flap under tension and the primary surgeon uses the skull base scissors to release the flap. In anterior skull base cases, the flap is placed in the nasopharynx during the resection. To close the defect, either intradural underlay fascia lata graft or a dural substitute such as the collagen matrix DuraGen (Integra Life Sciences) or Durepair (Medtronic) is used. This underlay graft should extend 5–10 mm beyond the bone edges of the defect and, as above, maintain smooth contact with the bony defect edges. The pedicled septal flap needs to be larger than the defect and overlap the mucosa free bony margins of the defect by at least 5 mm. If the septal flap from one side is not large enough, consideration can be given to using the opposite septal flap and resecting the septum. These flaps should then be placed side by side with minimal overlap over the bony defect. In some patients, this may still not allow complete coverage of the defect and a second layer of fascia lata is then used to

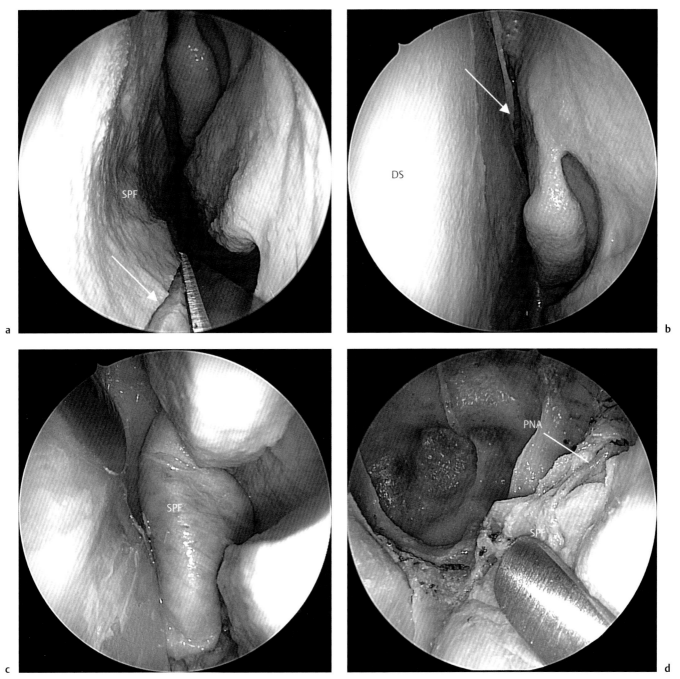

Fig. 20.21 In cadaver dissection (**a**) the inferior incision (*white arrow*) is taken back to the posterior choana. In (**b**) the superior incision (*white arrow*) and donor site (*DS*) of the septum is seen with the rolled septal pedicled flap (*SPF*) seen being pushed into the postnasal space. In (**c**) the septal pedicled flap (*SPF*) is rolled into the nasopharynx until reconstruction of the skull base. In (**d**) the postnasal artery (*PNA*) is seen entering the elevated septal pedicled flap (*SPF*).

create the second layer and may be bolstered by thin strips of fat on joining areas. The flap(s) are secured with Surgicel and sealed with a fibrin glue before being covered with Gelfoam and supported by a BIPP ribbon gauze nasal pack or, alternatively, an intranasal balloon inflated in the nasal cavity.

One of the morbidities associated with using the pedicled nasal septal flap is the crusting that happens on the donor site of the flap. To overcome this problem, we make a U-shaped incision on the opposite septal flap based anteriorly so that

the posterior portion of this mucosa can be swung around onto the opposite nostril and used to cover the donor site. This flap is secured with sutures at the beginning of the procedure (**Fig. 20.22**). At times the nose and nasal vestibule can dry out during the procedure, making the passage of instruments through this region difficult. To overcome this, we will place a rectangular piece of silastic over the columella with each tail going down the nostril and then place a through-and-through suture through the silastic and septum

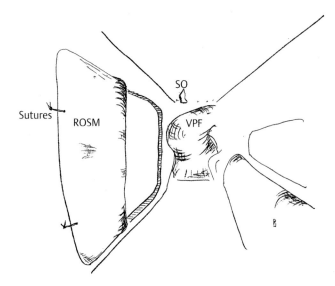

Fig. 20.22 The right-sided opposite septal mucosa (*ROSM*) is rotated from the right onto the left and secured anteriorly with sutures. This covers the donor defect and helps with the postoperative healing. *SO*, sphenoid ostium; *VPF*, vascularized pedicled flap.

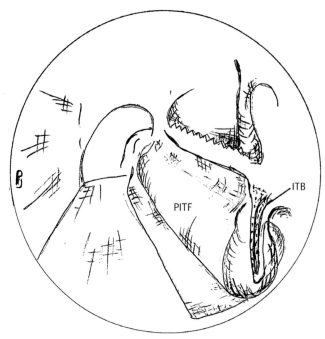

Fig. 20.23 The pedicled inferior turbinate flap (*PITF*) is raised by dissecting out the bone of the inferior turbinate (*ITB*) and raising adjacent nasal mucosa off the floor of the nose.

to keep the silastic in place. This helps with the passage of endoscopes and instruments and also protects the rotated and sutured septal flap.

In some patients, the tumor involves the septum or in revision patients where the septum has been resected or previously used, a septal flap is not available. In these patients, the pedicled inferior turbinate flap can be used as an alternative. It consists of the inferior turbinate and some adjacent floor of nose mucosa pedicled on a branch of the sphenopalatine artery that supplies the inferior turbinate through its posterior attachment. It is raised by performing a vertical incision down the anterior face of the inferior turbinate and then taking this incision onto the lateral nasal wall above the turbinate (the horizontal portion of the uncinate) and running this down the length of the turbinate (**Fig. 20.23**). At the posterior edge this is curved upward toward the sphenopalatine foramen to avoid cutting the artery supplying the flap. The anterior vertical cut is also brought around the anterior end of the turbinate onto the floor of the nose and taken posteriorly and curved up behind the posterior end of the inferior turbinate onto the lateral nasal wall (**Fig. 20.23**). The limitation of this flap is that it on average will only cover about 60% of the anterior cranial fossa. However, it will help bring vascularized tissue into the repair area and this with free grafts can be used to successfully close large defects in revision cases.

The anesthetist needs to be aware that as the patient is recovering from the anesthesia that he or she should be extubated while under relative deep anesthesia and a laryngeal mask inserted. This allows the patient to be ventilated without the need to use a facemask and also helps to ensure that the patient does not cough or strain during extubation which may precipitate intracranial bleeding and displacement of the reconstruction. The nasal pack is left in place for 1 week. The patient may be discharged with the pack in place and brought back for pack removal after 1 week.

◆ Case Examples and Surgical Technique

Anterior skull base midline meningiomas are one of the tumors that are suitable for a wholly endoscopic approach. These tumors arise from the dura and bone of the anterior skull base and may present late due to lack of symptoms. Often typical frontal lobe symptoms such as a subtle change in personality or inappropriate uncharacteristic behavior may be the only presenting feature. The intracranial pressure may be raised and the patient may complain of headaches. Meningiomas do have a tendency to recur after removal and recent papers discussing the high recurrence rate of sphenoid wing meningiomas concluded that tumor remnants left in the underlying bone were responsible for the recurrences.[7] The transnasal endoscopic approach overcomes this problem by removal of both the dura and underlying bone from which the tumor has arisen potentially lessening the possibility of recurrence after surgery.

Example 1

The first case example is of a young woman who presented with headache. A midline meningioma was diagnosed and initially was monitored with serial MRI scans but the tumor continued to grow (**Fig. 20.24**). She was offered both endoscopic and traditional external approach but chose to have an endoscopic resection.

The surgical plan for this patient was to do a bilateral complete sphenoethmoidectomy with exposure of the frontal ostia. It was not necessary to perform a frontal drillout

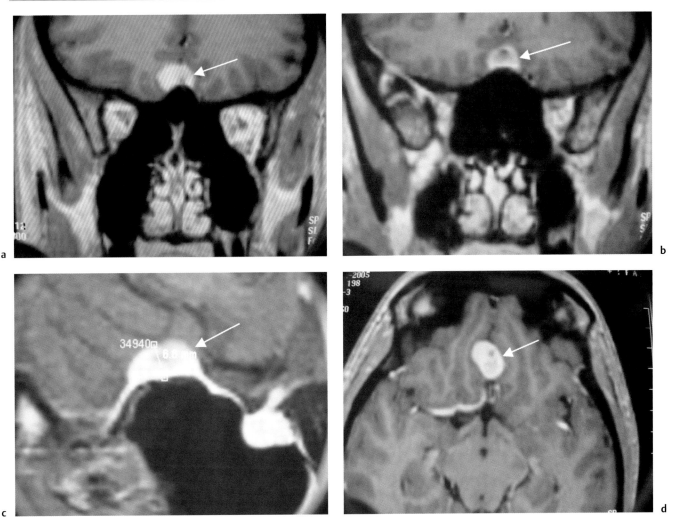

Fig. 20.24 (a,b) Coronal MRI scans in which the meningioma is indicated with a *white arrow*. (**c**) Parasagittal MRI scan in which the roof of the sphenoid is arched upward with the meningioma (*white arrow*) on its roof. (**d**) The meningioma is seen to push between the two cerebral hemispheres in this axial MRI.

procedure as the tumor was located in the posterior region of the anterior skull base. The posterior half of the septum was removed. The next step was to establish the extent of the tumor. With the aid of the computer-aided surgical (CAS) navigation system, the skull base osteotomies were marked out. The osteotomies were performed around the outside of the tumor using diamond burs and Kerrison punches. A combination of scalpel and endoscopic scissors were used to incise the dura allowing the tumor to drop into the nasal cavity. Arachnoid attachments were carefully dissected free of the tumor and the supplying blood vessels cauterized and divided. The entire tumor and attached dura were removed. The skull base was repaired using the previously described underlay and onlay layers of fascia lata, fibrin glue, and nasal pack. This was prior to the development of the pedicled septal flap. The patient was discharged the following day. Postoperative endoscopy shows a well-healed nasal cavity and skull base (**Fig. 20.25**) and follow-up MRI scans over the last 8 years have not shown any recurrence or residual tumor (**Fig. 20.25**).

Example 2

This elderly lady presented with memory loss and headaches. The large anterior cranial fossa meningioma had significant extension intranasally (**Fig. 20.26**). Note the calcification within the tumor and the different consistencies of the tumor in the nose and in the intracranial cavity. Also note that there was substantial brain edema around the intracranial tumor (**Fig. 20.26**).

The surgical approach for this patient was to perform bilateral maxillary antrostomies and complete sphenoethmoidectomies debulking the tumor during exposure of the sinuses. This debulking should be continued to where the skull base normally would be. An endoscopic frontal drill-out procedure was performed to expose the posterior wall of the frontal sinuses and the bone directly anterior to the tumor edge was removed. The inside of the tumor was carefully debulked, removing most of the inside of the tumor but retaining the outer shell. Once this had been completed, the surgical plane between the tumor and the anterior cerebral

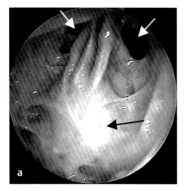 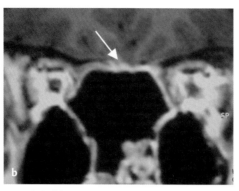 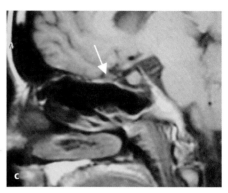

Fig. 20.25 (**a**) Endoscopic picture of the region of skull base reconstruction is indicated with a *black arrow*. Note the two frontal ostia anteriorly (*white arrows*). (**b**) Coronal MRI scan and (**c**) parasagittal MRI in which the region of skull base reconstruction and previous tumor is indicated with a *white arrow*.

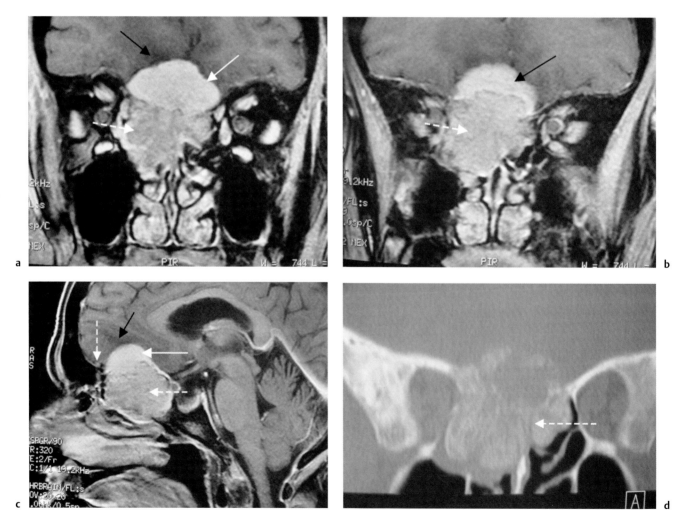

Fig. 20.26 In coronal MRI scans (**a,b**) and parasagittal MRI (**c**) the two consistencies of tumor are visible. The soft tumor is marked with a *solid white arrow*, whereas the calcified tumor is marked with a *broken white arrow*. In coronal CT scan (**d**) the calcified part of the tumor is clearly seen (*white broken arrow*).

Brain edema is indicated with a *solid black arrow* in (**a,c**). The other important feature seen in (**c**) is the close approximation of the tumor to the posterior wall of the frontal sinus (*broken white arrow*). This means that the anterior osteotomy should be through the posterior wall of the frontal sinus.

lobes was identified and the tumor carefully dissected away from the arachnoid. Neuropatties are placed where this dissection has been performed to maintain this plane and allow adjacent dissection to continue in the same plane. It also protected the underlying brain tissue from inadvertent damage. Any feeding vessels or veins draining from the tumor were cauterized with the suction bipolar forceps* (Integra) and divided. In this way, the tumor was progressively delivered into the nasal cavity until complete removal was achieved. The cavity was irrigated with warm lactated Ringer's solution and any bleeding vessels cauterized. The skull base was repaired in the manner previously described with two layers of fascia lata: the first placed as an underlay and the second as an overlay, followed by fibrin glue, Gelfoam, and a BIPP ribbon gauze nasal pack. Again, this case was done prior to the development of the pedicled septal flap. The pack was removed after 7 days. No lumbar drains were used. However, should a leak occur then a drain may be inserted.

Example 3

The third patient is a middle-aged man who presented with visual symptoms, headaches, and inappropriate euphoria. This midline olfactory groove meningioma was similar to the second case example but significantly larger and there was no nasal or sinus involvement (**Fig. 20.27**).

There are a number of ways that this meningioma could be tackled. The most common would be the bifrontal or pterional approaches.[13,14] The bifrontal approach gives good access to both sides but results in significant frontal lobe retraction and the important vascular structures are only approached late in the dissection.[13,14] The pterional approach[15,16] is rapid and requires ipsilateral frontal lobe retraction but the opposite frontal lobe does not need retraction and this has an advantage over the bifrontal approach. However, controversy exists as to whether it gives sufficient exposure to the contralateral side in patients with significant bilateral tumor extension.[15,16] In addition it allows access to the skull base vasculature relatively late in the dissection. The attraction of the transnasal approach is that the major arterial supply of the tumor, the anterior and posterior ethmoidal arteries, is ligated before

the tumor resection begins. In addition, the endoscopic approach removes the dura and underlying bone of the tumor, therefore theoretically lessening the chances of recurrence.[7] A significant advantage of this approach is the complete lack of brain retraction. The downside of the endoscopic approach is the ability of the surgeons to control significant bleeding from the arterial and venous bleeders. It is therefore important to evaluate the arterial blood supply of the tumor preoperatively with an angiogram and assess the arterial supply to the outer surface of the tumor—the so-called "peel" supply. If this is significant then the endoscopic approach may not be suitable. In addition, during this procedure any major feeding vessels from the external carotid artery such as the middle meningeal artery can be embolized.

Image guidance is essential for a patient such as this as it allows the tumor to be "seen" through the skull base so that the anterior osteotomy can be placed through bone directly adjacent to the tumor. Correct placement of the osteotomies allows the surgeon to identify the surgical plane between the outer surface of the tumor and normal brain tissue. This helps both with the removal of the core of the tumor while preserving the outer layer as well as when this outer layer is dissected from the arachnoid and brain. The standard preparation for resection of this tumor is bilateral maxillary antrostomies, complete sphenoethmoidectomies, and the endoscopic frontal drillout procedure of the frontal sinuses. Once this is complete, the anterior and posterior ethmoidal arteries are identified and ligated or cauterized and divided. The posterior osteotomies are performed with the diamond bur and the lateral osteotomies in the fovea ethmoidalis with either a diamond bur or Kerrison punch. The skull base is dropped into the nasal cavity after the fibrous attachment between the crista galli and falx is cut. It can then be removed from the nose and the base of the tumor exposed. In a tumor such as this, it is crucial that the tumor should be for the most part removed from the inside out thereby allowing the tumor to be collapsed inward on itself. If the tumor is soft this can be done with the skull base suction dissection instruments* (Integra) or with the 2.7-mm microdebrider blade. Great care must be taken when using the microdebrider blade with the intracranial cavity as it can be very aggressive when removing soft tissue. The suction should

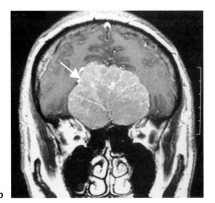
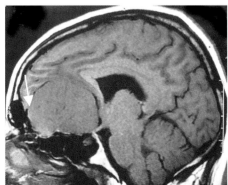
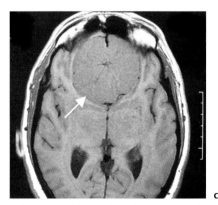

a,b   c

Fig. 20.27 (**a**) Coronal, (**b**) parasagittal, and (**c**) axial MRI scans in which the tumor is indicated with a *white arrow*. (**b**) Note how the tumor closely approximates the posterior wall of the frontal sinus.

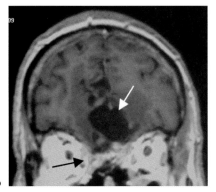 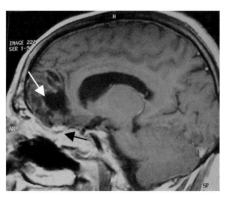 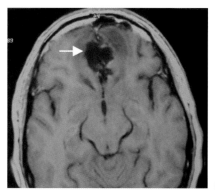

a,b

c

Fig. 20.28 (**a**) Coronal, (**b**) parasagittal, and (**c**) axial postoperative MRI scans; the region of where the tumor was resected is indicated with a *white arrow* and the reconstructed skull base with a *black arrow*.

be placed on a suction regulator to minimize the amount of tissue sucked into the cutting region. In addition, the oscillating speed of the blade should be below 1000 rpm and the entire extent of the blade should be visible during use. The blade is generally used facing superiorly so that the endoscope is looking at the opening when in use and the blade can be stopped if too much tissue is sucked into the opening or the tumor that is being resected is thought to contain a vessel. The second technique for removing the core of the tumor involves using the blades of the suction bipolar forceps to grasp the fibrous threads within the tumor and while gentle traction is placed on these, the bipolar is activated further shrinking the tumor and causing the tumor to collapse inward. Finally, new ultrasonic aspirators now have endonasal attachments (Cusa and Sonapet) which allow the inside of the tumor to be removed. This can be useful especially when there is bone inside the tumor as may be found in meningiomas. Once it is felt that only a relatively thin shell of tumor remains the surgical plane between the arachnoid and the brain is established and developed. A combination of malleable probes, suction Freer elevator, and neuropatties are used to mobilize the tumor from the brain. Vessels that cannot be mobilized off the surface of the tumor are cauterized with the bipolar forceps before being divided. In this patient, the surgery went relatively uneventfully until a relatively large vein draining the tumor into the inferior sagittal sinus was avulsed from the sinus. Ligar clips controlled the bleeding from the sinus and the remaining surgery was uneventful. This would not have been possible without two surgeons working simultaneously in the intracranial cavity. Skull base reconstruction was performed with an underlay and onlay fascia lata graft, fibrin glue, Gelfoam, and a BIPP nasal pack. Again, this case was done prior to the development of the vascularized pedicled septal flap. The pack was removed after 1 week. Postoperative MRI shows complete removal of the tumor (**Fig. 20.28**).

◆ Conclusion

Endoscopic transnasal intracranial surgery is a new and exciting development in skull base surgery. However, this surgery requires a high level of training and skill from both

the sinus surgeon and the neurosurgeon. In order to perform such surgeries, sinus surgeons and neurosurgeons need to form a skull base team. Such a team should develop their endoscopic skills by doing numerous endoscopic pituitary tumor dissections. As the level of expertise develops the team can tackle smaller selected intracranial tumors. Case selection and preparation are vitally important to the success of the surgery and the team should always be mindful that surgery with the highest likelihood of success and least morbidity should be chosen. One of the most important aspects of this surgery is the two-surgeon approach. Having two surgeons operating at the same time has huge advantages for both the ability of the surgeons to remove the tumor by placing traction on it and for the management of complications especially if significant hemorrhage occurs. The exact role of endoscopic cranial base resection in the management of malignancies is still not clear but it is likely that endoscopic techniques will increasingly play a role in the management of these patients. Finally, there is no substitute for a sound knowledge of anatomy and this chapter (and book) focuses on presenting the surgical anatomy in detail. This should be augmented with multiple cadaver dissections until the surgeons have extensive and detailed knowledge of the anatomy in this region.

References

1. Howard DJ, Lund VJ, Wei WI. Craniofacial resection for tumors of the nasal cavity and paranasal sinuses: a 25-year experience. Head Neck 2006;28(10):867–873

2. Batra PS, Citardi MJ, Worley S, Lee J, Lanza DC. Resection of anterior skull base tumors: comparison of combined traditional and endoscopic techniques. Am J Rhinol 2005;19(5):521–528

3. Castelnuovo PG, Belli E, Bignami M, Battaglia P, Sberze F, Tomei G. Endoscopic nasal and anterior craniotomy resection for malignant nasoethmoid tumors involving the anterior skull base. Skull Base 2006;16(1):15–18

4. Leong JL, Citardi MJ, Batra PS. Reconstruction of skull base defects after minimally invasive endoscopic resection of anterior skull base neoplasms. Am J Rhinol 2006;20(5):476–482

5. Buchmann L, Larsen C, Pollack A, Tawfik O, Sykes K, Hoover LA. Endoscopic techniques in resection of anterior skull base/paranasal sinus malignancies. Laryngoscope 2006;116(10):1749–1754

6. Snyderman CH, Kassam AB. Endoscopic techniques for pathology of the anterior cranial fossa and ventral skull base. J Am Coll Surg 2006;202(3):563

7. Hernesniemi J, Dashti R, Lehecka M, et al. Microneurosurgical management of anterior communicating artery aneurysms. Surg Neurol 2008;70(1):8–28, discussion 29

8. Uzün I, Gürdal E, Cakmak YO, Ozdogmus O, Cavdar S. A reminder of the anatomy of the recurrent artery of heubner. Cent Eur Neurosurg 2009;70(1):36–38

9. Pieper DR, Al-Mefty O, Hanada Y, Buechner D. Hyperostosis associated with meningioma of the cranial base: secondary changes or tumor invasion. Neurosurgery 1999;44(4):742–746, discussion 746–747

10. Zanation AM, Thorp BD, Parmar P, Harvey RJ. Reconstructive options for endoscopic skull base surgery. Otolaryngol Clin North Am 2011;44(5):1201–1222

11. Jardeleza C, Seiberling K, Floreani S, Wormald PJ. Surgical outcomes of endoscopic management of adenocarcinoma of the sinonasal cavity. Rhinology 2009;47(4):354–361

12. Hadad G, Bassagasteguy L, Carrau RL, et al. A novel reconstructive technique after endoscopic expanded endonasal approaches: vascular pedicle nasoseptal flap. Laryngoscope 2006;116(10):1882–1886

13. Hentschel SJ, DeMonte F. Olfactory groove meningiomas. Neurosurg Focus 2003;14(6):e4

14. Spektor S, Valarezo J, Fliss DM, et al. Olfactory groove meningiomas from neurosurgical and ear, nose, and throat perspectives: approaches, techniques, and outcomes. Neurosurgery 2005; 57(4, Suppl):268–280, discussion 268–280

15. Turazzi S, Cristofori L, Gambin R, Bricolo A. The pterional approach for the microsurgical removal of olfactory groove meningiomas. Neurosurgery 1999;45(4):821–825, discussion 825–826

16. Babu R, Barton A, Kasoff SS. Resection of olfactory groove meningiomas: technical note revisited. Surg Neurol 1995;44(6):567–572

21 Endoscopic Surgery of the Craniocervical Junction

◆ Introduction

Surgery on the craniocervical junction (CCJ) is complex due to its location behind the nasopharynx and difficulty of access through traditional techniques. The traditional approach has been the transoral approach.[1] This involves placing retractors in the mouth, opening the jaw, and retracting the tongue. Additionally, the soft palate is split and portions of the hard palate are resected, depending on the access required. The disadvantages of this approach are the need for a pre- and postoperative tracheostomy to secure the airway, contamination of the surgical field with oral bacteria, the potential postoperative dysfunction of the soft palate in swallowing and phonation, and the need to feed the patient through a nasogastric tube postoperatively.[2]

The endoscopic approach avoids these problems as the surgery site is out of the swallowing mechanism, swelling is usually limited and does not threaten the airway, and oral bacteria are avoided.[3]

◆ Pathology

There are a number of pathologies that can be addressed with this approach.

Rheumatoid Arthritis

The most common condition affecting the CCJ is the development of a rheumatoid pannus in patients with rheumatoid arthritis. The inflammatory process in the rheumatoid pannus causes ligament laxity, bone erosion, and then as the odontoid peg is no longer supported, it migrates into the brainstem causing compression by either direct pressure or by cervical subluxation.

Congenital Disorders

There are a number of congenital odontoid malformations, basilar invagination syndromes, and anomalies of the skull base that may affect the CCJ. Basilar invagination occurs when the tip of the odontoid moves more than 4.5 mm above a line drawn from the back of the hard palate to the base of the occiput (McGregor's line).[2]

Chordoma

Chordomas arise in the bone of the clivus and upper cervical spine from notochord remnants and are the most common tumor of the mobile spine.[2] These tumors rarely metastasize but are locally aggressive with bone destruction and neurologic involvement and complete resection with postoperative proton beam irradiation provides the best long-term survival.

Nasopharyngeal Carcinoma

These patients are treated initially with radiotherapy and usually respond well to this treatment. However, there is a small group of patients that fail multiple courses of radiotherapy and may need salvage surgery if the tumor involves this region. In addition, multiple courses of radiotherapy may result in radio-osteonecrosis of this region which in turn may require surgical debridement.

◆ Anatomy

The CCJ consists of the region of the upper spine (C1 and 2) and the skull base (occiput) that articulates with C1. C1 (atlas) does not have a vertebral body or spinous process which in

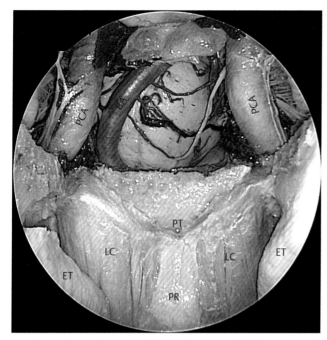

Fig. 21.1 Cadaveric dissection following the removal of the mucosa and pharyngobasilar fascia. The middle third of the clivus has been removed to reveal the pons. The longus capitis (*LC*) muscles insert broadly onto the floor of the sphenoid sinus (removed in this specimen). The pharyngeal raphe (*PR*) can be seen attaching to the pharyngeal tubercle (*PT*) of the occipital bone. *ET*, eustachian tube; *BA*, basilar artery; *PCA*, paraclival artery.

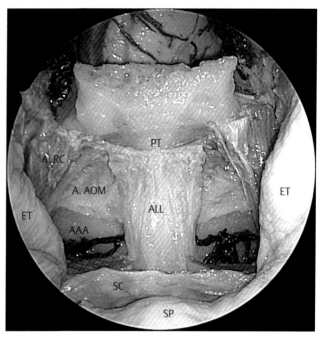

Fig. 21.2 Cadaveric dissection following the removal of the longus capitis muscles. This step reveals the anterior longitudinal ligaments (*ALL*), the anterior atlanto-occipital membrane (*A. AOM*), and the anterior rectus capitis muscle (*A. RC*). Note how the superior constrictor (*SC*) muscle finishes at the level of the soft palate (*SP*). *AAA*, anterior arch of the atlas; *ET*, eustachian tube; *PT*, pharyngeal tubercle.

turn allows significant movement between the atlas and the skull base. This movement accounts for over half of the head's axial rotation.[4] The atlas has two thick lateral masses that articulate with the occipital condyles. The odontoid peg is positioned where the vertebral body of the atlas would normally be and fixed to the clivus by the apical and alar ligaments. As most surgery in this region involves exposure and resection of the odontoid, the ligamentous attachments and layers of the CCJ are important to understand. When this region is approached anteriorly, the first layer encountered is the nasopharyngeal mucosa followed by the pharyngobasilar fascia, the longus capitis, and more inferiorly the longus coli muscles, atlanto-occipital membrane, anterior longitudinal ligament, atlanto-occipital ligaments, arch of the atlas, and odontoid peg (**Figs. 21.1, 21.2, 21.3,** and **21.4**). The peg is supported by the apical and alar ligaments which form a secure attachment to the occipital bone/clivus (**Fig. 21.5**). Posterior to the odontoid, the cruciate ligaments (vertical and horizontal elements) provide strong support for the odontoid and prevent posterior displacement (**Fig. 21.6**). The cruciate ligaments are commonly affected by the rheumatoid pannus and weakened by the associated inflammation. Behind the cruciate ligaments is the tectorial membrane (**Fig. 21.5**). In **Fig. 21.5** the anatomy is viewed from posterior with the tectorial membrane partially cut away to give a view of the cruciate ligaments. The superior aspect of the cruciate ligament is cut away to give a view of the apical and alar ligaments of the odontoid peg (dens). A parasagittal view is also provided demonstrating the layers from anterior to posterior in this complex area.

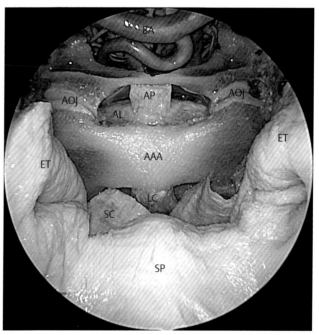

Fig. 21.3 Cadaveric dissection following the removal of the anterior atlantooccipital membrane, anterior longitudinal ligament, the longus capitis muscles, and the anterior rectus capitis muscles. This reveals the joint capsule of the atlanto-occipital joint (*AOJ*). This joint capsule has been removed to reveal the joint surfaces. The superior constrictor muscle (*SC*) has been split to show the insertion of the longus coli muscle (*LC*). The apical ligaments (*AP*) and alar ligaments (*AL*) can be seen clearly. *SP*, soft palate; *ET*, eustachian tube; *AAA*, anterior arch of the atlas; *BA*, basilar artery.

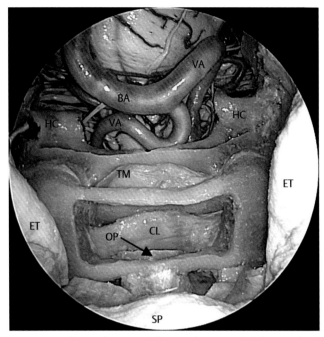

Fig. 21.4 Cadaveric dissection following the removal of the apical and alar ligaments, and the odontoid process has been drilled away (*OP*). This reveals the strong and thick transverse portion of the cruciform ligament (*CL*). Behind this is located the tectorial membrane (*TM*). *ET*, eustachian tube; *SP*, soft palate; *HC*, hypoglossal canal; *VA*, vertebral artery; *BA*, basilar artery.

and enter the upper cervical region and then pass behind the occipital condyles to join anterior to the medulla to form the basilar artery (**Figs. 21.8** and **21.9**). The vertebrobasilar junction is usually at the pontomedullary junction (**Fig. 21.8**). The main branch of the vertebral artery is the posteroinferior cerebellar artery (PICA) (**Fig. 21.6**).

◆ Preoperative Preparation

Preoperatively patients have both a CT scan and a MRI scan with contrast. This allows the soft tissue, bony landmarks, and vasculature to be accurately identified. The CT and MRI are merged on the image guidance machine (**Fig. 21.10**) and the toggle is used to move on a single image between bone windows and soft tissue windows. The contrast MRI also allows accurate identification of the vasculature so surgical approaches can be planned with minimum risk to the vasculature. The extent of resection of the anterior arch of the atlas and odontoid is decided on the scans and plans are made as to whether fixing of the CCJ is needed and if this is better done preoperatively or postoperatively. The thigh is prepared for harvesting of fat and fascia in case this may be needed in the reconstruction of the surgically created defect.

◆ Endoscopic Surgical Approach to the Odontoid Peg

The first step is to decide to what extent resection of the clivus is needed. In patients with a chordoma extending down into the atlas it may be necessary to resect the clivus from the floor of the pituitary fossa down to the base of the arch of the atlas (**Fig. 21.8**). If the pathology is an invagination of the odontoid, opening of the sphenoid may not be required and the resection can be limited to the nasopharynx. To maximize the access the inferior turbinates are lateralized or resected. To improve the postoperative healing, a pedicled septal flap is elevated and placed in an opened maxillary

As the intracranial cavity is approached the lower region of the brainstem and lower cranial nerves are exposed. The medullary pyramids face the clivus with the hypoglossal nerve arising from the upper medulla. This series of rootlets then converge on the hypoglossal canal which lies above the occipital condyles (**Figs. 21.6** and **21.7**). The accessory nerve has a cranial component whose rootlets hitch onto the vagus (**Fig. 21.6**). Its spinal portion arises from a series of rootlets from the lower medulla and upper spinal cord and then is the only cranial nerve to pass through the foramen magnum. The vertebral arteries pass lateral to the lateral masses in the axis

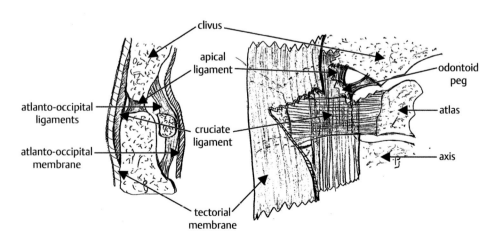

Fig. 21.5 An illustration of the craniocervical junction in the sagittal plane (*left*) and viewed from posterior with the tectorial membrane and cruciate ligaments partly cut away to reveal the underlying structures.

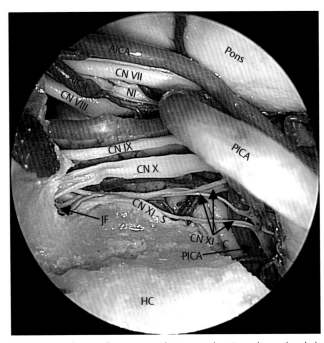

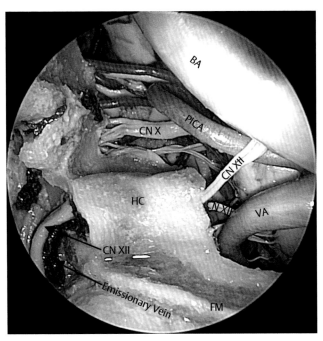

Fig. 21.6 Cadaveric dissection with image taken just above the skeletonized hypoglossal canal (*HC*) at the cerebellopontine angle. The anterior inferior cerebellar artery (*AICA*) can be seen intimately associated with the vestibulocochlear nerve (*CN VIII*), facial nerve (*CN VII*), and the nervus intermedius (*NI*). The posterior inferior cerebellar artery (*PICA*) can be seen running between the vagus (*CN X*) and spinal and cranial portions of the accessory nerves (*CN XI – S, CN XI – C*).

Fig. 21.7 Cadaveric dissection image showing the hypoglossal nerve exiting the hypoglossal foramen with its corresponding vein that communicates the internal jugular vein with the basilar plexus. *HC*, hypoglossal canal; *CN XII*, hypoglossal nerve and rootlets; *FM*, foramen magnum; *VA*, vertebral artery; *PICA*, posterior inferior cerebellar artery; *BA*, basilar artery; *CN X*, vagus nerve.

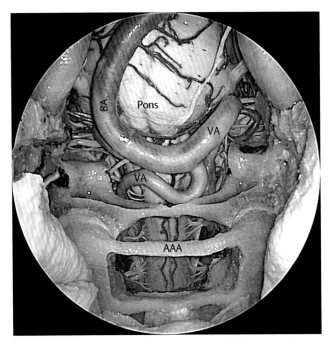

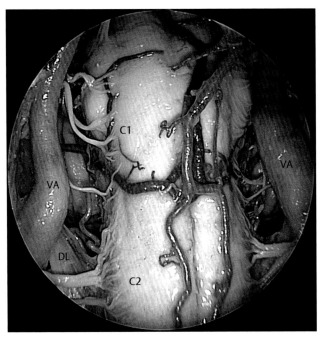

Fig. 21.8 Cadaveric dissection following removal of the tectorial membrane and the odontoid process. The anterior arch of the atlas has been drilled away centrally to reveal the upper cervical spinal cord behind. C1 and C2 spinal nerves can been seen clearly. *AAA*, anterior arch of atlas; *VA*, vertebral artery; *BA*, basilar artery.

Fig. 21.9 Cadaveric dissection image shows the close-up view of the upper cervical spinal cord. The image clearly shows the C1 and C2 nerve rootlets, the dentate ligaments (*DL*), and the vertebral artery (*VA*) as it enters the foramen magnum. *ASA*, anterior spinal artery.

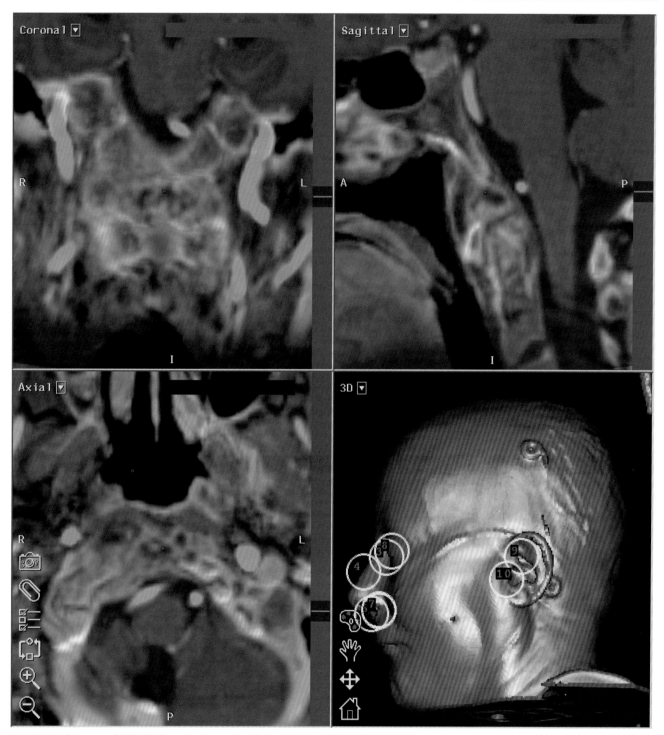

Fig. 21.10 This merged CT/MRI shows the tumor (*red dot*) at the base of the clivus and abutting the atlas and odontoid peg in the region of the craniocervical junction in a coronal, sagittal, and axial plane. Note the contrast in the vessels allowing clear identification of the major vessels.

sinus to move it out of the operative field. If the region to be resected is extensive then bilateral pedicled septal flaps are harvested. A posterior septectomy is performed and where only one septal flap has been raised, the mucosa from the opposite posterior septal region is folded anteriorly to cover the donation site of the pedicled septal flap and secured anteriorly with sutures.

Image guidance is used to map out the cervical carotid arteries to ensure that they are not in the surgical field. In addition, the clivus, anterior arch of the atlas, and body of the axis are identified. The arch of the atlas is at the most caudal region that can be reached through the transnasal approach. If it is necessary to increase the caudal exposure, the posterior superior edge of the hard palate can be drilled away but care

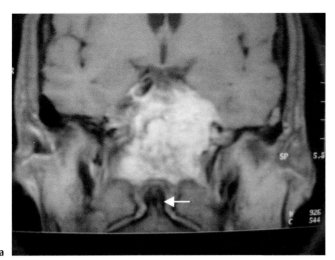
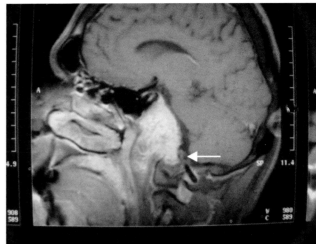

a   b

Fig. 21.11 A large clival chordoma with involvement of the entire clivus and extending inferiorly into the craniocervical junction abutting the atlas and odontoid peg (*white arrow*).

should be taken to preserve the oral mucosa under the hard palate. The next step is to remove the mucosa and longus capitis muscles over these structures as far lateral as the eustachian tubes (as this is usually medial to the carotids) until the anterior longitudinal ligament and the atlanto–occipital membrane are identified. No attempt is made to raise a flap as doing this is difficult and the raised flap compromises the access. Instead, the Coblater or unipolar diathermy is used to remove these structures down to and including the atlanto-occipital membrane. The bone of the anterior arch of the atlas and the odontoid is exposed. A high-speed drill is used to remove the bone of the anterior arch up to the lateral masses. This increases the exposure of the odontoid peg (dens). To begin the odontoid resection, the superior aspect of the dens is exposed by cutting the apical ligament. Care should be taken not to open the dura. This allows the dens to be removed from top down by using a high-speed drill to gently remove the center of the dens, leaving a posterior egg shell behind. This egg shelled bone is then carefully dissected free of the alar ligaments and cruciate ligament. Traction is placed on the bony fragments to lessen the intradural compression during dissection. The bony fragments and any associated rheumatoid pannus is dissected free of the tectorial membrane. In some patients, the pannus may contribute to the compression so this should be removed until underlying pulsatile dura is seen ensuring a complete decompression. The defect is covered with the pedicled septal flap with the edges of the flap covered with a layer of Surgicel (Ethicon; Somerville, NJ) and fibrin glue. No other packing is placed.

Other pathologies can also be addressed in this area. In some patients clival chordomas may localized to the CCJ and the surgical access is similar to what has been described above (**Fig. 21.10**). In this patient, the chordoma is at the lower end of the clivus and involves the arch of the atlas and extends laterally to the occipital condyles. In **Fig. 21.11** a much larger chordoma extends from the base of the pituitary all the way to the atlas and involves the atlas and upper aspect of the odontoid peg. This patient would require a full clival exposure and a CCJ exposure to ensure complete resection of the tumor.

◆ Key Points

- Multiple different pathologies occur in the region of the CCJ.
- Imaging with both CT and MRI is important for assessment of the pathology, vasculature, and for planning of the surgical approach.
- A decision needs to be made before surgery as to the need of cervical fixation either pre- or postsurgery.
- A pedicled septal flap is raised before a posterior septectomy is done.
- All soft tissues and ligaments anterior to the peg and arch of the atlas are removed.
- The peg and anterior arch of the atlas are removed with a high-speed drill with the posterior wall egg shelled before being dissected free.

References

1. Hadley MN, Spetzler RF, Sonntag VK. The transoral approach to the superior cervical spine. A review of 53 cases of extradural cervicomedullary compression. J Neurosurg 1989;71(1):16–23
2. Wu JC, Mummaneni PV, El-Sayed IH. Diseases of the odontoid and craniovertebral junction with management by endoscopic approaches. Otolaryngol Clin North Am 2011;44(5):1029–1042
3. Kassam AB, Snyderman C, Gardner P, Carrau R, Spiro R. The expanded endonasal approach: a fully endoscopic transnasal approach and resection of the odontoid process: technical case report. Neurosurgery 2005;57(1, Suppl)E213, discussion E213
4. Cardosa ACC, Brock R, Martins C, de Alancastro LP, Rhoton AL. Microendoscopic anatomy of the craniocervical Junction. In: Stamm A, ed. Transnasal endoscopic skull base and brain surgery. Thieme New York; 2011

22 Carotid Artery and Major Vascular Injury during Endoscopic Surgery

◆ Introduction

The incidence of injury to the internal carotid artery (ICA) during ESS is very low with only 29 cases having been described in the literature.[1] Injury during endoscopic skull base surgery is, however, more common with an incidence during pituitary surgery of around 5% and higher in parasellar and post fossa surgery.[1] One of the limitations of endoscopic skull base surgery for tumors involving the carotids has been the ability of the surgeon to endoscopically control and repair major vascular hemorrhage. Major vascular injury has a significant and probably underestimated mortality of 15% and permanent morbidity of 26%.[1] Significant tumor involvement of the major vasculature has in the past been considered a relative contraindication to the endoscopic approach. However, with training courses on animals duplicating the conditions of vascular rupture during surgery,[2] skills have been developed that allow skull base teams to tackle such cases.

◆ High-Risk Patients

Patients at high risk are patients with previous radiotherapy, hormone-secreting pituitary tumors particularly prolactinomas, and growth hormone–secreting tumors. Acromegalic patients will at times have ectatic carotids often with the tumor in contact or surrounding the carotid.[3] Any tumor including meningiomas, clival chordomas, and craniopharyngiomas that contacts or envelop the carotids places the patient at higher risk during dissection of the tumor.[1]

◆ Management

Surgical Field

A major vascular injury creates the most challenging surgical field possible in endoscopic surgery. The high-volume and high-pressure blood flow quickly contaminates the end of the endoscope leaving the surgeon without a view.[4] No safe maneuvers can be performed if the surgeon cannot see. It is usually not possible for the surgeon to both obtain a surgical view and perform an effective maneuver if he/she is alone. The two-surgeon approach allows one surgeon to control the blood stream and direct it away from the endoscope and this allows the second surgeon to obtain sufficient view to perform the maneuvers necessary for achieving hemostasis.[4] There are a number of principles for surgical field control. First, two large bore (10–12 French) suctions are needed and if available the endoscope should have a lens cleaning system that enables the end of the endoscope to be washed immediately if it is contaminated. This means that the endoscope does not be need to be removed to clear the view. The first step is to decide which nostril to place the endoscope. Usually the blood stream is directed predominantly into one side of the nose[4] (**Fig. 22.1**).

This should be assessed and the endoscope should be placed down the opposite nostril. The second surgeon should place the suction down the side of major flow while the primary surgeon places the endoscope and second suction down the opposite nostril. The primary surgeon should push the pedicled septal flap out of the way and clear the nostril of blood ahead of the endoscope. We have found that in these situations the flap floats and if only one suction is used it quickly becomes blocked as the flap is sucked into the end of the suction and the surgical field is lost. Once the flap is pushed into the nasopharynx, the second surgeon can place their large bore suction directly over the bleeding vessels and guide the blood stream into their suction, thereby providing the primary surgeon with the visualization necessary to perform the surgical maneuver for hemostasis (**Fig. 22.2**). In **Fig. 22.2** the patient had a large posterior fossa meningioma with the left vertebral artery pushed by the tumor onto the right side and partially encased by the tumor. The Sonopet (Stryker; Kalamazoo, MI) was being used to debulk the tumor when the vertebral artery was touched with subsequent bleeding. Note how the suction is positioned directly over the bleeding vessel (*white arrow*) and how it was able

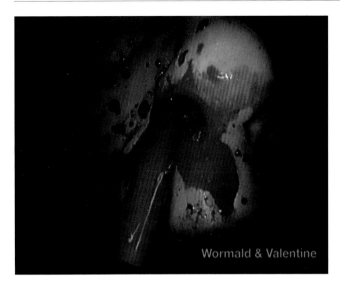

Fig. 22.1 The vascular stream can be seen coming predominantly out of the right nostril. When an endoscope is placed in the nose it should be placed down the left nostril to avoid instant contamination of the end of the scope with blood.

to collect all the blood from the vessel while the muscle graft was maneuvered to be placed onto the vessel.

If the endoscope and the suction are placed down the same nostril when this guiding of the blood stream is attempted, the blood stream will often track alongside of the suction with immediate soiling of the endoscope and loss of the surgical field (**Fig. 22.3**).

Hemostasis

Muscle Patch

In the past, the first response of surgeons in this very challenging situation was to attempt to pack the bleeding vessel

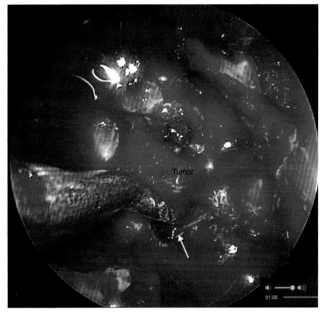

Fig. 22.2 This image shows a large posterior fossa meningioma (*tumor*) with a large suction placed just above a bleeding vertebral artery—blood stream indicated by the *white arrow*. The suction is "hovering" above the bleeding vessel and collecting all the blood allowing the lesion to be seen.

to achieve hemostasis. Raymond et al[5] reviewed 12 cases in which a carotid injury had occurred. In eight of the 12, the nasal packing resulted in complete occlusion of the ICA, four had stenosis of the ICA, and one patient partial occlusion of the middle cerebral artery as well as the ICA. The authors concluded that overpacking contributed to both the morbidity and mortality of the patients.[5] In skull base surgery there is often wide exposure of the surgical field with a large amount of brain and associated critical vessels such as the basilar and brainstem perforators from the exposed circle of Willis. Packing in this situation can contribute

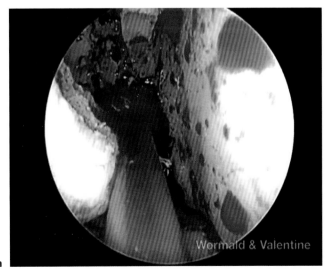
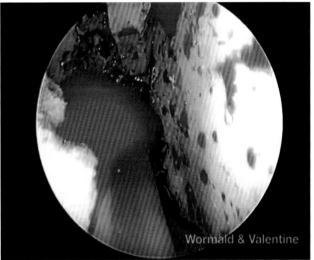

a   b

Fig. 22.3 (a) The suction and endoscope are placed in the same nostril attracting the vascular stream to the suction. (b) The vascular stream tracks up the suction and will soil the endoscope with loss of vision.

significantly to the morbidity and even mortality of the patient and should only be done on the bleeding vessel alone rather than on the surgical area being operated upon. In our department, we have developed an animal model of carotid artery injury and assessed the various materials commonly available for management of a significant vascular injury. These included oxidized cellulose, thrombin-gelatin matrix, and crushed muscle patch. Valentine et al[2] showed the only effective agent was crushed muscle which succeeded in achieving hemostasis in all cases. The other materials did not achieve hemostasis with resultant exsanguination of the animal model. The techniques of using the muscle patch repair is for the muscle to be harvested from either the thigh (usually pre-prepared in skull base cases for taking of a fascia lata graft) or from the sternomastoid muscle in the neck. A 2 cm × 1.5 cm × 1 cm piece of muscle is harvested and then crushed between two metal kidney dishes. The primary surgeon uses a Blakesley forceps to guide the muscle patch toward the bleeding vessel. The Blakesley should not be closed over the muscle patch but the jaws of the instrument should remain open with the muscle patch folded into the jaws. If the Blakesley is closed around the muscle patch, it becomes very difficult to remove the Blakesley from the vascular lesion without disrupting the muscle patch (**Fig. 22.4**). We have found that in a few of the injuries that we have managed that it is almost impossible to remove the Blakesley without there being a re-bleed if the Blakesley was closed at the time of positioning the muscle against the vascular lesion. Once the muscle patch is ready for positioning, the second surgeon keeps the surgical field visible by continually guiding the blood stream up the large bore suction. The suction is hovered just above the site of injury. If the suction gets too close it will suck onto the wall of the vessel and result in loss of the surgical field. If the suction is too far away from the lesion then all the blood is not collected from the lesion and again the surgical field is lost. These techniques are now taught in our workshops where the sheep animal model of carotid injury is used[6] with the nasal model to re-create exactly the clinical situation with the very challenging surgical field and teach how to maintain the surgical field and be able to place the muscle patch and achieve hemostasis. Such courses are recommended as the skills attained in this way will more effectively allow surgeons faced with this very difficult situation to achieve better outcomes for their patients.

Direct Vascular Repair

In the situation where there has been considerable dissection of the vasculature and the vascular lesion is not enclosed by bone or in a difficult to access location, direct repair of the injury is possible. We have developed in conjunction with Integra a series of endoscopic vascular clamps that can be endoscopically placed (**Fig. 22.5**). These clamps have been designed to side clamp the vessel lesion while still allowing patency of the vessel during suturing of the lesion (**Fig. 22.5**). The AnastoClip device (LeMaitre Vascular Inc; Burlington, MA) is a rapid vessel closure system (**Fig. 22.6**) which everts the vessel lesion edges without penetrating the vessel wall (**Fig. 22.7**). The clips need to be placed tightly together along the entire length of the lesion in the vessel wall.

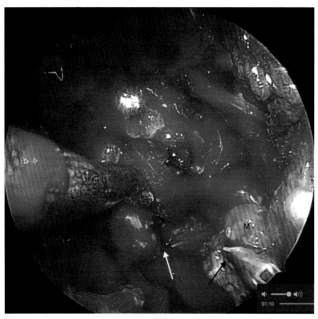

Fig. 22.4 This is the same patient as in **Fig. 22.2** with the suction still hovering above the bleeding vessel (*white arrow*). The muscle patch (*M*) is approaching the lesion held by the Blakesley. The Blakesley jaws are closed (*black arrow*) which will make removal of the forceps without dislodgement of the muscle patch very difficult once hemostasis is achieved.

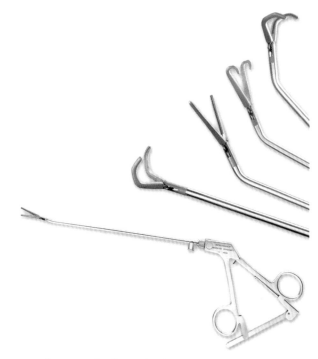

Fig. 22.5 The series of endovascular clamps, clip appliers, and suturing forceps* developed in conjunction with Integra to manage vascular injuries during endoscopic skull base surgery.

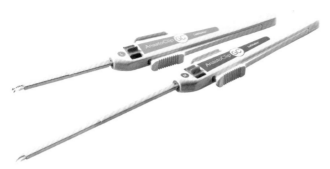

Fig. 22.6 The AnastoClip device (LeMaitre Vascular) used for primary vessel closure once the vessel walls are approximated with either a vascular clamp or aneurysm clip. (Image courtesy of LeMaitre Vascular.)

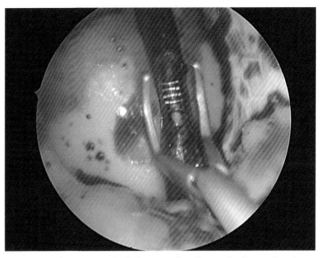

Fig. 22.8 After removal of the vascular clamp the lesion has been successfully closed with the AnastoClips maintaining perfusion through the vessel.

Recently, a longer endoscopic applicator (15 cm) has been developed to facilitate use in the endoscopic skull base environment. Instead of the vascular clamps placed on the lesion, an aneurysm clip can be applied (**Fig. 22.8**). Once the aneurysm clip is in place, the AnastoClips can be placed onto the vessel wall for final closure (**Fig. 22.9**). If the bleeding vessel is entirely endocranial then the aneurysm clip can be left as the definitive closure technique for the lesion. These techniques are technically demanding and should be practiced on the animal model courses before being attempted on patients. Laws et al[7] have also described direct repair of a vascular lesion but again it is stressed that to do this requires considerable technical skill, the correct equipment, experience, and training.

Intravascular Techniques

In some patients, it may not be possible to achieve hemostasis and the patient should be immediately transferred to the endovascular suite for either stenting, balloon occlusion, or coiling. Stenting is the preferred technique but can be very difficult in the anterior genu of the cavernous carotid. Distal migration may also occlude the ophthalmic artery with subsequent blindness. A balloon occlusion should ideally be done with an awake patient to test to see if there is sufficient collateral circulation to allow perfusion of that side of the brain without neurological deficit. The balloon occlusion test (BOT) is usually performed for 30 minutes and if there are no neurological sequelae the vessel can be occluded. This is not possible in the emergency situation where vascular control has not been achieved and occlusion techniques may be the only way that the patient's life can be saved. In addition, there is 4% risk of a stroke in the 30 days after stent placement.[8] Antiplatelet therapy may be needed for up to 3 months after placement.[9]

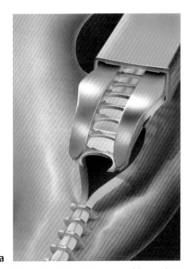

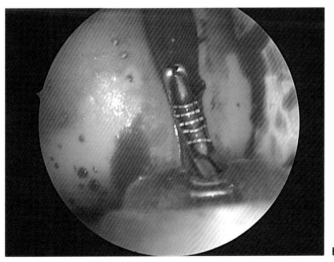

a   b

Fig. 22.7 (**a**) Illustration of how the AnastoClips evert the vessel wall edges to approximate the edges as a primary closure technique. (Image courtesy of LeMaitre Vascular.) (**b**) The AnastoClips are placed close together while the lesion edges are approximated by a vascular clamp which side clamps the vessel while still allowing perfusion through the vessel.

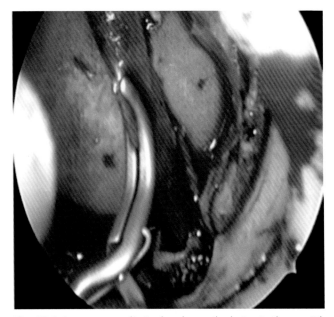

Fig. 22.9 An aneurysm clip is placed over the lesion in the carotid. Although narrowed, there is still perfusion through the vessel.

◆ Postoperative Complications

Once hemostasis has been achieved and the surgery completed, the patient should be transferred directly to the endovascular suite for an angiogram. The repair is assessed and if necessary further endovascular intervention can be performed. The most common postoperative complication is the formation of a pseudoaneurysm and this occurs in up 60% of patients.[1] A pseudoaneurysm is a defect through all layers of the vessel wall with flow of blood into a contained space outside the walls of the vessel. The aneurysm commonly forms in the first 6 weeks postsurgery but can form even years later. If the immediate postoperative angiogram is normal, the patient is monitored in intensive care until the packing is removed and a further angiogram is performed usually a week later. If this is normal the angiogram is repeated again at 6 weeks, 3 months, and 1 year. If a pseudoaneurysm is detected, it is treated by either stent graft placement or, if this is not possible, by coiling the aneurysm opening or occluding the vessel either with coiling or balloons. Coiling the aneurysm opening has a higher complication rate as the pseudoaneurysm does not have a wall against which the coil can sit and rupture may still occur.[10] Coiling the aneurysm opening

is reserved for patients who fail the balloon occlusion test as extracranial/intracranial carotid artery bypass surgery has a high complication rate and is the only alternative. The other major complication is a carotid-cavernous sinus fistula (CCF) which occurs between the carotid defect and cavernous sinus. The endovascular treatment is the same as for a pseudoaneurysm. However, in this situation, detachable balloons may be used to occlude the fistula while maintaining parent vessel patency.

◆ Major Vessel Injury Management Training

As major vessel injury is the next major frontier for endoscopic surgeons, the availability of realistic animal model training in the management of this significant complication is a major advance. Adelaide now runs these courses twice a year and encourages skull base teams (ENT and neurosurgeon) to attend and learn the techniques of surgical field management, muscle patch, and direct vessel suturing (www.adelaidesinussurgery.com).

References

1. Valentine R, Wormald PJ. Carotid artery injury following endonasal surgery. Am Clin N Am 2011; 44(5): 1059–79
2. Valentine R, Boase S, Jervis-Bardy J, Cabral DD, Robinson S, Wormald PJ. The efficacy of hemostatic techniques in the sheep model of carotid artery injury. Int Forum Allergy Rhinol 2011;1(2):118–122
3. Hatam A, Greitz T. Ectasia of cerebral arteries in acromegaly. Acta Radiol Diagn (Stockh) 1972;12(4):410–418
4. Valentine R, Wormald PJ. Controlling the surgical field during a large endoscopic vascular injury. Laryngoscope 2011;121(3):562–566
5. Raymond J, Hardy J, Czepko R, Roy D. Arterial injuries in transsphenoidal surgery for pituitary adenoma; the role of angiography and endovascular treatment. AJNR Am J Neuroradiol 1997;18(4):655–665
6. Valentine R, Padhye V, Wormald PJ. Simulation training for vascular emergencies in endoscopic sinus and skull base surgery. Otolaryngol Clin North Am 2016;49(3):877–887
7. Laws ER Jr. Vascular complications of transsphenoidal surgery. Pituitary 1999;2(2):163–170
8. Wholey MH, Wholey MH, Jarmolowski CR, Eles G, Levy D, Buecthel J. Endovascular stents for carotid artery occlusive disease. J Endovasc Surg 1997;4(4):326–338
9. Leung GK, Auyeung KM, Lui WM, Fan YW. Emergency placement of a self-expandable covered stent for carotid artery injury during transsphenoidal surgery. Br J Neurosurg 2006;20(1):55–57
10. Higashida RT, Halbach VV, Dowd CF, Barnwell SL, Hieshima GB. Intracranial aneurysms: interventional neurovascular treatment with detachable balloons—results in 215 cases. Radiology 1991;178(3):663–670

Index

Note: Italic *f* and *t* indicate figure and table, respectively.